Clinical Diagnosis
of Atherosclerosis

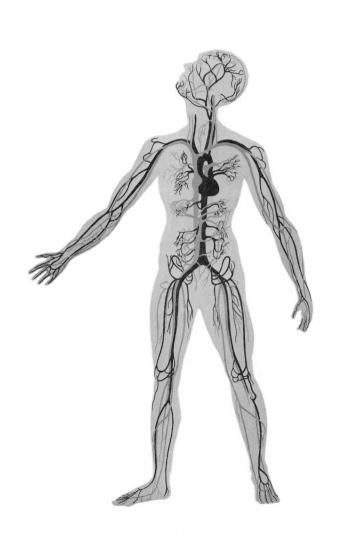

Clinical Diagnosis of Atherosclerosis
Quantitative Methods of Evaluation

Edited by

M. Gene Bond
William Insull, Jr.
Seymour Glagov
A. Bleakley Chandler
J. Fredrick Cornhill

With 103 Figures

Springer-Verlag   New York   Heidelberg   Berlin

M. Gene Bond, Ph.D., Associate Professor of Comparative Medicine, Bowman Gray School of Medicine, Wake Forest University, Winston-Salem, North Carolina 27103, U.S.A.

William Insull, Jr., M.D., Department of Medicine, Baylor College of Medicine; Director, Lipid Research Clinic, Methodist Hospital, Houston, Texas 77030, U.S.A.

Seymour Glagov, M.D., Professor of Pathology, Pritzker School of Medicine, University of Chicago; Autopsy Service, University of Chicago Hospitals and Clinics, Chicago, Illinois 60637, U.S.A.

A. Bleakley Chandler, M.D., Professor and Chairman, Department of Pathology, Medical College of Georgia, Augusta, Georgia 30912, U.S.A.

J. Fredrick Cornhill, D. Phil., Associate Professor of Surgery, Laboratory of Experimental Atherosclerosis, Ohio State University, College of Medicine, Columbus, Ohio 43210, U.S.A.

Sponsoring Editor: Chester Van Wert
Production: Anthony Buatti

Library of Congress Cataloging in Publication Data
Main entry under title:
Clinical diagnosis of atherosclerosis.
    Includes index.
    1. Atherosclerosis—Diagnosis.   I. Bond, M. Gene.
[DNLM: 1. Arteriosclerosis—Diagnosis.   WG 550
C641 1982]
RC692.C54   1982   616.1'36'075   83-382
ISBN 0-387-90780-7

Typed by the Bowman Gray School of Medicine, Winston-Salem, North Carolina
Printed and bound by Halliday Lithograph, West Hanover, Massachusetts
Printed in the United States of America

9 8 7 6 5 4 3 2 1

ISBN 0-387-90780-7   Springer-Verlag   New York   Heidelberg   Berlin
ISBN 3-540-90780-7   Springer-Verlag   Berlin   Heidelberg   New York

Contents

Part 4
Summary   549

Preface

This volume is the product of a February 1982 conference, cosponsored by the American Heart Association, the National Institutes of Health, and the Bowman Gray School of Medicine, which examined techniques for delineating quantitatively the natural history of atherosclerosis. Against the background of current pathologic and clinical knowledge of atherosclerosis, invasive and noninvasive evaluative methods now in use and under development are surveyed in depth.

Correlative clinicopathologic studies of atherosclerosis pose special questions with respect to both luminal and plaque characteristics that are addressed in this volume. An old observation, based on the examination of arterial casts, suggested that the so-called nodose lesion of atherosclerosis may be at first flattened into the wall of a weakened, dilated artery, rather than raised into the lumen. This is now fully confirmed in vivo by ultrasonic and other imaging techniques. The morbid anatomist is challenged anew to describe lesions as they are likely to occur in vivo. To achieve closer correlation with natural conditions, perfusion fixation of arteries under arterial pressure is becoming more widely used and has already demonstrated more valid quantitation of the composition and configuration of lesions.

While the noninvasive methods of B-mode and Doppler ultrasound are suitable only for the clinical study of superficial arteries, such as the carotid or femoral, the new and relatively noninvasive procedure of intravenous digital subtraction angiography can be effectively used for the examination of deep systems, such as cerebral vessels. The application of nuclear magnetic resonance and positron emission tomography to the metabolic evaluation of lesions and to the assessment of blood flow is just beginning to unfold. Unlike noninvasive methods, the invasive technique of direct arterial angiography is usually employed after the appearance of symptoms, when the disease has reached an advanced stage at the site of involvement.

With such rapid strides in technology taking place, it is apparent that a revolution in the ability to measure the progression and regression of atherosclerotic lesions is at hand. Noninvasive approaches have the potential of achieving an economy of scale by sequentially following precisely located lesions in individuals on therapeutic regimens, thus obviating the need for large, enormously costly and complicated clinical trials. Moreover, the opportunity to discover and trace the evolution of lesions by these means in asymptomatic but high-risk populations will allow for early intervention. At the same time, this will underscore the often ignored fact that atherosclerosis is an insidious disease that progresses silently for years before becoming overtly manifest in its advanced stages.

The technology discussed herein may itself open new avenues for investigating the pathogenesis of atherosclerosis. Witness the remarkable demonstration by pulsed Doppler ultrasound of the whirlpool effect that disturbed blood flow produces in the carotid sinus, where atherosclerosis is so common. Witness the demonstration by B-mode ultrasound of the jerking arterial pulsations that rub together opposing lesions of the carotid artery, an area of high risk for the development of ulcerative plaques and mural thrombosis. Observations like these have added a new dimension to the study of thromboarterial disease.

The concluding chapters find an urgent need for pathologists and clinical investigators to develop acceptable reference standards for the measurement of lesions in vivo and ex vivo. Concepts of progression and regression of lesions must be carefully defined and made open ended to allow for multiple and additional methods of assessment by quantitative morphometry. This volume reflects the success of the conference, which did much to fulfill an initial challenge: "If by joint efforts image and tissue morphologists are to succeed in arriving at a reproducible means of quantitating lesions in the living subject, they must understand each other and know precisely what is and what is not being measured."

A. Bleakley Chandler

Acknowledgments

The conference on Quantitative Evaluation of Atherosclerosis and the publication of this volume were made possible by support from the following organizations and from private industry.

The Council on Arteriosclerosis of the American Heart Association
The National Heart, Lung and Blood Institute
The Bowman Gray School of Medicine of Wake Forest University

American Cyanamid Company
Boehringer Ingelheim Limited
Burroughs Wellcome Company
Carolina Medical Electronics
Ciba-Geigy Corporation
H.R.L., Incorporated
Hoffman-LaRoche Incorporated
Lilly Research Laboratories
Merck, Sharp & Dohme
Merrell Dow Pharmaceuticals Incorporated
Revlon Health Care Group
A.H. Robins Company
Sandoz, Incorporated
Schering Corporation
G.D. Searle and Company
Smith Kline Corporation
The Upjohn Company
Warner-Lambert Company

The Organizing Committee and the editors of this volume gratefully acknowledge their debt of gratitude to the following individuals: Dr. Sheldon A. Schaffer for local arrangements; Sarah Johnston, Office of Information and Publications, Bowman Gray School of Medicine, for brochure preparation; Mrs. Hugh B. Lofland for her excellent editorial assistance; Mrs. Shirley Pegram, Ms. Maria F. Hiller, and particularly Mrs. Lona Ellis for preparation of the final manuscripts; Ms. Hermina Trillo, Mrs. Jean Gardin, Ms. Sharon Wilmoth, Mrs. Dianna Swaim, and Ms. Loren Bynum for their invaluable assistance during the Workshop. Particularly, the cochairmen of the Workshop wish to acknowledge their debt of gratitude to Mrs. Janet Kaduck Sawyer, whose exceptional skill and effort resulted in a well-organized meeting and in the preparation of this book.

The members of the Organizing Committee also gratefully acknowledge the permission granted by W. L. Gore and Associates, Inc. to use "The Vascular Man" as the symbol for this symposium.

Contributors

Organizing Committee

Chairmen

M. Gene Bond, Ph.D., Department of Comparative Medicine, Bowman Gray School of Medicine, Wake Forest University, Winston-Salem, North Carolina

William Insull, Jr., M.D., Department of Medicine, Baylor College of Medicine; Lipid Research Clinic, Methodist Hospital, Houston, Texas

Members

Robert W. Barnes, M.D., F.A.C.S., F.A.C.C., Department of Surgery, Medical College of Virginia, Virginia Commonwealth University; Noninvasive Peripheral Vascular Laboratory, Medical College of Virginia; Department of Vascular Surgery, McGuire VA Medical Center, Richmond, Virginia

David H. Blankenhorn, M.D., Department of Medicine, Atherosclerosis Research Division, University of Southern California School of Medicine, Los Angeles, California

A. Bleakley Chandler, M.D., Department of Pathology, Medical College of Georgia, Augusta, Georgia

J. Fredrick Cornhill, D.Phil., Laboratory of Experimental Atherosclerosis, Ohio State University College of Medicine, Columbus, Ohio

Assaad S. Daoud, M.D., Department of Pathology, Albany Medical College, Union University, and Laboratory Service, VA Medical Center, Albany, New York

Seymour Glagov, M.D., Department of Pathology, Pritzker School of Medicine, University of Chicago; Autopsy Service, University of Chicago Hospitals and Clinics, Chicago, Illinois

James F. Greenleaf, Ph.D., Department of Biophysics and Medicine, Biodynamics Research Unit, Mayo Foundation, Rochester, Minnesota

C. Alex McMahan, Ph.D., Department of Pathology, University of Texas Health Sciences Center, San Antonio, Texas

C. Richard Minick, M.D., Department of Pathology, Cornell University Medical College, New York, New York

William P. Newman III, M.D., Department of Pathology, School of Medicine, Louisiana State University Medical Center, New Orleans, Louisiana

Sheldon A. Schaffer, Ph.D., Medical Research Division, American Cyanamid Company, Pearl River, New York

D. Eugene Strandness, M.D., Department of Surgery, University of Washington School of Medicine; University Hospital, Seattle, Washington

Robert W. Wissler, M.D., Ph.D., Department of Pathology, University of Chicago, Chicago, Illinois

Participants

Mark L. Armstrong, M.D., F.A.C.P., Department of Medicine, Cardiovascular Division, University of Iowa College of Medicine; University Hospital, Iowa City, Iowa

Marshall R. Ball, M.D., Department of Radiology, Bowman Gray School of Medicine, Wake Forest University, Winston-Salem, North Carolina

Ralph W. Barnes, Ph.D., Department of Neurology, Bowman Gray School of Medicine, Wake Forest University, Winston-Salem, North Carolina

James B. Bassingthwaighte, M.D., Ph.D., Center for Bioengineering and Biomathematics, University of Washington School of Medicine, Seattle, Washington

Errol M. Bellon, M.D., Department of Radiology, Case Western Reserve University School of Medicine; Cuyahoga County Hospital, Cleveland, Ohio

Alan Berson, Ph.D., Devices and Technology Branch, Division of Heart and Vascular Diseases, National Heart, Lung and Blood Institute, Bethesda, Maryland

Thomas F. Budinger, M.D., Ph.D., Department of Medical Research, Donner Laboratory; Department of Bioinstrumentation, Electrical Engineering and Computer Sciences, Lawrence Berkeley Laboratory, University of California, Berkeley, California

Bill C. Bullock, D.V.M., Department of Comparative Medicine, Bowman Gray School of Medicine, Wake Forest University, Winston-Salem, North Carolina

Anthony J. Comerota, M.D., Department of Surgery, and Vascular Laboratory, Temple University Hospital, Philadelphia, Pennsylvania

Jerry G. Davis, B.S.E.E., Department of Biomedical Engineering, Clinical Research Division, Lovelace Medical Foundation, Albuquerque, New Mexico

Ralph G. DePalma, M.D., Department of Surgery, George Washington University, Washington, D.C.

James A. DeWeese, M.D., F.A.C.S., Department of Surgery, Division of Cardiothoracic Surgery, University of Rochester School of Medicine and Dentistry, Rochester, New York

Marlowe W. Eldridge, M.S.M.E., Research Division, Lovelace Medical Foundation, Albuquerque, New Mexico

Titus C. Evans, Jr., M.D., Ph.D., Department of Internal Medicine, Mayo Medical School; Division of Cardiovascular Disease and Internal Medicine, Mayo Clinic, Mayo Foundation, Rochester, Minnesota

Domenick J. Falcone, Ph.D., New York Hospital-Cornell Medical Center, New York, New York

C. Miller Fisher, M.D., Department of Neurology, Harvard Medical School, and Massachusetts General Hospital, Boston, Massachusetts

Lloyd D. Fisher, Ph.D., Department of Biostatistics, School of Public Health; Coronary Artery Surgery Study Coordinating Center, University of Washington, Seattle, Washington

Katherine E. Fritz, Ph.D., Department of Pathology, Albany Medical College, Union University; Atherosclerosis Research Laboratory, VA Medical Center, Albany, New York

Edward Ganz, M.D., Donner Laboratory, University of California, Berkeley, California

Don P. Giddens, Ph.D., School of Aerospace Engineering, Georgia Institute of Technology, Atlanta, Georgia

E. Richard Greene, Ph.D., Department of Medicine, University of New Mexico School of Medicine; Department of Physiology and Biophysics, Clinical Research Division, Lovelace Medical Foundation, Albuquerque, New Mexico

David P. Hajjar, Ph.D., New York Hospital-Cornell Medical Center, New York, New York

Elmer C. Hall, Ph.D., Department of Biometry, Emory University School of Medicine, Atlanta, Georgia

Gary J. Harpold, M.D., Department of Neurology, Bowman Gray School of Medicine, Wake Forest University, Winston-Salem, North Carolina

M. Daria Haust, M.D., F.R.C.P.(C), Departments of Pathology, Paediatrics, and Obstetrics and Gynaecology, University of Western Ontario; Department of Pathology, Children's Psychiatric Research Institute, London, Ontario

Ruth Hegyeli, M.D., Division of International Programs, National Heart, Lung and Blood Institute, Bethesda, Maryland

William Hollander, M.D., Department of Medicine and Biochemistry, Boston University School of Medicine, Boston, Massachusetts

Barbara B. Hrapchak, Ph.D., Department of Biochemistry, Chemical Abstracts Services, Columbus, Ohio

John Jarmolych, M.D., Department of Pathology, Albany Medical College, Union University; Anatomic Pathology Section, Laboratory Service, VA Medical Center, Albany, New York

J. Ward Kennedy, M.D., Department of Cardiology, University of Washington; Department of Medicine, Division of Cardiology, Cardiovascular Disease Section, Seattle VA Hospital, Seattle, Washington

Thomas Killip, M.D., Department of Medicine, Henry Ford Hospital, Detroit, Michigan

Raelene L. Kinlough-Rathbone, M.D., Department of Pathology, McMaster University, Hamilton, Ontario

Robert S. Lees, M.D., Department of Cardiovascular Disease, Massachusetts Institute of Technology; Division of Peripheral Vascular Disease, New England Deaconess Hospital, Boston, Massachusetts

Martin Lipton, M.D., Department of Radiology, University of California Medical Center, San Francisco, California

William M. McKinney, M.D., Department of Neurology, Bowman Gray School of Medicine, Wake Forest University, Winston-Salem, North Carolina

Gardner C. McMillan, M.D., Division of Heart and Vascular

Diseases, National Heart, Lung and Blood Institute, Bethesda, Maryland

Fernando G. Miranda, M.D., University of New Mexico Medical School; Depatment of Neurosciences, Lovelace Medical Center, Albuquerque, New Mexico

Michael B. Mock, M.D., Division of Cardiovascular Diseases and Internal Medicine, Mayo Clinic, Mayo Foundation, Rochester, Minnesota

Brian R. Moyer, M.D., Department of Biomedicine, Donner Laboratory, University of California, Berkeley, California

J. Fraser Mustard, M.D., Ph.D., F.R.C.P.(C), Department of Pathology, McMaster University, Hamilton, Ontario

P. David Myerowitz, M.D., Department of Surgery, Division of Cardiothoracic Surgery, University of Wisconsin School of Medicine, Madison, Wisconsin

Theron W. Ovitt, M.D., Department of Radiology, University of Arizona Health Sciences Center, Tucson, Arizona

Marian A. Packham, Ph.D., Department of Biochemistry, University of Toronto, Toronto, Ontario

Rodolfo Paoletti, M.D., Universita di Milano, Instituto di Farmacologia e di Farmacognosia, Milano, Italy

David C. Price, M.D., Department of Biomedicine, Donner Laboratory, University of California Medical Center, San Francisco, California

John M. Reid, Ph.D., Department of Electrical and Computer Engineering, College of Engineering, and Biomedical Engineering and Science Institute, Drexel University, Philadelphia, Pennsylvania

Richard W. St. Clair, Ph.D., Department of Pathology, Bowman Gray School of Medicine, Wake Forest University, Winston-Salem, North Carolina

Janet K. Sawyer, B.S., Department of Comparative Medicine, Bowman Gray School of Medicine, Wake Forest University, Winston-Salem, North Carolina

Colin J. Schwartz, M.D., F.R.A.C.P., Department of Pathology, University of Texas Health Sciences Center, San Antonio, Texas

Robert H. Selzer, M.A., M.S., Observational Systems Division, Jet Propulsion Laboratory, California Institute of Technology; Southern California School of Medicine, Pasadena, California

Donald M. Small, M.D., Biophysics Institute, Boston University School of Medicine, Boston City Hospital; University Hospital, Boston, Massachusetts

Merrill P. Spencer, M.D., Institute of Applied Physiology and Medicine, Department of Clinical Physiology, Providence Medical Center; Vascular Laboratory, Northwest Hospital, Seattle, Washington

David S. Sumner, M.D., Department of Surgery, and Peripheral Vascular Service, Southern Illinois University School of Medicine, Springfield, Illinois

James F. Toole, M.D., LL.B., Department of Neurology, Bowman Gray School of Medicine, Wake Forest University; North Carolina Baptist Hospital, Winston-Salem, North Carolina

Dragoslava Vesselinovitch, D.V.M., Specialized Center of Research on Arteriosclerosis, Department of Pathology, Pritzker School of Medicine, University of Chicago Medical Center, Chicago, Illinois

Wyatt F. Voyles, M.D., Clinical Research Division, Lovelace Medical Foundation, Albuquerque, New Mexico

John Watson, Ph.D., Devices and Technology Branch, Division of Heart and Vascular Diseases, National Heart, Lung and Blood Institute, Bethesda, Maryland

David A. Waugh, M.D., Biophysics Institute, Boston University School of Medicine, Boston, Massachusetts

Christopher P. L. Wood, M.B., B.S., F.R.C.S., Department of Radiology, Clinical Research Centre, Northwick Park Hospital, Harrow, England

Yukio Yano, M.D., Department of Biomedicine, Donner Laboratory, University of California Medical Center, San Francisco, California

Christopher K. Zarins, M.D., Department of Surgery, Pritzker School of Medicine, University of Chicago; Department of Vascular Surgery, University of Chicago Medical Center, Chicago, Illinois

Michael A. Zatina, M.D., Department of Surgery, University of Chicago Medical Center, Chicago, Illinois

1

Workshop Overview

D. Eugene Strandness

The amount of effort expended in the study of atherosclerosis is impressive. While progress is being made, the problems are so complex it is difficult to know exactly where to apply our greatest energies. If we were to approach this disease strictly from an epidemiologic standpoint, we would be forced to conclude that this may be the most common self-inflicted disease in our society. This would have to be true if we accept the observations that cigarette smoking and dietary fat are the most important risk factors yet identified.

An interesting fact to emerge is the observation that the mortality rate from ischemic heart disease appears to be on the decline (1). Between 1968 and 1976, death from cardiovascular disease decreased 21-39%, depending upon sex and racial group. This is an impressive accomplishment by any standard, and certainly suggests that progress is being made, but the question is where? While a host of people are lining up to take the credit, it is not clear what factors are responsible for this improvement. This dilemma highlights the problems the medical community faces in attempting to quantitatively document not only the presence of atherosclerosis, but also those factors responsible for this apparent change in the natural history of the disease. Clearly, we must be able to define some objective endpoints that are uniquely associated with atherosclerosis and that can be shown to change in a predictable manner as the disease progresses or regresses.

The quantitative evaluation of this disease will mean different things to different people. Those specialty groups that have an interest in the problem of atherosclerosis are very diverse (Fig. 1). While each of these specialty groups tends to focus on different aspects of the problem, each contributes in a unique way to our understanding of the disease and its clinical expression.

It would be ideal if there were a specific arterial site easily accessible, amenable to repetitive studies, and representative of the disease involvement in all of the major vascular beds. In order to qualify for such attention, the lesion development would have to be responsive to all those risk factors we might attempt to modify. Unfortunately, there is probably no such arterial segment, although this possibility should be discussed.

Grossly and microscopically, the complicated plaque appears to be the same regardless of its site of origin. However, we now know there are differences among arteries particularly with regard to related risk factors, that lead preferentially to the development of atherosclerosis in the certain vascular beds. In addition, the mechanisms that lead to the commonly observed clinical events vary in different segments of the arterial tree.

For example, in the extracranial arterial circulation, the clinical expression of disease appears to be more dependent on the anatomic nature of the plaque than on the extent to which it narrows the artery. It is now recognized that loss of endothelial continuity over the plaque with ulceration is probably the single most important factor in the release of emboli which result in transient ischemic attacks and strokes.

In contrast, reduced perfusion from high grade stenoses and occlusions are the most common factors responsible for ischemia and tissue death when atherosclerosis involves the arterial supply to the limbs. While emboli can occur from ulcerated plaques in

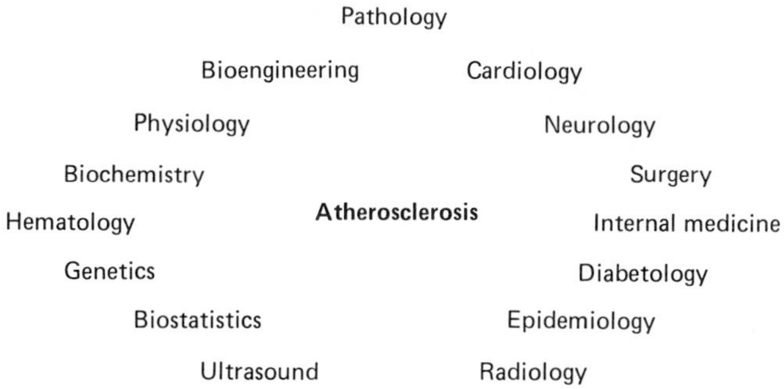

Pathology

Bioengineering   Cardiology

Physiology   Neurology

Biochemistry   Surgery

Hematology   **Atherosclerosis**   Internal medicine

Genetics   Diabetology

Biostatistics   Epidemiology

Ultrasound   Radiology

Fig. 1 Spectrum of specialties that have an interest in the problems of atherosclerosis.

the legs, this phenomenon does not account for the most commonly observed clinical events. Thus, it appears that the direction of research should be tailored to each of the major arterial beds affected by atherosclerosis. This greatly complicates the problems since differing technologies will have to be developed to meet these challenges.

Another serious problem is the point in time that physicians have the opportunity to make the diagnosis. By the time the patient appears with symptoms, the disease has, with rare exceptions, reached an advanced stage at the site of involvement. Thus, in a real sense, we are always looking at the disease at the least desirable point in time. Pathologically, the offending lesion(s) is usually the complicated plaque which may in addition have a superimposed thrombus which extends for varying distances. Thus, it will be important not only to deal with atherosclerosis as the primary event but also take into account the fact that secondary events such as thrombosis occur, which make the objective evaluation of the disease even more difficult. Let us then turn to the three vascular regions of major clinical importance and address the problems as they currently appear.

The coronary circulation stands first in importance and complexity. These arteries are not only deeply placed within the mediastinum but are continually in motion. The only method currently in widespread use that is capable of describing their morphology is selective coronary arteriography. In fact, it is the only diagnostic test available which permits a glimpse of the coronary anatomy in its entirety. Unfortunately, because of the cost, discomfort, and morbidity, it is not a procedure which readily lends itself to repetitive use. Furthermore, there appear to be inherent problems in objectively documenting the extent of narrowing produced by the plaques. Unfortunately, atherosclerosis does not produce axisymmetric lesions with predictable surface characteristics. This fact is recognized by everyone who deals with the disease directly, and it complicates attempts to quantitate cross-sectional area reduction on the basis of arteriographic images, even when taken in multiple planes.

Isner et al. (2) examined the problem of judging the degree of narrowing of the left main coronary artery by cineangiography. Their studies compared the results observed at necropsy in 28 patients who had angiography performed within 40 days of death. Surprisingly, they found that quantification of lesions with less than 90% luminal diameter reduction may often be impossible. If this is in fact true, we are faced with a serious problem in attempting to use methods such as this for documentation of both progression and regression of atherosclerotic plaques. As will be discussed, this difficulty is not unique to the coronary arteries, or to this form of imaging.

Cardiologists have long recognized that arteriography, while an essential method for obtaining a firm diagnosis, does have shortcomings. It provides very little information concerning myocardial function, information which is essential for many clinical decisions, including an evaluation of the results of therapy. For this reason a great deal of effort has been expended in developing methods of evaluating both global and regional myocardial performance. These techniques have made it possible to document changes in ventricular perfusion and function, but it is not always feasible to determine with certainty the basis for the change. This is a problem which plagues all of the functional tests currently in use. While it may be reasonable to assume that worsening is in some way secondary to disease progression, the converse may not hold true.

Finally, with regard to the heart, there is now good evidence that secondary events such as thrombosis play an important role in both acute and chronic myocardial ischemia. There is no doubt that progressive arterial narrowing can and will impair perfusion largely on the basis of mechanical factors. However, it is now clear that the final event preceding the development of a myocardial infarct is often thrombosis with total occlusion. Although the two processes are closely interrelated, it will be important to be able to make this distinction in documenting the natural history of atherosclerosis in the coronary arteries.

Our understanding of the pathogenesis of stroke has undergone dramatic changes over the past 20 years. There is good evidence that artery-to-artery emboli from the extracranial arterial system are among the most common causes of transient ischemic attacks and strokes (3). There is also reasonably good evidence that these emboli arise from ulcerated areas on the surface of the plaque that have reached this stage by loss of endothelial coverage. Thus the developing plaque at the carotid bifurcation, for reasons that are poorly understood, undergoes degenerative changes leading to the lesion that places the patient at risk. This is important because it is likely that this change within the plaque is more important and predictive of future events than is the degree of arterial narrowing it produces.

The carotid artery in the neck is an intriguing site with regard to prospective studies. This area is easily accessible to ultrasonic methods and presents the opportunity not only of studying its geometry and flow patterns but also of characterizing the material that constitutes the plaque. Furthermore, disease once identified may, in theory, be followed repetitively to evaluate the natural history of atherosclerosis in this arterial segment. In fact, it is now possible using existing technology to

detect carotid bifurcation disease, which we don't know how to
treat. While this fact produces a dilemma for the medical community, it also provides a unique opportunity for those scientists
interested in the relationship between carotid bifurcation
disease, risk factors, and clinical sequelae.

Arteriography has become the definitive diagnostic test for
atherosclerosis. Selective, multiplanar studies make it feasible
to define the location and severity of involvement from the level
of the aortic arch to the brain itself. The technique remains a
"gold standard" of sorts as long as the demands placed on it are
not too rigorous. For studies at a single point in time, it meets
the needs of the clinician quite well. However, if one looks to
the method as a possible technique for monitoring atherosclerosis
progression and regression, problems become apparent.

The carotid bifurcation is a very complex anatomic unit. The
bulb is the most common site of involvement, but the plaques that
develop are not axisymmetric, are of varying length, and have
markedly different surface characteristics. Thus, it is not surprising that there is also considerable intra- and interobserver
variability when arteriography is used in estimating the degree of
narrowing. Chikos et al. (4) examined this problem in 128 selective carotid arteriograms. It was apparent that estimating percent
stenosis to the nearest 5% is beyond the resolution of the method.
Classification of the percent stenosis into five groups (0, 1-9,
10-49, 50-99, and 100% stenosis) resulted in an intraobserver
agreement of 74%, which increased to 80% when reader pairs were
used. While digital subtraction angiography will be useful in
studying patients with suspected carotid artery disease, it will
be plagued with the same problem.

If we accept the hypothesis that artery-to-artery emboli are
the most common cause of stroke, then defining the surface characteristics of the plaque may be of greater importance than assessing the degree of diameter reduction. While this problem would
appear to be simpler given current imaging methods, even here

there are some questions. Edwards et al. (5) compared the documentation of ulceration as noted by arteriography with the surgical examination of the excised plaque. In only 12 of 20 cases (60%) in which an ulcer was found in the surgical specimen was it observed in the preoperative arteriographic studies.

Claims have been made that high resolution ultrasonic scanning systems may be better than angiography in defining the presence of an ulcer in the carotid bulb. While this may in fact be true, prospective trials will have to be done to verify this assertion. The possibility of bias is always a problem in studies of this type, particularly if the same individuals involved in interpreting the ultrasonic scan also participate in evaluating the surface characteristics of the excised lesions.

The final, major area prone to develop atherosclerosis is the peripheral arterial system. Numerous clinical and pathological studies have provided information on the common sites of occurrence and the types of lesions that are found. The clinical sequelae of atherosclerosis in this area are largely secondary to reduced perfusion, which is the result of high grade stenoses and occlusions. While emboli from ulcerated plaques can occur, they do not constitute the problem seen in the carotid system.

The disease in the limbs develops at a relatively slow rate, but is often present at multiple arterial sites. Loss of the limb secondary to gangrene is the terminal expression of the disease, but is relatively uncommon. The rate of limb loss in nondiabetic patients with atherosclerosis is about 1% per year (6). In the presence of diabetes, this increases five-fold (7). It is now clear that the disease may progress simultaneously at more than one arterial site with only minimal changes in the patient's status. This is possible because of the available collateral circulation, which regularly develops in response to arterial narrowing and occlusion.

The clinical presentation of the disease is usually straightforward and easily recognized by an experienced physician. The

development of rather simple, noninvasive tests has been an
invaluable aid not only in verifying the clinical impression but
also in providing objective information on the extent of the
involvement and its severity. These tests have also found a place
in documenting changes that occur secondary to disease progression
and following arterial reconstruction. While these tests provide
sensitive methods of documenting changes in perfusion, they will
not be specific in indicating the basis for the change.

It is now feasible to examine the entire length of the arterial system by arteriography. This method provides a "road map" for
the surgeon but is not considered necessary for diagnostic purposes. Slot et al. (8) have also examined the problem of using
single-plane images for estimation of the degree of arterial
narrowing. These authors found that short of total occlusion, the
interobserver agreement in estimating the degree of narrowing was
extremely poor for nearly all visualized arterial segments from
the level of the aorta to the lower leg.

While many peripheral arterial sites are available and accessible to such methods as ultrasound, no systematic studies have
been done to evaluate their potential utility. While such studies
are certainly feasible, it is necessary to decide where to look
as well as to ascertain those changes that will be important for
quantification of atherosclerosis.

Where then do we start? It would certainly be presumptuous for
me to make any suggestions in this regard. Perhaps it would be
wise for each of us to approach this serious health problem as if
it had just been discovered. While this is not possible, it does
have some merit, particularly if we want to minimize any possible
bias in the conclusions that might be reached. However, it must
be remembered that, regardless of our own attitudes, more questions
remain than there are available solutions. If nothing else is
accomplished, the program will familiarize each of us with the
tools currently in use and on the horizon and with how their
potential can be realized in the years to come.

REFERENCES

1. Stern MP (1979) The recent decline in ischemic heart disease
   mortality. Ann Intern Med 91:630-640
2. Isner JM, Kishel J, Kent KM, Ronan JA Jr, Ross AM, Roberts WC
   (1981) Accuracy of angiographic determination of left main
   coronary arterial narrowing. Angiographic-histologic correlative analysis in 28 patients. Circulation 63: 1056-1065
3. Mohr JP, Caplan LR, Melski JW, Goldstein RJ, Duncan GW,
   Kistler JP, Pessin MS, Bleich HL (1978) The Harvard Cooperative Stroke Registry: A prospective registry. Neurology 28:
   754-762
4. Chikos PM, Fischer L, Hirsch JH, Harley JD, Thiele BL,
   Strandness DE Jr (to be published) Observer variability in
   evaluating extracranial carotid artery stenosis.
5. Edwards JH, Kricheff II, Riles T, Imparato A (1979) Angiographically undetected ulceration of the carotid bifurcation
   as a cause of embolic stroke. Radiology 132: 369-373
6. Boyd AM (1962) The natural course of arteriosclerosis of the
   lower extremities. Proc R Soc Med 55: 591-593
7. Silbert S, Zazeela H (1958) Prognosis in arteriosclerotic
   peripheral vascular disease. JAMA 166: 1816-1821
8. Slot HB, Strijbosch L, Greep J (1981) Interobserver variability in single plane aortography. Surgery 90: 497-504

2

Quantitating Atherosclerosis
Problems of Definition

SEYMOUR GLAGOV AND CHRISTOPHER K. ZARINS

Techniques for evaluating the effects of atherosclerosis on the circulatory system in the living subject have evolved rapidly and in parallel with improved modes of medical and surgical therapy. In addition to means for assessing altered flows and pressure gradients, and reductions in tissue perfusion at various sites, methods have been developed for visualizing and characterizing the arterial deformations generally responsible for these dysfunctions. As methods for lesion characterization in the living subject improve and enter into wider use, it becomes increasingly evident that we must seek more detailed and precise correlations between the disease process as it appears on gross and microscopic examination of vessel samples and the images and numerical data produced by each of the available clinical modes of lesion detection. There are several compelling reasons for this. First, it is self-evident that controversies regarding the relative accuracy, sensitivity and specificity of each of the detection methods can ultimately be resolved only by quantitative comparisons of the images with the actual, corresponding lesions. Secondly, we have entered an era in which we wish to follow the disease process sequentially in each of the major arterial beds in order to assess

The work presented here was supported by grants HL 15062-10 and NSF CME 7921551.

the effects of preventive and therapeutic measures on the progression, retardation, arrest, or reversal of specific lesions and of
the generalized disease. To these may be added the need to discern
whether clinical interventions affect the composition and integrity of lesions. The recent decrease in mortality attributable
to atherosclerotic cardiovascular disease may be due, at least in
part, to control of the clinical risk factors thus far identified
(1), but it is also conceivable that some pharmacological agents
or vigorous therapeutic regimens designed to retard plaque growth
and enhance plaque regression, as well as mechanical dilations
designed to enlarge arterial lumens, could produce changes in
plaque consistency or configuration that favor potentially lethal
plaque disruptions and thromboses. Thus, although it remains
essential to continue to locate stenoses and to determine the
absolute diameter, length, and number of stenoses which correspond
to symptom-producing changes in flow profile and distal perfusion,
the next phase of correlative study must also enable us to quantitate the evolution of the atherosclerotic process itself in both
symptomatic and asymptomatic individuals.

WHAT SHOULD BE MEASURED?

Quantitation of atherosclerosis should ideally be concerned with
four related, but distinguishable, anatomic manifestations of
lesions, i.e., extent, severity, lesion composition, and complication. These features are shown semidiagrammatically in Fig. 1.
By *extent* of disease, we mean the mass or bulk of atherosclerotic
intimal tissue accumulated in a specified artery or artery segment, in a regional arterial system, or in the entire arterial
tree. The location under study must be defined as precisely as
possible, for generalized disease may be distributed in a variety
of patterns so that advanced disease in one artery does not
necessarily indicate that other vulnerable vessels of the same
individual are similarly involved (2). Estimates by gross grading
or by planimetry, of the proportion of luminal surface area
covered by lesions may provide reasonable approximations of extent

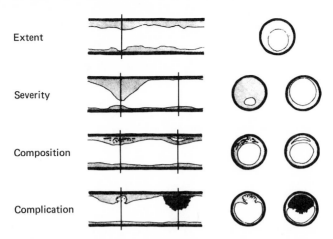

Fig. 1 Semidiagrammatic representation of quantifiable aspects
of atherosclerotic lesions. Each feature is illustrated by a
vessel segment in longitudinal cross section. Vertical lines
identify levels of the transverse cross sections shown at the
right. The shaded areas are intimal lesions. *Extent* is a measure
of the bulk of atherosclerotic intimal tissue in a specified
artery segment, branch, or arterial tree. *Severity* is an evaluation of the degree to which the lumen is narrowed. *Composition*
deals with differences in concentration and distribution of the
cellular and matrix constituents of lesions; the plaque on the
left is dense and fibrocalific (a "hard" lesion), while the lesion
on the right has a loose semi-solid center or core (a "soft"
lesion). *Complication* is concerned with secondary disruptions,
losses of cohesion and accretions, which are manifested as plaque
hemorrhages, ulcerations (lesion shown on the left), and thromboses (lesion shown on the right).

for some purposes, but such procedures do not usually take account
of the thickness of lesions and are therefore not really quantitative determinations of the volume of disease tissue present. By
severity of disease, we mean the degree to which the disease has
narrowed arterial lumens and compromised flow. Although extensive
disease is often associated with multiple stenoses, widely patent
arteries may develop focal severe narrowings, particularly at
geometric sites of predilection. Severity may be quantitated from
angiograms with respect to absolute diameter and length of each
stenosis and with respect to the number of stenoses in a given
vessel or arterial tree. Usually severity is expressed as percent
stenosis, on the basis of estimates derived by comparing specific

narrowings to nearby or immediately adjacent, presumably spared, regions.   Such estimates may be quite misleading as indices of either lesion size or extent of disease, as discussed by Zarins et al. in Chap. 13; this becomes apparent from consideration of the features evident on histologic sections as outlined below.
By *lesion composition* we mean the nature, consistency, and distribution of usual lesion components, including calcification.   In general, calcification of plaques correlates best with age and presumably therefore with age of the lesions (3).   By *complication*, we mean evidence that a lesion is fragmented, disrupted, hemorrhagic, ulcerated, or thrombotic, i.e., that there has been a potentially ominous departure from the usual cohesive organization of the lesion.

Although many severely stenotic atherosclerotic lesions are smooth-surfaced and free of luminal irregularities or disruptions, moderately stenotic lesions may become complicated, particularly by ulceration and/or thrombosis.   Some qualification must therefore be introduced with regard to the use of the term "severity" to categorize degree of stenosis or obstruction to flow at the site of a lesion.   In common usage, "severity" usually connotes gravity of a disease, i.e., the degree of potential, imminent, or actual morbidity.   Indeed, a high degree of stenosis can interfere with perfusion in the absence of sufficient collateral supply, and is a potential site of total occlusion.   The presence of multiple, marked stenoses in one or more arteries is particularly serious. Nevertheless, a moderate degree of stenosis, one that may be considered to be compatible with adequate flow, may still pose a serious threat of sudden obstruction or occlusion, at the lesion by disruption, hemorrhagic expansion, or thrombosis, or distal to the lesion by embolization of plaque material or thrombus formed at the lesion.   Thus, if we use the term "severity" to indicate severity of stenosis, we will in most instances be able to relate degree and number of stenoses to the clinical findings, especially for coronary and peripheral vascular disease, but we must also

realize that any lesion is a potential threat to the circulation
by way of local thrombosis and distal embolization, especially
in relation to cerebrovascular disease as pointed out by Dr.
Strandness in Chap. 1.

LESION CONFIGURATION AND TOPOGRAPHY: USUAL METHODS OF
SPECIMEN PREPARATION

In order to establish a sound basis for correlating the disease
process with images produced by modern imaging techniques, the
anatomic pathologist must meet the challenge of the contrast
angiographer and the ultrasonic arteriographer and seek to describe and measure lesions as they are likely to appear in vivo.
The cardiovascular pathologist in particular must be prepared to
furnish accurate qualitative and quantitative descriptions of
vessels and lesions in each of the major vascular distributions
and to become increasingly conversant with the techniques developed by clinicians and engineers to characterize vessel anatomy
and pathology in the living subject. Examination of an excised
endarterectomy specimen, such as the one shown in Fig. 2, containing part or all of an intimal lesion, may be useful for
confirming clinical evidence that a stenosis or obstruction was
due to atherosclerosis and/or thrombosis and may yield valuable
information concerning plaque consistency and the distribution of
plaque components, but it will permit only a very limited quantitative correlation with the diagnostic image. Nor will examination
of excised and undistended arteries by the usual longitudinal or
transverse sectioning methods provide adequate data for comprehensive quantitative correlation. In the usual longitudinally opened
and flattened preparations of undistended arteries, atherosclerotic lesions appear on the luminal surface as flat plaques,
elevated plaques, or encrustations. When the plaques are flat and
do not project from the luminal surface they usually appear as
pale or yellow specks, spots or linear streaks, often in irregular
longitudinal arrays. These are the so-called fatty streaks, an
example of which is shown in Fig. 3. Gelatinous lesions and other

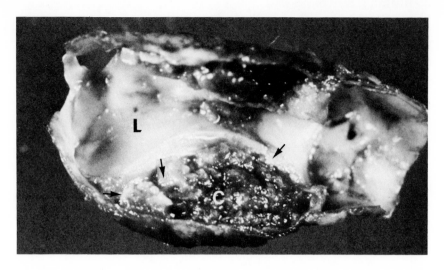

Fig. 2   An endarterectomy specimen removed from the carotid bulb.
The smooth luminal surface (L) overlies densely calcific zones
(arrows) of the underlying intimal mass which includes the friable
core (C) and remnants of the arterial wall.   Qualitative assessments of lesion composition and complication are possible from
such material, but quantitation of lesion features is limited.

relatively flat intimal changes have also been described as early
or potential sites of plaque formation.   When intimal plaques in
fresh or immersion-fixed arteries project from the luminal surface
as raised plateaus or mounds, they are frequently discrete, well
demarcated, and oval, with their long dimensions oriented in the
direction of flow.   Typical appearances of such plaques are shown
in Fig. 4A, B.   The luminal surfaces of such lesions are often
smooth, glistening, and white, and the immediately underlying
tissue is indurated and rigid, in marked contrast to the supple,
uninvolved or fatty-streaked luminal surface.   These are the
so-called fibrous, or pearly, raised plaques.   With more extensive
disease, lesions tend to become confluent and appear to be increasingly elevated.   Plaques then appear to be nodular and to
have more irregular margins.   Ulcerations with or without
prominent thrombi may complicate and disrupt all or part of a
raised plaque, exposing friable or pultaceous, granular, yellow,
or hemorrhagic material.

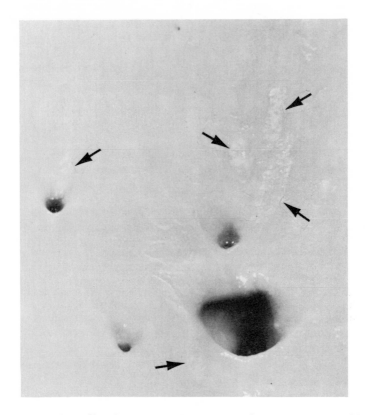

Fig. 3   Immersion-fixed aorta.   Fatty streaks appear as yellow
or pale linear surface markings (arrows), usually aligned longitudinally in the direction of flow.

In transverse cross sections of undistended vessels, fatty
streaks and other flat intimal changes result in little or no deformation of the vessel lumen, but the raised plaques are usually
perceived as eccentric, relatively flat, or convex intimal deposits
bulging into the lumen.   Such a cross section is shown in Fig. 5A.
A typical advanced raised plaque consists, on transverse cross
section, of a so-called necrotic center or core and an overlying
band of tissue, termed the fibrous cap.   The necrotic center is
usually a conglomerate of several components and may include cells,
cell debris, formed matrix fibers, and other extracellular proteins
derived from cells or plasma, lipids in amorphous and/or crystalline form within and outside of cells, and calcific deposits.

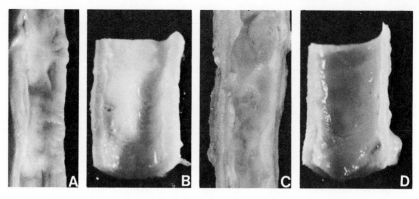

Fig. 4 Lesions viewed en face in longitudinally opened superficial femoral arteries. A: Unfixed postmortem specimen.
Confluent plaques appear as nodular mounds, bulging from the
luminal surface. B: Immersion-fixed artery. A discrete fibrous lesion stands out as a distinct raised plaque with a sharply
defined edge. C: Pressure-fixed vessel. Confluent plaques
appear as intimal thickenings and luminal narrowings, but not as
nodular bulges which would appear convex or transverse cross
section. D: Pressure-fixed vessel. The surface of a discrete
lesion is concave and its margins appear only as an indistinct
transition in surface color and consistency. Under these conditions fibrous plaques usually do not have raised edges.

Since many plaques show little or no evidence of necrosis at the
time of histologic examination, the topographic term "core" for
this portion of a lesion may be a more appropriate general desig-
nation than "necrotic center." Such terms as "fibrous," "fibrocalcific," "lipid-rich," and "cellular," are expressions of the
predominant or most impressive component feature of a particular
lesion and are not mutually exclusive descriptions. The fibrous
cap is neither amorphous nor necrotic, but consists of matrix
fibers and cells and may also contain calcific material. A
relatively uninvolved portion of artery wall lying opposite a
prominent lesion in such a preparation may be pictured as maintaining a concave luminal shape. Because the lesion tends to
bulge into the lumen and the remaining less involved media is
considered to have been concave, the lumen on a transverse cross
section of an undistended artery is often represented as a crescentic or bowed cleft or slit. When vessel lumens are occasionally

seen end-on in contrast angiograms or in transverse cross-sectional
scans, bulging lesions and slit-like lumens are rarely encountered.
Nor are they frequent when vessels are fixed while distended at
physiologic intraluminal pressures (see Chap. 13). The principal
reason for these apparent discrepancies is that release of normal
distending pressure before fixation often causes the intact portion
of the artery wall to recoil, flatten or collapse, and the more
rigid plaque to buckle, giving rise to bulging, convex lesion
configurations and narrow, slit-like lumens on transverse cross
sections, and to raised lesion edges in longitudinally opened
preparations.

The classical methods for displaying and describing lesions
in freshly opened or immersion-fixed arteries have served in the
past as a basis for illuminating general lesion composition, for
characterizing lesion distribution, and for estimating the proportion of the intimal surface covered by grossly evident lesions.
They have also enabled pathologists to quantitate the relative
abundance of the various types of lesions and to assess the
proportion of lesions showing disruptive complications. They
may however, be inadequate, if not misleading, as a basis for
quantitative validation of clinical estimates of severity of
stenosis, for characterizing lesion configuration and organization, or for assessing the true extent of disease. In view of
these considerations, it may be useful, as we embark on a critical
review of current methods for the quantitative evaluation of
atherosclerosis, to identify the anatomical features of lesions
and the distribution of lesion components, not as they appear in
usual representations, but as these are likely to appear under
conditions of normal intraluminal distending pressures.

LESION CONFIGURATION AND TOPOGRAPHY: CONDITIONS OF
NORMAL PRESSURE DISTENTION

When arteries are fixed while normal intraluminal distending
pressures are maintained, the overall configuration of lesions
as well as the transverse cross-sectional topography of lesion

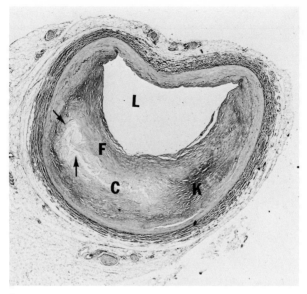

A

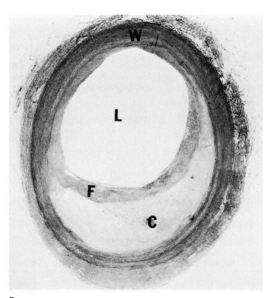

B

Fig. 5 A: Transverse cross section of an immersion-fixed coronary
artery. A raised plaque appears as a somewhat irregular projection
covered by a fibrous cap. The lumen cross section is nearly
crescent-shaped. Labels indicate the necrotic center or core of
the lesion (C), fibrous cap (F), lumen (L), calcification (K) and
cholesterol crystals (arrows). B: Transverse cross section of a

components are usually quite different from those shown in usual illustrations of undistended vessels. The most striking feature of lesion configuration on transverse cross sections of most normally distended arteries is the preservation of a circular or slightly oval, more or less symmetrical lumen, regardless of the size of the intimal lesion (Fig. 5B). The lesion is most often a gradual widening of the intima with wedge-shaped edges and a con- cave luminal surface, and its luminal surface tends to remain more or less regular except where a lesion is complicated by ulceration and/or thrombosis. Even under such conditions, the underlying atherosclerotic lesion will still usually maintain an overall crescent shape on cross section with a concave interface between lesion and thrombus. Thus, observed en face from within the lumen (Fig. 4C and D), the margins of most uncomplicated lesions do not appear as abruptly elevated edges, but as transitions in color and consistency of the intima. Early experimental lesions, similar to human fatty streaks, examined in the distended state at high magnifications show surface irregularities and crevices corre- sponding to the contours of the immediately underlying spherical intimal foam cells, but no evident elevated edges (4). Where fibrous caps have formed, luminal surfaces remain smooth on gross and light microscopic inspection, although there may be changes in orientation and juxtaposition of overlying endothelial cells. The fibrous cap is therefore not usually a superimposed irregular or dome-like deposit on the lesion (Fig. 5A), but a concave covering with about the same curvature as the adjacent uninvolved media. Thus, when circular, the lumen of a normally distended, uncompli- cated atherosclerotic artery is usually circumscribed by the intima and media of the relatively uninvolved sector and the adjacent, contiguous, concave fibrous cap of the lesion (Fig. 5B).

---

pressure-fixed carotid artery. The lumen (L) is very nearly circular and is defined by the more intact portion of the arterial wall (W) and the concave fibrous cap or channel (F). The core (C) of the lesion appears to be sequestered to one side by the well- organized fibrous cap.

It should also be noted that undistended vessels with advanced disease may also show circular or oval lumens on cross section and little surface deformation. This finding usually corresponds to the presence of encircling, rigid fibrocalcific lesions which will not alter greatly in configuration upon release of intraluminal pressures. These features may help to explain why correlations between angiograms and postmortem findings in undistended specimens are best for the most severely advanced lesions (see Chap. 12). The reported angiographic underestimations of narrowings by less advanced lesions may in many instances actually reflect postmortem overestimations due to measurements on collapsed or partially distended vessels.

In addition, pressure fixation preserves vessel geometry at branch ostia, bifurcations, and curves, revealing lesion localizations that are more accurate than those noted in freshly opened or immersion-fixed arteries (5). Even when vessels are fixed while distended, ostia of branches and normal curvatures may be deformed if vessels are opened by a single longitudinal incision and flattened. Two parallel cuts which "bivalve" the vessel and conserve wall curvature and ostial geometry result in configurations that are quite different from those seen in flattened material (6,7).

The internal elastic lamina (IEL) marks the inner limit of the media and can usually be traced around the entire circumference of the vessel. It lies beneath the endothelium in the spared segment of the vessel wall and continues beneath the lesion, i.e., between the thickened intima and the media. It corresponds to the original boundary between intima and media before the lesion developed, but is not necessarily a reliable index of the original luminal diameter, for vessels tend to dilate with age and apparently also in association with the formation of atherosclerotic lesions (8) (Chap. 19). In distended normal arteries the IEL is straight, not wavy (9), but beneath lesions the IEL may be irregularly undulated, atrophic, and discontinuous, suggesting that the lesion, and particularly the fibrous cap, rather than the underlying media,

sustains the distending tension. Further support for splinting of
the underlying media by the lesion is suggested by the frequent
presence of a straightened, neoformed elastic lamina beneath the
endothelium covering the fibrous cap. An example is shown in Fig.
6A. The media underlying the lesion may be well preserved but may
not be of the same curvature as the lumen even in pressure-fixed
vessels (Fig. 6B). Lesions may therefore vary widely in size,
i.e., in mass and volume, for any given decrease in lumen diameter
as the underlying media may bulge outward as if to accommodate the
lesion and conserve lumen cross-sectional area. The composition
and organization of the necrotic center or core, and of the immediately surrounding reactive connective tissue of the thickened
intima, vary considerably from lesion to lesion but both the
composition and the distribution of the components appear to be
independent of lesion size. Calcification occurs most frequently
in central portions of the lesion core in association with the
debris of past degeneration or fibrosis (Fig. 6A) but is also
found in denser masses and plates about the necrotic center both
deep to the lesion and on the luminal side. In general, the
constituents of the core tend to be arranged symmetrically on
transverse cross sections of distended vessels, but lesions may
occasionally be asymmetrical composites of juxtaposed crescentic
zones of different composition (Fig. 6B). There is little information concerning the microanatomic distribution and organization
of lesion components in longitudinal cross sections, for lesions
have been characterized almost exclusively on transverse cross
sections.

The standard descriptive terms "raised plaque," "fibrous cap,"
and "necrotic center" for characterizing atherosclerotic lesions
will no doubt continue to be employed. We must however, realize
that these terms originated as descriptions of lesion features in
collapsed arteries. The raised plaque does correspond to the
abnormal atherosclerotic intimal thickening, distinguishable from
the surrounding arterial tissue, but viewed from the lumen in most

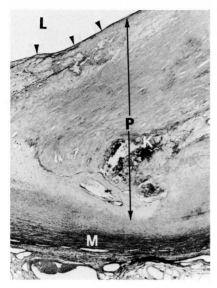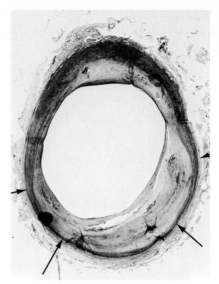

A   B

Fig. 6 A: High magnification of a fibrocalcific lesion in a
pressure-fixed internal carotid artery. The precise location of
the original internal elastic lamina at the margin between the
media (M) and the intimal plaque (P) is no longer clear. A newly
formed continuous and straight elastic lamina (arrowheads) is
evident at the luminal limit of the fibrous cap. The lumen (L)
is seen upper left, calcification (K) is visible. B: Transverse
cross section of a pressure-fixed internal carotid artery. The
lumen remains circular, while the lesions are associated with
bulges in the underlying media (arrows).

distended arteries, its edges are not normally raised. In this

sense the term "raised plaque" may be a bit of a misnomer. The

fibrous cap is most often actually a fibrous channel modeled to

continue the curvature of the adjacent artery wall, while the

necrotic center is a dystrophic core, morphologically resembling

a torpid, metabolic or chemical injury, more or less isolated from

the lumen by the fibrous cap (channel). The necrotic center or

core of the lesion may be static, progressive, organizing,

degenerating, or involuting, depending on its stage of evolution

at the time we see it. Absence, minimal formation or disintegra-

tion of a fibrous cap would tend to expose the necrotic center

material or, in the extreme situation, to cause the lesion to
appear as a grumous, greasy, friable excoriation. The predominance
of such material would make a lesion soft in contrast to the hard,
rigid, and brittle consistency of a fibrocalcific lesion with an
intact fibrous cap.

Thrombi in distended vessels are observed in several forms:
first, as organizing, smooth-surfaced, relatively uniform masses,
entirely or almost entirely plugging the lumen, or adherent to the
lesion surface and crescent-shaped, similar in surface configuration to the lesion and the adjacent wall. Organized thrombi of
the latter type may actually be difficult to distinguish from the
associated lesions into which they have been incorporated.
Second, thrombi appear as layered structures with a gradient of
increasing organization from the irregular lumen to the underlying
atherosclerotic lesion. This picture is characteristic of the
thrombi which form in abdominal aortic and iliac aneurysms. The
third morphologic appearance is the most complex and includes
associated evidences of lesion disruption, fragmentation, and
hemorrhage. Such thrombi may be quite fresh and demonstrably
associated with gaps or ulcerations of the fibrous cap and continuous with necrotic center material, some of which may be extruded
into the lumen. A thrombus of this type is shown in Fig. 7.

DO SOME LESIONS FORM CONVEX BULGES INTO THE LUMEN ON
TRANSVERSE CROSS SECTIONS?

Although atherosclerotic lesions usually appear as eccentric deposits on cross sections of arteries, advanced lesions in relatively
small vessels such as the coronary arteries, may occupy the entire
circumference before occlusion occurs. Presumably, a progressing
lesion enlarges in both longitudinal and circumferential directions
and encirclement would tend to occur as soon as the circumferential
expanse of the lesion is equal to the circumference of the vessel.
The lesion would still be expected to be thickest where it started
and render the lumen eccentric with respect to the media. If

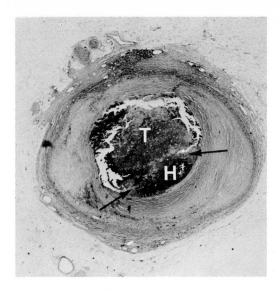

Fig. 7 Thrombus associated with plaque. A thrombus (T) associated with a disruptive plaque hemorrhage (H) in an atherosclerotic
coronary artery. Organization is noted where the thrombus is
adherent (arrow) to the artery wall.

lesions originated nearly simultaneously and progressed at similar
rates in different sites, encirclement would be expected to occur
first in small arteries and later, or not at all, in larger vessels.
Some evidence has been presented that human lesions cover intimal
surfaces most rapidly where they develop earliest (10), but we
lack precise quantitative data, based on the examination of distended vessels, concerning relative rates of growth of individual
lesions in longitudinal, circumferential, and radial directions
and in different sites. In any case, radial projection of a
lesion into the lumen need be only slightly greater than one-third
of its circumferential encroachment for occlusion to precede
complete encirclement and only somewhat greater than this in its
central portion for the transversely sectioned luminal surface of
the lesion to become convex. Lesion complication as well as
overriding of adjacent lesions would tend to produce asymmetric,
irregular, and convex lesion cross sections. Since most lumens
remain circular and eccentric with respect to the area outlined by

the media, even in the presence of large lesions, it is reasonable to assume that, on the average, circumferential and longitudinal growth of individual plaques is more than three times greater and more rapid than central extension into the lumen during lesion evolution. Nevertheless, it is possible that lesion enlargement radially into the lumen could, under certain circumstances, be much greater than one-third of circumferential or longitudinal enlargement. In such a case a lesion could indeed bulge into the lumen on transverse section and cause the lumen to be crescent-shaped or slit-like. Rapid lesion formation before the fibrous cap is well-formed, swelling of a lesion due to insudation of plasma components with or without plaque disruption, rapid cell proliferation, hemorrhage into a plaque, or organizing thrombosis could all conceivably result in such formations. The coronary arteries, subjected as they are to marked excursions of flow velocity during the cardiac cycle and to mechanical torsions and bucklings due to the motion of the heart, could be placed at relatively high risk for plaque complications and variations in plaque configuration. Elevated heart rates could tend to accentuate such changes. A distinction has been drawn between coronary artery lesions which are "eccentric," i.e., associated with partially preserved artery walls and nonaxisymmetric lumens, and lesions which are "concentric," i.e., completely encircling, with or without axisymmetric lumens (11,12). Inferences have been drawn that these configurations have pathogenetic and/or prognostic significance. The extent to which coronary artery plaques are indeed "eccentric" as opposed to "concentric" or encircling, or tend to bulge into the lumen on transverse cross section under conditions of normal distending pressure are therefore problems worthy of careful quantitative study. The relative incidence of such manifestations elsewhere in the arterial tree and the relation of such differences in configuration to extent of disease and to lesion location, composition, and complication in the course of lesion, will also require clarification.

LESION FEATURES REVEALED BY CLINICAL IMAGING TECHNIQUES

We may now consider briefly which of the morphologic features of
lesions, as they appear in distended arteries, are likely to be
identified by several current modes of in vivo imaging.

Contrast angiography provides a longitudinal display of the
vascular lumen. In a strict sense the lesion itself is not
revealed by this method, only its luminal outline. Differences in
lumen diameter are demonstrable but little information is available concerning the true extent of disease or the composition of
lesions, for neither lesion size nor the degree of encumbrance of
the original lumen area, as defined by the IEL, can be appreciated.
With sufficient resolution, and favorable projections, irregularities of the luminal surface are revealed. These may correspond
to ulcerations and/or thrombi but may also represent complex
configurations where adjacent lesions are in close approximation
or override one another. Detection of thrombi will also depend on
the type of thrombus present. Small ulcerations with small thrombotic deposits may be symptomatic, particularly in the carotid
vessels, but may go undetected by usual angiographic methods.
Organized and organizing thrombi, with conservation of the lumen,
tend to conform to lesion shape and are difficult to distinguish
from an underlying atherosclerotic plaque. Thrombi with a gradient
of organization from lumen to plaque and those associated with
disintegration of the plaque are likely to present the most
irregular surfaces and should be detectable, but because plaques
and thrombi are most often eccentric, demonstration is critically
dependent on proper projection of the image. Although most lumens
are circular and have relatively smooth surfaces, absolute luminal
dimensions may be incorrectly estimated on single projections,
because lesions are usually eccentric, but particularly when
conditions do arise, spontaneously or by intervention, to alter
lesion configurations and render lumens oval or slit-like.
Estimates of degree of narrowing can be made only by comparison of
a selected stenosis with the diameter of a presumably uninvolved

adjacent vessel segment. Since atherosclerosis tends to be a diffuse process, the portion of the vessel adjacent to a marked narrowing is likely to be diseased as well. What is referred to as the percent stenosis by the angiographer is actually the percent difference in lumen diameter, or in calculated lumen area, between markedly narrowed and nearby least narrowed points. It does not, however, follow from these considerations that narrowing with respect to original IEL diameter is regularly underestimated, in view of the evidence that atherogenesis may be associated with enlargement of the affected vessel at least during early stages of the disease (8). Widely patent and/or tortuous arteries, extensively involved by intimal and/or medial disease, may have even larger than normal luminal diameters, while in adjacent locations, intimal plaque formation has overtaken the widening tendency and produced stenosis. Sequential studies designed to follow lesion progression or regression over relatively long time spans by contrast angiography are limited to evaluation of changes in lumen diameter and configuration. These are at best only approximate indices of lesion size, for they do not take into account true lesion volumes and depend on the accuracy with which projections can be precisely reproduced in successive examinations. Thus, from angiograms, we may obtain information on absolute luminal dimensions (severity) and intimal irregularities (complication), depending on the projections examined, but little information concerning the volume (extent) or three-dimensional configuration of lesions. Except for relatively large calcifications, little can be learned about the consistency or composition of lesions and even calcifications are obscured by the contrast medium.

Ultrasound techniques allow characterization of flow by means of the Doppler effect, providing clinically useful information concerning the location and degree of stenoses (severity). Utilizing continuous wave signals, changes in flow velocity, and disturbances in flow velocity, profile can be detected. High grade stenoses or total obstructions are detected in vessels

accessible to the probe but lesser stenoses may be overlooked.
Sensitivity may be somewhat better in exposed vessels. Estimates
of stenosis based on determinations by spectral analysis can be
related to relatively small decreases in lumen diameter, on the
order of 25%, but are subject to error in relation to branch
angles, bends, departures from axisymmetry of lesions and other
geometric variables. This technique alone does not permit characterization of lesion composition, complication, or extent of
disease, except that multiple stenoses in one or more vessels can
be detected and changes with time in both number and severity of
stenosis may be estimated. Use of pulsed signals and range-gating
permits analysis of Doppler frequency shifts at selected sampling
sites within the flow stream and may therefore be used to generate
a flow image of the lumen as well as information concerning the
diameter and position of the artery. Ideally, such an ultrasound
arteriographic image has the same advantages and disadvantages as
a contrast angiographic image, except that the Doppler imaging
technique is not invasive. Calcifications may result in ultrasound imaging problems due to acoustic shadowing.

Pulse-echo ultrasonography, particularly in the form of B-mode
scans may be used to produce longitudinal or cross-sectional
images of arteries at a series of levels. Reflection of the sound
waves responsible for the production of the images occurs at
boundaries between tissues of different density. Lumens are
readily distinguishable from artery walls, for the density of the
blood column differs from that of the surrounding arterial tissues.
It is therefore possible to ascertain lumen size and the precise
position and configuration of a lesion with respect both to vessel
circumference and to longitudinal location along the vessel. For
sequential studies of stenoses, problems of reproducing precise
projections may therefore be obviated, for three-dimensional
representations are possible. Since it is noninvasive, the method
lends itself to epidemiologic and screening studies which could
include large numbers of asymptomatic patients, as well as both

symptomatic and asmptomatic patients subjected to regimens designed to arrest or reverse the disease. Improvements in sensitivity and specificity should enable us to distinguish differences in sonic impedance among media, lesion necrotic center, calcifications, fibrous cap, and thrombus. B-mode cross-sectional images would then be nearly equivalent to histologic sections and lesion area could be integrated over a given artery length to give lesion volume.

Displays in real time reveal features of artery deformation and wall motion in the course of the cardiac cycle and in relation to manipulation. Cyclic variations in arterial curves and branch angles as well as differences in distensibility could both be related to vessel wall composition and to plaque localization and consistency. Cyclic displacements of attached intraluminal masses would be expected to be associated with thrombi. Ultrasound imaging therefore holds out the possibility of assessing true extent and localization of disease, severity of stenosis, lesion composition, ulceration, and the state of thrombi (complication), as well as the effects of disease on the mechanical properties of the artery wall. With multiplex systems that provide, in addition to images, information concerning flow velocity at any point and spectral analysis of flow disturbances, data can be obtained simultaneously concerning the hemodynamic consequences of visualized lesions. Comparisons can also be made among different arteries in the same individual to illuminate the hemodynamic factors which may govern the differential localization, configuration, composition, and complication of atherosclerotic lesions.

SUMMARY

Continued quantitative investigation of the distribution, volume, and spatial organization of lesions and lesion components, based on appropriate studies of pressure-fixed postmortem vessels, is essential in order to provide both contrast and ultrasound angiographers with a more accurate grasp of the range of lesion configuration and composition at various stages of lesion evolution. Quantitative correlations of these findings with in vivo angiograms and with postmortem angiograms of vessels distended during angiography (see Chap. 13), are essential if we are to use present imaging methods to greatest advantage and if we are to evaluate and validate future attempts to improve accuracy, sensitivity, and specificity. Experimental models, particularly those utilizing nonhuman primates, should continue to be especially valuable for such investigations. Such models permit controlled, sequential studies of the entire arterial system and may be designed to deal with specific questions and permit access to vessels under study for direct visualization and biopsy. Semiquantitative comparisons will have to be replaced by precise quantitation of both images and anatomic specimens. Quantitative comparisons of lesions with images must also take into account the inevitable shrinkages which accompany fixation and processing for histologic examination (3,13). Quantitation from histologic sections will require the utilization of planimetry to measure size, shape, and orientation of lesions and their components. Tedious point counting will have to be replaced for many purposes by the more efficient computer-assisted contour tracing and densitometry techniques that are already available (8,14,15).

Studies thus far indicate that under conditions of normal pressure distention, most uncomplicated lesions are mainly eccentric or non-axisymmetric intimal deposits with luminal surface configurations that tend to conform to the curvature of affected arteries. Lumen transverse cross sections are most often circular or oval and are defined by the relatively uninvolved sector of the artery wall and the fibrous cap, as though a modeling process, concurrent with lesion evolution, had resulted in substitution to some degree of the fibrous cap for the media at the site of the lesion and in attempted sequestration of the necrotic center (core) away from the lumen. Advanced, encircling ("concentric") fibrocalcific lesions may retain in vivo lumen dimensions in the

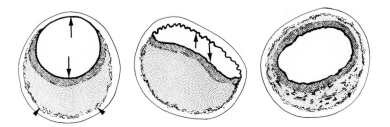

Fig. 8 Semidiagrammatic representation of lesion configurations
in various types of preparations. A: Pressure-fixed artery with
partially intact wall ("eccentric" lesion). Lesion surface is
concave and the lumen is circular. The boundary between lesion
and media is marked by a greatly altered transitional zone (arrowheads), which replaces the original internal elastic lamina. The
internal elastic lamina at the uninvolved portion of wall (upward-
pointing arrow) is discrete, taut, and continuous with the newly
formed elastic lamina (downward-pointing arrow) of the fibrous
cap. Such preparations are likely to provide reasonably accurate
quantitative estimates of lumen area, lesion configuration, and
lesion composition. B: Immersion-fixed, collapsed artery with
partially intact wall. The plaque tends to bulge into the lumen
and the lumen is crescent-shaped. The internal elastic lamina
(upward arrow) at the uninvolved but collapsed wall is undulated,
but the elastic lamina (downward arrow) over the fibrous cap may
remain more or less straight due to support by the underlying,
rigid fibrous cap. Such preparations may lead to underestimates
of lumen area and incorrect interpretations of plaque configuration. C: Immersion-fixed artery with a circumferential "hard"
fibrocalcific lesion. A rigid encircling ("concentric") lesion
may maintain the lumen in a more or less circular configuration
despite the absence of distending pressure during fixation.
Measurements of lumen area on transverse cross sections of
immersion-fixed arteries with advanced, encircling fibrous lesions
may therefore correspond more closely to in vivo angiographic
estimates than measurements made on immersion-fixed vessels with
smaller or nonencircling lesions of the type shown in B.

absence of distending pressure, but lumens associated with smaller

and softer lesions are not maintained. The original lumen, prior

to lesion formation, is defined by the original IEL with the

reservation that enlargement of vessels with age and in associa-

tion with lesion formation may render this a poor approximation.

These features are summarized semidiagrammatically in Figs. 8 and

9. Lesions vary in complexity with no simple relationship between

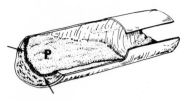

Fig. 9   Cutaway semidiagrammatic view of an atherosclerotic artery
segment under conditions of normal pressure distention.   The
luminal aspect of the lesion (P) is concave, the transition between artery wall and lesion is gradual, and the lesion edge is
wedge-shaped.   The fibrous cap (arrows) with its overlying elastic
lamina and the adjacent artery wall delineate the luminal channel.

lesion complexity and either lesion size or lumen size.   Thrombi
are associated with a variety of morphologic appearances including
lesion disruption, but may be organized and incorporated into
lesions, thereby contributing to lesion complexity.

   We should strive to maintain a clear and consistent operational
terminology, not only with respect to lesion configuration and
topography but also in relation to the quantifiable aspects of
atherosclerosis.   We have suggested that the terms "extent" for
lesion bulk, "severity" for degree of lumen compromise, "composition" for the nature and distribution of lesion constituents, and
"complication" for lesion disruptions, hemorrhages, and thromboses,
be used for measurements of the disease process and be specified
whenever possible.   Each of these features has a distinct clinical
implication and represents a particular correlative imaging
problem.

   We have tried in this presentation to focus on terms and definitions as we use them in referring to atherosclerotic disease and
to lesions and images of lesions.   If the joint efforts of image
and tissue morphologists are to succeed in identifying the directions which are to be taken in order to arrive at reproducible
means for quantitating the disease in the living subject, we must
understand one another and know precisely what we are, and are not
measuring.   We must also know how well we are doing at present.

REFERENCES

1. Levy RI (1981) Declining mortality in coronary heart disease. Arteriosclerosis 1:312-325
2. Glagov S, Rowley DA, Kohut RI (1961) Atherosclerosis of human aorta and its coronary and renal arteries. Arch Pathol 72:558-571
3. Rifkin RD, Parisi AF, Folland E (1979) Coronary calcification in the diagnosis of coronary artery disease. Am J Cardiol 44:141-147
4. Taylor K, Glagov S, Lamberti J, Vesselinovitch D, Schaffner T (1978) Surface configuration of early atheromatous lesions in controlled-pressure perfusion-fixed monkey aortas. Scan Electron Microsc 2:449-457
5. Zarins CK, Taylor KE, Lundell MI, Glagov S (1978) Aortic ostial morphology and the localization of atherosclerotic lesions: preliminary observations. In: Nerem RM, Cornhill JF (eds) The role of fluid mechanics in atherogenesis. Proc Specialists Meeting, Columbus, Ohio. Ohio State University, 5-1 to 5-4
6. Roach MR, Hinton P, Fletcher J (1978) Artefacts of localization of atherosclerosis in pinned aortas. Atherosclerosis 31:1-10
7. Zarins CK, Taylor KE, Bomberger RA, Glagov S (1980) Endothelial integrity at aortic ostial flow dividers. Scan Electron Microsc 3:249-254
8. Bond MG, Adams MR, Bullock BC (1981) Complicating factors in evaluating coronary artery atherosclerosis. Artery 9:21-29
9. Wolinsky H, Glagov S (1964) Structural basis for the static mechanical properties of the aortic media. Circ Res 14:400-413
10. Avtandilov GG (1963) Effect of age on dynamics of development of atherosclerosis of the aorta and coronary arteries (planimetric investigations). Arkh Patol 25:21
11. Roberts WC (1977) Coronary heart disease. A review of abnormalities observed in the coronary arteries. Cardiovasc Med 2:29-49
12. Roberts WC (1975) The coronary arteries in coronary heart disease. Morphologic observations. Pathobiol Annu 5:249-282
13. Wolinsky H, Glagov S (1967) A lamellar unit of aortic medial structure and function in mammals. Circ Res 20:99-111
14. Wissler RW, Vesselinovitch D, Schaffner TJ, Glagov S (1980) Quantitative rhesus monkey atherosclerosis progression and regression with time. In: Gotto AM, Smith LC, Allen B (eds) Atherosclerosis V. Springer-Verlag, New York , pp 757-761
15. Glagov S, Grande T, Vesselinovitch D, Zarins CK (1981) Quantitation of cells and fibers in histologic sections of arterial walls: Advantages of contour tracing on a digitizing plate. In: McDonald TF, Chandler AB (eds) Connective tissues in arterial and pulmonary disease. Springer-Verlag, New York, pp 57-99

Part 1

Critical Review of Current
and Prospective Quantitative
Methods for Evaluating
Atherosclerosis

Introduction

ROBERT W. BARNES AND JAMES F. GREENLEAF

The purpose of the first session of this workshop is to review those existing and potential techniques for quantitative evaluation of atherosclerosis. Specifically each presentation includes a brief description of the basic principles of the method in terms understandable to the nonexpert. The fundamental assumptions inherent in using the technique are described. Emphasis is placed upon the requirements necessary for precise and accurate measurements, including calibration techniques. The limitations or technical problems associated with the method are reviewed. The evidence for reliability, including repeatability, variability, sensitivity, specificity, and predictive value of the technique is presented. Finally the recommendations for future research and development of each method, including the needs for contributions from related or differing disciplines, are discussed.

The session is introduced by an overview of the state of the art of image analysis. The paper by Dr. Selzer describes methods for quantitative imaging from angiograms in which the accuracy obtained by using computerized techniques is shown to be two to three times better than that obtained by visual evaluation. In addition, it is shown that increases in precision and accuracy by using the computer can greatly decrease the number of subjects required to obtain desired confidence levels in the results. In addition, it is stated that hardware necessary for obtaining

quantitative measurements from these images is becoming more and
more inexpensive and widely available and can be used for analysis
of video formats which are obtained by nuclear magnetic resonance
(NMR), ultrasound, x-ray angiography, and other imaging modalities.
The problem of measuring alterations in lumen size or the effects
of atherosclerosis in three dimensions from computer assisted
tomographic images was not addressed.

Dr. Cornhill reviews current and future techniques of morphologic analysis of atherosclerotic lesions.

The biochemical dynamics of atherosclerotic lesions are reviewed
by Drs. Small and Waugh.

The role of contrast arteriography in quantitative evaluation
of experimental atherosclerosis is reviewed by Dr. DePalma. Using
both canine and primate models, serial arteriograms were obtained
to evaluate progression and regression of atherosclerotic lesions
in the carotid bifurcation, thoracic aorta, abdominal aorta, and
the superior and inferior mesenteric, lumbar, and spermatic
arteries. Arteriography proved to be highly specific but relatively insensitive to lesions that frequently caused arterial
bulging without lumen encroachment. Such arterial dilatation
associated with atherosclerosis is not widely appreciated because
of frequent failure to fix arterial specimens at physiologic
intraluminal pressure, a point that is emphasized by Dr. Zarins
in a subsequent session of this workshop.

The principles, limitations, and clinical application of digital
subtraction angiography are reviewed by Dr. Ovitt. This modality
is currently experiencing widespead interest and early clinical
trial. The advantages of providing conventional contrast images
from intravenous injections, which may be performed on an outpatient basis, are obvious attributes contributing to the proliferation of this technique. However, problems with the method
remain, including reduced resolution compared to intraarterial
study, motion artifacts, overlapping images, large doses of
contrast and limited numbers of views and size of field with

current techniques. Nevertheless digital subtraction techniques will play an important role in morphologic imaging for both initial diagnostic screening and follow-up studies in peripheral arterial and carotid atherosclerosis. The feasibility of reliably imaging coronary arteries or coronary bypass grafts with this technique remains to be established.

The role of Doppler ultrasound for both qualitative and quantitative evaluation of atheroslerosis is reviewed by Dr. Greene and associates. Continuous wave Doppler ultrasound is the most simple, versatile, and inexpensive technique to screen patients for atherosclerosis of peripheral and cerebral arteries. However, previous techniques have frequently been qualitative and subject to experience by the examiner. Refinements in frequency analysis, using real-time sound spectral displays and computer processing techniques, permit more quantitative and sensitive detection of arterial flow disturbances. Such Doppler spectral analyses have also increased the diagnostic accuracy of Doppler or B-mode arterial imaging techniques. Further modification of existing instruments may permit quantification of peripheral arterial blood flow or cardiac output as well as interrogation of flow abnormalities of deeper visceral arteries, such as the renal, hepatic or mesenteric arteries, or portal vein.

The paper by Dr. McKinney describes the quantitative capabilities of B-mode imaging in measuring atherosclerosis, primarily by presenting a series of images of the carotid artery in which lesions and other pathologies were demonstrated using high resolution B-mode imaging. The ease of B-mode imaging and the noninvasiveness of ultrasonic methods were seen to be a great advantage over other techniques for preliminary studies into the extent of atherosclerotic disease in the carotid artery. Whether or not quantitative measurements could be obtained with B-mode imaging procedures and the consistency and confidence in such measurements were not discussed; however, the clinical usefulness of such images was described.

Dr. Budinger described the imaging capabilities of single photon radioisotopic imaging, positron emission imaging, and NMR methods. It appears as though some form of antibody imaging can be developed to obtain specific images of developing lesions in the arterial system; however, the specific intensity of such techniques at the site of interest is not yet demonstrated to be sufficient to obtain a useful image. Dr. Budinger estimates that sensitivity can be increased one hundred-fold with specially designed positron emission cameras and the use of short half-life isotopes. The use of nuclear magnetic resonance imaging was stated to be capable of imaging, but would require topical application of the measurement field in addition to very high frequencies for adequate signal noise ratio. Whether such problems as FR absorption in the body can be solved under such circumstances is yet to be determined.

The problem of quantifying the atherosclerotic lesion itself using noninvasive and external applications of energy for imaging is still unsolved. It appears as though images of the lumen or the blood column within the artery are less useful intrinsically, although easier to obtain, than images of the lesion itself. It appears clear that ultrasonic imaging is incapable of such mea- surements except in the most superficial arteries, while nuclear magnetic imaging may be capable of obtaining higher-resolution images but also in peripheral arteries. Isotopic methods will give low resolution by perhaps semi-quantitative information on the distribution of injury or altered diffusion characteristics of the arterial wall, and in exceptional instances could present a measure of the plaque itself.

3

Atherosclerosis Quantitation by Computer Image Analysis

ROBERT H. SELZER

Existing methods to quantify atherosclerosis in living persons directly from arterial images have virtually all been developed for use with conventional angiograms for the obvious reason that practical alternative methods for arterial visualization have not been available. As will be described later in this session, a number of important new noninvasive imaging techniques have emerged recently, which will provide additional possibilities for lesion quantitation. Intravenous digital radiography, for example, can be used to visualize most of the major arteries except the coronaries, and ultrasound systems are available for routine carotid artery imaging. Experimental ultrasound systems are under development that may be capable of imaging deeper arteries including the coronaries. Imaging systems using nuclear magnetic resonance have successfully visualized arteries in small animals and phantoms that simulate arteries in the millimeter range (1). While these noninvasive methods appear very likely to be used for quantitative lesion assessment in the near future, relatively

The portion of the work described in this paper that was performed at the Jet Propulsion Laboratory of the California Institute of Technology and at the University of Southern California School of Medicine was supported in part by grants HL-14138, HL-23619, HL-23807, and contract HV-7-2930 from the National Heart, Lung, and Blood Institute and by funding from the NASA Office of Life Sciences.

little quantitative experience has been gained to date. Conversely, computer methods to quantify atherosclerosis from conventional selective angiograms have reached a stage of relative
maturity, in which their use in clinical studies is practical and
on-going. The intent of this paper is to outline lesion quantitation methods using the angiographic techniques for illustration
and to discuss some of the physical factors, performance measurements, and image analysis problems that have common applicability
to both invasive and noninvasive imaging.

An image analysis system to quantify atherosclerosis can be
used in at least two somewhat different ways: to evaluate individual patients with symptomatic disease or to assess lesion
change in clinical trials. For individual evaluation, the size
and location of major obstructive lesions are of primary importance, while for clinical trial purposes, changes in both obstructive and early disease throughout the artery may need to be
determined. Emphasis in this paper will be on automated change
detection for clinical trials. The implication of this approach
is that greater stress will be placed on the role of measurement
precision, rather than accuracy, and relatively abstract methods
to measure changes in lumen geometry will be discussed that have
little or no application to individual patient evaluation for
the purpose of therapy. Indirect methods for detecting changes
in lumen geometry such as those based on analysis of flow or
perfusion are beyond the scope of the discussion. Similarly,
visual assessment techniques are not evaluated.

In the next section, the problem of deciding what information
should be extracted from serial artery images to assess change
is discussed; following that a method is described to determine
the influence of measurement precision on clinical trial design.
Existing quantitative lesion assessment methods are illustrated
with examples of selective femoral and coronary angiograms analysis. Finally, image acquisition and processing hardware for
quantitative arterial analysis are discussed.

THE LESION QUANTITATION PROBLEM

The most commonly used visual estimator of atherosclerosis from
angiograms is simple stenosis, defined as the maximum percent
arterial narrowing within a specified length of vessel. Stenosis
appears easy to measure and easy to interpret, but a strong case
can be made that it is a poor estimator of atherosclerosis.
Consider the illustration in Fig. 1, where arterial segments with
vastly different amounts of atherosclerosis are described by the
same stenosis value. In addition, the variability of stenosis
measurement can be quite high, particularly when diffuse disease
is present, because of the difficulty of establishing the normal
or nondiseased lumen dimension. Among film readers, variation in
selecting the normal reference area has been identified as a major
cause of interobserver error (2). Comparable problems occur for
computer-measured stenosis, but to a lesser degree. If the
objective is to measure vessel change from serial images, the need
for a normal area measurement might be eliminated by direct

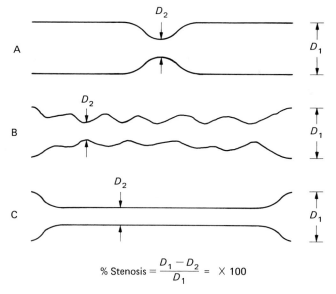

$$\% \text{ Stenosis} = \frac{D_1 - D_2}{D_1} = \times 100$$

Fig. 1   Vessel outlines indicating identical stenosis values for
arteries with varying amounts of disease.

measurement of lesion size change. However, the following conditions would have to exist:

1. Replicable exposure geometry
2. Controllable vasospasm and vasodilation
3. Correction for arterial pulsation effects
4. Discrete and symmetric lesions.

Conditions 1 and 2 can be achieved by careful angiographic
procedures. If pulsation size changes are significant--Sandor (3)
found changes of 2-7% in the coronary arteries of dogs--phase
matching of serial frames can be used. Condition 4 presents
greater problems, since lesions are frequently complex and asymmetric as indicated by the postmortem femoral casts in Fig. 2.

The necessity for lesion symmetry can be overcome by radiographic methods based on quantitative densitometry of iodine X-ray
absorption that make it possible to compute true arterial cross-
sectional area and thus incremental lumen volume changes (4,5).
Ultrasound and NMR generate individual cross-sectional images
directly, but methods must be developed to accumulate adjacent
sequences of cross sections in order to determine lesion change
along several centimeters of an artery.

One conclusion of the above discussion is that for image-based
quantitation, atherosclerosis probably has to be represented by a
continuous computer measure that reflects lumen geometry along the
length of the artery. An example of a somewhat abstract quantity
that correlates with atherosclerosis is the relative irregularity
of the detected edges of an arterial image, which might be
estimated by computing the average difference between the edge
coordinates detected originally and a smoothed (filtered) version
of the points.
An example is illustrated in Fig. 3 using the difference between
two filters. Many other methods to quantify irregularity are
possible, such as Fourier analysis and polynomial curve fitting.
Selection of a particular approach depends on factors such as the
correlation of the measurement with atherosclerotic change, the
computational difficulty, and the robustness of the measurement.
This latter factor is discussed in the following section.

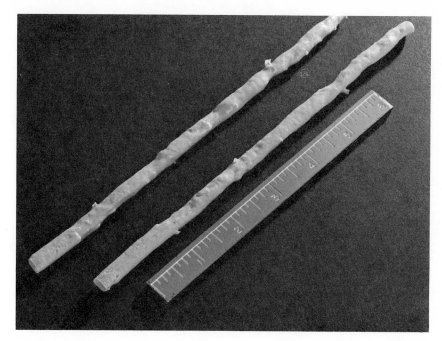

Fig. 2   Femoral artery casts (scale in inches).

MEASUREMENT VARIABILITY AND TRIAL DESIGN

Before specific methods for lesion change estimates are described, it is useful to consider the influence of measurement variability on trial design. When serial images are used to assess arterial lesions as an endpoint for randomized trials of therapy, the power of the study in detecting a treatment effect depends on the number of subjects randomized, the interval between images, and the magnitude of the effect on atherosclerosis expected from the treatment. Two other important considerations are the variability of lesion measurement and the natural variability of atherosclerotic change in the population from which the trial subjects are drawn.

Suppose the rate of atherosclerosis change is estimated by a quantity derived from the serial images, either by computer or visual processing. An example might be the measured percent

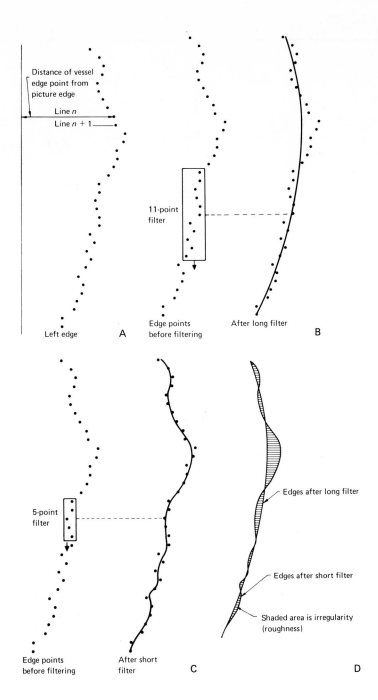

Distance of vessel
edge point from
picture edge

Line *n*
Line *n* + 1

Left edge   A

11-point
filter

Edge points
before filtering

After long filter   B

5-point
filter

Edge points
before filtering

After short
filter   C

Edges after long filter

Edges after short filter

Shaded area is irregularity
(roughness)

D

stenosis change per year. As described by Blankenhorn and Brooks
(6), the relationship between the number of subjects required in
a trial and the other design factors mentioned above is shown in
the equation below.

$$N = \frac{K}{\delta^2}\left[PPV + \left(\frac{Mp}{D}\right)^2\right]$$

(1)

where

      K = constant dependent on the desired statistical power and
          significance level for the trials,
      δ = expected percent rate of change of atherosclerosis due
          to the treatment,
    PPV = patient-to-patient percent variance of atherosclerosis
          change without treatment.
    Mp = the percent measurement precision, and
      D = the trial duration.

The expected percent change due to the treatment, δ, is
determined (or at least can be estimated) once the treatment is
selected. PPV, the normal patient-to-patient variability of the
rate at which atherosclerosis changes without treatment, can only
be estimated for the general population and may be large. Screening of potential study subjects by noninvasive methods to decrease
this variability could have a major impact on the size of clinical
trials. The measurement precision, Mp, is closely dependent on
image quality and, as described below, can be used as one means
of comparison of the various invasive and noninvasive arterial
assessment methods.

An obvious difficulty in using this equation is that relatively little is known today about the size of treatment effects and
population variance. However, using estimates derived from recent
trials in which quantitative assessment methods were employed,
some insight into the relative defects of measurement precision

Fig. 3   (Opposite)   Example of roughness calculation using two
filters. A: Representation of detected vessel edge points. B:
Application of first filter designed to follow vessel curvature
but to ignore localized irregularity caused by lesions.   C:
Application of second filter designed to follow edge deviation
caused by lesions but to suppress edge scatter caused by random
noise.   D: Superimposed edges after filtering. The shaded
difference area is a measure of relative edge roughness.

can be gained. Consider a trial design in which PPV = 14.1, as
estimated at USC from angiographic analysis of 217 femoral segments in serial films of 79 patients, treatment effect δ = 2%
change per year, significance level α = .05, power β = .90
(K = 21.02). Then, from equation (1), for a 1-year trial,

$$N = \frac{21.01}{4} (14.1 + Mp^2) \hspace{3cm} (2)$$

From (2), the relationship between measurement precision and
the required number of trial subjects can be calculated.

Mp (%)	Number of Trial Subjects
2	95
4	158
6	263
8	410
10	600

Thus, each 2% additional measurement error increases the size
of the trial by approximately 50%. Alternatively, if the number
of subjects is fixed at 95 and the duration of the test computed,
we obtain

Mp (5)	Test Duration (years)
2	1
4	2
6	3
8	4
10	5

Thus each 2% adds a year to the required trial time if the
specified significance level and power are to be achieved.

FEMORAL ANGIOGRAM ANALYSIS

The first computer effort to quantify lesion change from serial
angiograms was initiated in 1971 by USC and JPL and involved
measurement of changes in edge irregularity of the femoral artery
as recorded on annual angiograms. As shown in Fig. 4A, the
computer was programmed to find the edges of the artery as those
points along lines perpendicular to the vessel image where the

film density change was greatest (7). A smooth, tapered cylinder, designed to simulate the normal arterial lumen, was "best fit" to the detected edges, as shown in Fig. 4B and the average difference between the cylinder and the edges computed. In a postmortem validation study using this and other algorithms, edge irregularity was found to be significantly correlated with atherosclerosis (8). In two subsequent clinical studies involving approximately 150 subjects, the rate of change of edge irregularity was measured from serial femoral angiograms and used as a clinical endpoint. An overall measurement precision of approximately 4% was achieved (6,9,10).

The precision of the angiographic quantitation methods is strongly dependent on image noise and contrast. In one study which examined the relationship between edge scatter and vessel image contrast in intravenous carotid angiograms, the edge scatter was determined to be inversely proportional to contrast at correlation levels over 90% (11).

Quantitation techniques based on edge information in angiograms are relatively easy to compute, but have the undesirable property of being sensitive to rotation. To solve this problem, a technique developed by Hila (4) to determine arterial diameter by densitometric analysis of the angiographic shadow was adapted by Crawford et al. (5) to compute lumen chord length in the direction of the x-ray beam at every point of the vessel image. Since the cross-sectional area of the vessel is the sum of chord lengths perpendicular to the vessel, a profile of area variation along the vessel can be calculated and a rotation-invariant measure of disease generated. This technique was tested in phantoms and cadavers and found to measure chord lengths with an accuracy of 2-7%, depending on vessel size. The method has not yet been used in a clinical study.

Efforts are currently underway by Kaminuma and Yamazaki in Tokyo and by Erikson in Stockholm to implement computer femoral angiogram analysis, but clinical results have not yet been reported.

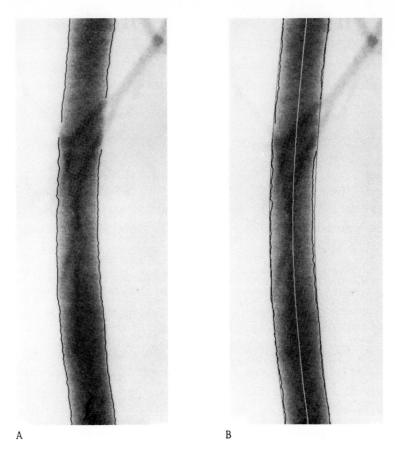

A   B

Fig. 4 Computer processed femoral angiograms. A: Display of
computer-detected edges. B: Display of computer estimate of
normal lumen.

These techniques are applicable with little modification to
other major arteries such as the carotid. Similar quantitative
methods can be implemented on digital radiographic systems and
preliminary studies have been published by Kruger and coworkers
(12,13). The combination of low preenhancement image contrast
plus the additive noise from image subtraction may make it more
difficult to achieve measurement precision for intravenous angiograms as low as that possible with selective angiograms, but this
factor will have to be weighed against the simplicity and decreased risk of intravenous methods.

CORONARY ANGIOGRAM ANALYSIS

Several instrumental procedures have been developed for coronary
angiograms; these include use of a caliper on magnified projection
images of the film (14), a viewing telescope that projects cross-
hairs onto images of the film (15), and semiautomated computer
procedures. A feature common to all of these is that a human
observer must inspect the image and estimate the location of the
vessel edge. The most advanced semiautomated method is that of
Brown and coworkers (16), in which coronary lesions are traced
from two perpendicular projected views using a hand-held stylus
connected to a computer. The views are registered by the computer,
stenosis computed using an assumption of elliptical cross sections
and various physiological parameters computed such as the
Poiseuille resistance of the measured segment. This technique,
with reported standard deviation in stenosis change measurement
in the range of 7-9% represents a substantial improvement over
the 15-25% precision reported for visual assessment techniques.

A procedure for computer measurement of coronary angiograms
has been developed by a USC/JPL team in which the degree of human
intervention is limited to selection of the vessel segment to be
analyzed and to providing an approximate indication of the vessel
midline. The computer is programmed to locate the vessel edges
in the image and to compute stenosis and other measures of irregularity that reflect the degree of atherosclerosis. In a manner
similar to the femoral analysis, the edges are determined as the
maximum gradient measured along a series of straight lines approximately perpendicular to the indicated vessel midline (Fig. 5).

After the edges for all lines have been located, a new midline to the vessel that follows the overall vessel curvature is
determined by smoothing the midpoints of the paired edges. The
computer estimate of the normal or predisease lumen location,
also shown in Fig. 5, is obtained by translating the smooth
midline outward in both directions a distance of d/2, where d is
the 90th percentile of all measured diameters for a given vessel

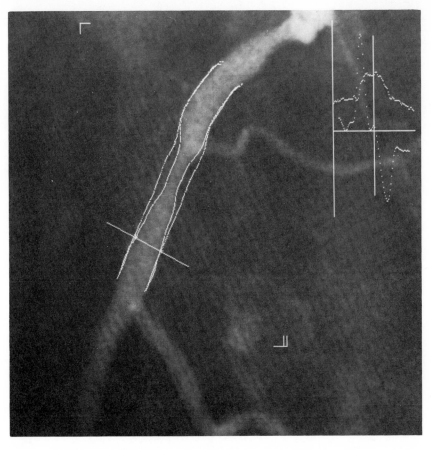

Fig. 5 Computer processing of angiogram of right coronary artery.
A sample intensity profile line and the computed gradient curve
are shown in the upper right corner of the frame.

segment. A tapered version (not shown) of the normal computer
lumen estimate is also generated in order to account for decrease
in arterial caliber associated with branches.

A small pilot study was conducted on serial cineangiograms of
men with premature atherosclerosis (17). Five smokers and five
nonsmokers (or exsmokers) were selected from a pool of 54
subjects. The two groups were matched for age, total plasma
cholesterol, relative body weight, and systolic blood pressure.
For the 51 lesions analyzed, human panel evaluation and computer

measurements of mean diameter of stenosis were in good agreement (29.1% vs 29.6%). Correlation between smoking and the rate of atherosclerosis increase based on diameter stenosis change was found, but the significance of the difference was marginal (p = .068). Another computer measure called edge angularity that utilizes all of the segmental edge information was also significantly correlated with smoking (p = .036). Our initial estimate of measurement precision is approximately 4% for detection of individual lesion change.

Automated coronary analysis is a rapidly expanding field. A nonexhaustive search revealed at least nine groups, listed in Table 1, that have active development projects using methods similar to those described above (18-21,25).

IMAGE ACQUISITION AND THE COMPUTER INPUT

Almost all work to date to quantify atherosclerosis by computers has relied on digitized film data for image input. For some of the newer noninvasive modalities, film is replaced by video recording, which makes the computer transfer of images relatively difficult, while for other modalities the image generation process is itself digital, which minimizes problems associated with computer input. A somewhat oversimplified discussion of image acquisition and computer input for the various imaging methods is given below.

Conventional Angiograms

A block diagram for image acquisition, recording, and digitizing for conventional (arterial-injection) angiography is shown in Fig. 6A. The image intensifier of the angiographic system usually exposes film, but with some systems the output is viewed by a television camera whose output is recorded on video disk or tape. A variety of devices including mechanical scanners, laser scanners, and television cameras equipped with video digitizers are used to

Table 1. Partial listing of research centers in automated coronary image analysis.

Investigators	Institution	Input to Computer	Measurements	Approach
Sandor et al. (3)	Harvard Univ., Boston	35 mm film	Diameter vs time	Edge detection
Brown et al. (16)	University of Washington, Seattle	Edge coordinates	Stenosis Poiseuille resistance Pressure drop	Manual edge tracing
Cashin et al. (17)	JPL, USC, Pasadena	35 mm film	Stenosis Area loss Volume loss "Roughness"	Edge detection and densitometry
Alderman et al. (18)	Stanford Univ., Palo Alto	35 mm film	Stenosis	Computer edge detection
Reiber et al. (19)	Erasmus Univ., Rotterdam	35 mm film	Stenosis	Computer edge detection
Kishon et al. (20)	Tel Aviv Univ., Tel Aviv	35 mm film	Stenosis	Densitometry
Barth et al. (21)	Institute for Biomedical Technology, Stuttgart	35 mm film	Stenosis	Computer edge detection
Siebes et al. (25)	Max-Planck-Inst., Bad Mauheim	Edge coordinates	Stenosis Pressure drop	Manual edge tracing

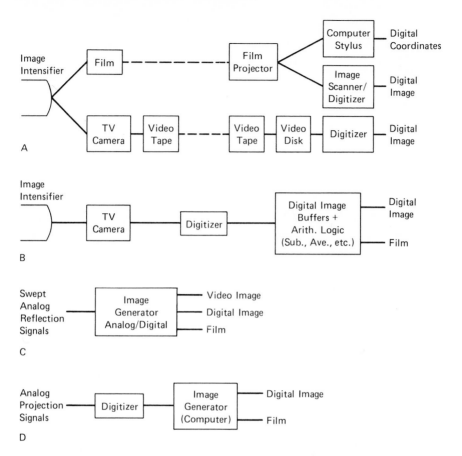

Fig. 6 Image recording and digitizing for invasive and noninvasive arterial imaging modalities.

convert the film image to numerical format for computer analysis.
It is possible to digitize video signals for a few frames directly
from the playback of a video tape recorder, but practical problems
in matching high video data rates to the input speed and internal
storage capacity of most computers usually make the use of an
intermediate video disk necessary.   The actual process of image
digitizing requires from 1/30 of a second to several minutes,
depending on the type of device, the required signal-to-noise
ratio, and the spatial resolution.   In some applications, as
previously described, instead of digitizing the entire image
a stylus is used to trace important features whose coordinates

are transmitted to the computer. In Fig. 6A, dashed lines
represent physical and time separation of the image acquisition
and the digitizing systems.

Digital Radiography

Digital radiographic systems (which probably should be called
digital intravenous angiography systems, since they are used
almost exclusively for venous-injection contrast studies), are
shown in Fig. 6B. A small number of images are digitized directly from the video camera signal and processed for enhancement purposes using frame subtraction, averaging, and other
operations in real time. Thus the digital image is available
for subsequent quantitative analysis, and if film is generated
for long-term storage, it is derived from the digital image.
A number of linear scanning systems in which the patient is
exposed to a thin, fan-shaped x-ray source have also been developed and used for direct digital recording. The exposure time
for these systems is currently somewhat long to be effective for
angiography.

   Most digital radiographic systems can only generate and store
a small number of sequential images because the digital data
rates are too high for existing computer storage devices.
Special-purpose high-speed digital disk systems, high-bandwidth
video tape recorders, and very large solid state memories have
been assembled that overcome this problem for either low-speed,
high-resolution recording (5 frames per second, 500 lines per
frame) or high-speed, low-resolution recording (30 frames per
second, 128 lines per frame).

Ultrasound

For ultrasound systems, a 2-dimensional image is generated that
represents reflection signals along a series of lines defining a
plane through the object. As indicated in Fig. 6C, image generation

is analog, digital, or hybrid, and for some existing commercial
systems the output picture is available as a video signal in
digital form or on film. For some commercial systems, a redigi-
tizing process similar to that shown in Fig. 6A must be employed
because the digital signal is not available. The problems of
matching video-rate data output to computer storage devices exist
for ultrasound as well as for digital radiographic systems.

Nuclear Magnetic Resonance and Computer Tomography

As shown in Fig. 6D, NMR and computerized axial tomography generate two-dimensional digital images from a series of one-dimensional
"projections" using computers that are built-in to the imaging
instrument. Commercial NMR imaging systems expected to be available in 1982 will be equipped with relatively powerful computers
to perform the image reconstruction. These computers will be
capable of postreconstruction image analysis, but to date, NMR
arterial imaging and measurement is at an early stage of development (1). Except for the DSR x-ray tomographic system of the Mayo
Clinic (22), arterial imaging by computerized axial tomography
systems has not been accomplished because of low imaging speed
and low spatial resolution.

THE IMAGE PROCESSING SYSTEM

The development of automated methods to measure coronary artery
dimensions from angiograms, which began in 1977, has accelerated
in the last two years, partly because improved and less expensive
computing and digitizing systems have become available. Some of
the recent technological and marketing developments in the image
processing field can be illustrated by comparing a system for
coronary analysis assembled at JPL over a period of seven years
with hardware available today. The USC/JPL coronary image analysis system includes a DEC PDP 11/45 computer, a De Anza IP 5500
image array processor which serves as an interactive picture

display, and a computer-controlled Vanguard film transport in which the optical projection system has been replaced with a Vidicon TV camera/digitizer. The image array processor consists of four picture-sized buffer memories, a very high-speed arithmetic logic unit that makes it possible to perform buffer-to-buffer arithmetic operations in one video frame time (1/30 sec) and a video signal digitizer. The state of the art in image processing is strongly oriented toward solid state image memories such as those contained within the De Anza IP 5500.

Procurement costs of this system over a 6-year period have been $300,000. Four or five companies are currently selling complete image processing systems packaged in desk-size consoles for less than $100,000 that have enough computing capability for coronary artery analysis. To illustrate a specific area in which cost changes have taken place, in 1974 a 512 x 512 image memory array cost $4000 per bit-plane, or $32,000 for an eight bit-plane image buffer. Today, the 512 x 512 memory cost is $500 per bit-plane and is declining.

At this time cineangiographic film appears to be the best storage medium for coronary artery images that are to be subjected to quantitative analysis. Video recording or direct digitizing of the signal from a television camera that views the image intensifier output from an angiographic system can be used to capture coronary artery images, but both methods have drawbacks in terms of computer measurements. The process of video recording, playback, and digitizing, even with a video disk and no video tape in the link, is likely to produce an excessively noisy digital image. Playback noise can be reduced by repetitive digitizing but recording noise cannot be overcome. Direct digitizing from the camera video decreases the noise, but as previously indicated, the technology for storing a high-speed sequence of digital images is not readily available. Improvement of the signal-to-noise ratio of the recorded analog signal by the technique of real-time predye

subtraction and iodine residual amplification as described by
Mistretta (23) is not applicable to arterial-injection angiograms
because the iodine signal before amplification is nearly full-
scale. In addition, the quantitation methods are degraded by
the added random noise associated with image subtraction.

Repetitive digitizing of a film image will minimize noise
induced by the digitizer, and while film also contains noise, it
is generally lower than that for recorded video. Another reason
for the use of film in quantitative coronary artery analysis is
to achieve the high spatial resolution needed to obtain high
measurement precision.

SUMMARY

Published data on the precision of measurement for detecting
atherosclerosis change from selective angiograms are still very
limited because many of the studies are at an early stage. The
initial estimates of coronary processing error of 7% for semiautomated analysis and 4% for automated analysis are encouraging
when compared to errors greater than 15% reported for visual
evaluation methods. Measurement variability of 3.7% for femoral
analysis has been estimated and comparable results should be
anticipated for carotid analysis.

To this author's knowledge, human coronary artery images of
sufficient quality for quantitative analysis have not been obtained by intravenous contrast angiography. Limited success in
intravenous coronary imaging in dogs has been reported (24), but
quantitative analysis remains to be accomplished. Quantitative
measurements of atherosclerotic change in peripheral arteries
using digital radiography are under development, and estimates of
measurement variability can be anticipated soon. In one study of
intravenous carotid film angiography in dogs, measurement precision was estimated at 8-12% (11).

Quantitative change measurement based on arterial image
geometry has yet to be reported for other noninvasive modalities,

but studies comparing ultrasound and angiographic measurement
of carotid disease are underway.

Noninvasive images will likely produce higher measurement
variability when subjected to quantitative procedures when compared to that produced by invasive images, but the adverse effects
on trial design that result from high measurement variability may
be more than offset by the decreased risk and cost of noninvasive
imaging and by the opportunity to pre-screen trial subjects in
order to decrease patient-to-patient variance of selected subjects.

REFERENCES

1. Crooks L, Sheldon P, Kaufman L, Rowan W, Miller T (1982)
   Quantification of obstructions in vessels by nuclear magnetic
   resonance (NMR). IEEE Trans Nucl Sci NS-29
2. Zir LM, Miller SW, Densmore RE, Gilbert JP, Harthorne JW
   (1976) Interobserver variability in coronary angiography.
   Circulation 53:627-632
3. Sandor T, Spears JR, Paulin S (1981) Densitometric determination of changes in the dimensions of coronary arteries.
   Soc Photo-Opt Instr Eng Dig Radiog 314:263-272
4. Hilal SK (1966) Determination of the blood flow by a radiographic technique. AJR 96:896-906
5. Crawford DW, Brooks SH, Barndt R, Blankenhorn DH (1977)
   Measurement of atherosclerotic luminal irregularity and
   obstruction by radiographic densitometry. Invest Radiol
   12:307-313
6. Blankenhorn DH, Brooks SH (1981) Angiographic trials of
   lipid-lowering drugs. Arteriosclerosis 1:242-249
7. Selzer RH, Blankenhorn DH, Crawford DW, Brooks SW, Barndt R Jr
   (1976) Computer analysis of cardiovascular imagery.
   Proceedings of the CALTEC/JPL Conference on Image Processing
   Technology, Data Sources and Software for Commercial and
   Scientific Applications, Pasadena, California, pp 6-1-6-20
8. Crawford DW, Brooks SH, Selzer RH, Barndt R Jr, Beckenbach ES,
   Blankenhorn DH (1977) Computer densitometry for angiographic
   assessment of arterial cholesterol content and gross pathology
   in human atherosclerosis. J Lab Clin Med 89:378-392
9. Blankenhorn DH, Brooks SH, Selzer RH, Barndt R Jr (1978) The
   rate of atherosclerosis change during treatment of hyperlipoproteinemia. Circulation 57:355-361
10. Brooks SH, Blankenhorn DH, Chin HP, Sanmarco ME, Hanashiro PK,
    Selzer RH, Selvester RH (1980) Design of human atheroscle-
    rosis studies by serial angiography. J Chronic Dis 33:347-357

11. Blankenhorn DH, Brooks SH, Chin HP, Crawford DW, Hestenes JD, Selzer RH (1981) Atherosclerosis assessment by angiographic image processing and ultrasound. Annual report NHLBI Contract N01-HV-7-2930, p 50

12. Kruger RA (1981) Estimation of the diameter and iodine concentration within blood vessels using digital radiography devices. Med Phys 8:652-658

13. Kruger RA, Mistretta CA, Riederer SJ (1981) Physical and technical considerations of computerized fluoroscopy difference imaging. IEEE Trans Nucl Sci NS-28:205

14. Rafflenbeul W, Smith LR, Rogers WJ, Mantle JA, Rackley CE, Russell RO Jr (1979) Quantitative coronary arteriography. Coronary anatomy of patients with unstable angina pectoris reexamined 1 year after optimal medical therapy. Am J Cardiol 43:699-707

15. Gensini GG, Kelly AE, Da Costa BDB, Huntington PP (1971) Quantitative angiography: the measurement of coronary vasomobility and the intact animal and man. Chest 60: 522-530

16. Brown BG, Bolson E, Frimer M, Dodge HT (1977) Quantitative coronary arteriography. Estimation of dimensions, hemodynamic resistance, and atheroma mass of coronary artery lesions using the arteriogram and digital computation. Circulation 55: 329-337

17. Cashin WL, Brooks SH, Blankenhorn DH, Selzer RH, Sanmarco ME (submitted for publication) Computerized edge tracking and lesion measurement in coronary angiograms; A pilot study comparing smokers with non-smokers.

18. Alderman EL, Berte LE, Harrison DC, Sanders W (1981) Quantitation of coronary artery dimensions using digital image processing. Soc Photo-Opt Instr Eng Dig Radiog 314:273-278

19. Reiber JHC, Booman F, Hong ST, Slager CJ, Schuubiers JCH, Gerbrands JJ, Meester GT (1978) A cardiac image analysis system. Objective quantitative processing of angiocardiograms. Proceedings of Conference on Computers in Cardiology, September 12-14, Palo Alto, California. Computers in Cardiology, IEEE catalog No.78CH 1391-2C, 239-242

20. Kishon Y, Yerushalmi S, Deutsch V, Neufeld HN (1979) Measurement of coronary arterial lumen by densitometric analysis of angiograms. Angiology 30:304-312

21. Barth K, Decker D, Faust V, Irion KM (1981) Die automatische erkennung und messung von stenosen der herzkranzgefasse im digitalen rontgebild. Digital Signal Processing Conference, Göttingen

22. Robb RA, Ritman EL (1979) High speed synchronous volume computed tomography of the heart. Radiology 133:655-661

23. Mistretta CA, Crummy AB (1981) Diagnosis of cardiovascular disease by digital subtraction angiography. Science 214: 761-765

24. Cornelius NH, Selzer RH, Hsia SS, Blankenhorn DH, Crawford DW (1981) Computer enhancement of intravenous coronary angiograms. Clin Res 29:76-A

25. Siebes M, Kirkeeide R, Gottwick M, Stammler G, Winkler B, Schaper W (1981) Computergestutzte Geometriebestimmung und Berechnung der Druckaball - Fluss-Verhältnlsse von anglografisch dargestellten Modellstenosen. Biomed Tech Bd 26 - Erganzungsband September

DISCUSSION: THOMAS F. BUDINGER

The tools that Dr. Selzer applies to invasive angiography are valuable assets to noninvasive angiography techniques. The new tools available are X-ray computed tomography, emission tomography, NMR, and digital subtraction angiography, while ultrasound and conventional angiography are now considered "older techniques."

We heard earlier that the techniques Dr. Selzer uses are not able to measure anything other than the degree of patency of an artery. But the impression that we might have here is that we learn little from contrast angiography with respect to the site of the lesion and the composition of the lesion. I want to emphasize the fact that the methods Dr. Selzer pioneered at the Jet Propulsion Laboratory are now applicable to evaluating the new tools that show composition; we are going to hear more about those tools, for instance, those that can tell us something about the fatty composition down to 200 μm.

What is perhaps more important than evaluating the composition of the lesion is to be able to quantitate with the same class of tools the moment-to-moment changes (kinetics) of the accumulation of antibodies, platelets, etc. in the arterial wall. The techniques of Dr. Selzer are needed to quantitate these parameters. One of his concluding statements is that the hardware to do the image processing is available at almost any institution. The hardware that is likely to be available in the next two years will make the man-machine interaction--tasks, automatic edge detection, and image enhancement--very easy to accomplish. The great progress made with computer tools in trying to quantify angiographs provides a valuable starting point in quantifying the new modes for imaging.

4

Morphology
Morphometric Analysis of Pathology Specimens

J. Fredrick Cornhill and M. Gene Bond

One of the major limitations in understanding the morphological changes that occur during atherosclerosis initiation, progression and regression, has been the relative lack of precise quantitative methods for establishing the extent, severity and topographical distribution of lesions. The most commonly used methods for determining atherosclerosis involvement within an arterial segment have been based on visual estimation. Atherosclerotic arteries, for instance, have been graded on arbitrary sliding scales representing increasing involvement, i.e., grade 1, 2, 3, 4, etc, relative descriptions, i.e., mild, moderate, severe, etc., on estimates of percent surface area containing lesions, and on the basis of percent "lumen stenosis" from cross-sectional histological slides. These methods are adequate for testing hypotheses that are aimed at determining large differences in the amount of atherosclerosis either between or among groups or within individual groups of subjects. However, these methods are considerably less sensitive in describing smaller or more subtle differences.

In recent years with the increasing availability of computers and computer-assisted image processing, quantitative morphometric techniques have been developed for evaluating atherosclerotic lesions. These include methods for studying extent and topographical localization of the disease on the luminal surface of arteries, the measurement of lesion involvement from cross-sectional histological material and quantifying of various tissue and cellular components using transmission and scanning electron microscopy.

SURFACE MEASUREMENTS

Quantitative measurements of atherosclerosis surface characteristics are important in defining the extent of disease, as well as determining factors operable at the level of the artery wall that affect lesion initiation, progression and regression. What are thought by many investigators to be the early forms of atherosclerosis, i.e., the relatively flat sudanophilic lesions, have been shown to be associated with ostia in young human beings, and also in several animal models including pigeons, rabbits, swine and nonhuman primates. A polar coordinate method has been applied to measuring these specific ostial lesions (1). To use this technique the vessel is opened longitudinally, fixed and processed in a saturated sudanophilic stain to demonstrate lipid accumulation. The centroid of the ostia is placed at the polar coordinate origin and oriented so that 0 degrees corresponds to a known anatomical or physiological landmark, e.g., blood flow direction (Fig. 1). The ostia is traced and the distance between the ostial lip and the edge of the lesion is measured at different radial angles, and then the data are plotted on rectangular coordinates (Fig. 2). The method is easily computerized using digitizers interfaced with computers or image analysis systems, and enables investigators to quantitate specific ostial lesions, and to produce mean composite images representative of entire populations. Applications of this technique have been used in topographic studies of sudanophilic ostial lesions (2), in studies of atherosclerosis progression and regression in the diet-induced, hypercholesterolemic rabbit model (3,4), in studies of naturally occurring lesions in the White Carneau pigeon (5), and in studies of aortic ostial lesions in human fetuses and children (6).

There are several limitations in the polar coordinate method for evaluating atherosclerosis associated with ostia. The method

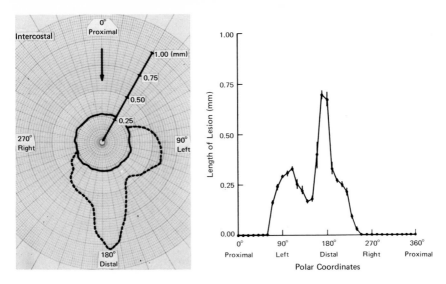

Fig. 1   Polar coordinate and rectangular coordinate graphs of an intercostal artery and associated lesion. In the polar coordinate drawing, the sudanophilic lesion on the aortic wall (broken line) is distal to the intercostal ostia (solid line). In the rectangular coordinate graph, the mean length and the standard error of the mean of the lesion on the aortic wall (i.e., differences between broken and solid lines) has been plotted against the polar coordinate angle; relative maxima occur at 100° and 170°. (From Ref. 2.)

per se is limited to examining only lesions associated with ostia, and only the early, relatively flat lesions most typically diagnosed as fatty streaks. Another method however, to be discussed, has been developed to effectively measure and map the more severe lesions on the entire arterial surface. The polar coordinate method is most easily applied to arteries that are removed in the fresh state, opened longitudinally, immersion fixed and then processed with a stain to demonstrate lipid. Artifacts, such as contraction when the artery is dissected free from its adventitial attachments, changes in ostial size due to lack of pressure fixation, and shrinkage artifacts resulting from immersion fixation or tissue processing through gross stains, may potentially affect linear measurements from the ostial centroids. Nevertheless, if the assumptions and limitations of the method are clearly understood by investigators, polar coordinate techniques should prove

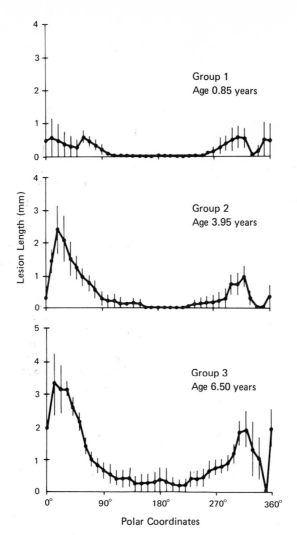

Fig. 2 Rectangular coordinate plot of the length of the celiac
sudanophilic lesion of the White Carneau pigeon as a function of
polar coordinate angle. Zero degrees and 360° are proximal (i.e.,
upstream) of the celiac ostia, and 180° is distal (i.e. downstream). Lesions develop initially in the proximal region and
then grow radially with some limited circumferential growth in
the distal region with increasing age. (From Ref. 5.)

to be a useful and powerful method for describing localization and
extent of atherosclerosis in predilective regions of the artery
wall, and for potentially establishing the morphologic correlates
induced by hemodynamic stress.

Other methods have been developed that allow investigators to measure the surface characteristics of larger arterial segments, and from the raw data to reconstruct probability maps of single or multiple types of atherosclerotic lesions. A computer-drawn topographic representation of the distribution of sudanophilic lesions in the opened human basilar artery is presented in Fig. 3. Using this method, photographs of flattened arteries are analyzed for the presence or absence of lesions, that either are or are not stained, at approximately 1000 identical sites on all vessels. The probability of a lesion being present at each site is then determined, and a probability map constructed for an artery normalized for size. In Fig. 3, areas having the highest probability for the occurrence of atherosclerosis are the proximal and ventral parts of the artery, while the distal and dorsal regions have the lowest probability for the occurrence of atherosclerosis.

The method of determining topographic probability from a standard vessel is produced by normalizing arterial length and width and is limited to short arteries or to arterial segments with relatively simple geometries. The technique cannot be applied to arteries with more complicated geometries such as the thoracic aorta, where simple normalization of vessel length and width potentially can obscure important spatial variations in lesion distribution. A general technique however, has been developed in which a biological image is divided into multiple triangular sections with the vertices of each triangle being anatomical landmarks such as ostia (8). Using linear transformations the data may be applied to a standard coordinate system which overcomes the problems of local and global variation in shape and size among specimens. With the data transformed to a standard coordinate system, and with the use of image segmentation algorithms (9), it is possible to produce quantitative probability maps that represent the spatial variation of sudanophilic lesions within populations of arteries. A computerized, image processed representation of sudanophilic lesions in thoracic aortas of cholesterol-fed mini-pigs is presented in Fig. 4. This probability

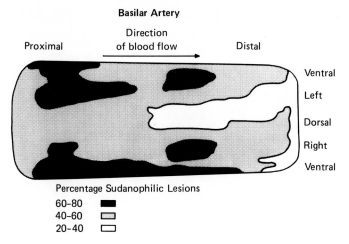

Fig. 3 Computer drawn and smoothed topographic representation of the average location of sudanophilic lesions in the human basilar arteries. (From Ref. 7.)

map, derived from several arterial segments, indicates that atherosclerosis is not uniformly distributed over the entire surface of the vessel, but rather, that there is a strong spatial dependence with the highest probability for disease to be associated with large ostia such as those of the brachiocephalic and subclavian arteries, and in the region of the ligamentum arteriosum. In the ostial regions, the highest probability for the occurrence of atherosclerosis was observed in the area immediately lateral to the leading edge of flow dividers. The second region of highest probability was found immediately proximal to the inflow track of the ostia. Areas immediately distal to the larger ostia were relatively free from disease. The outer curvature of the aortic arch, the portion from which the brachiocephalic and left subclavian arteries arise, had a much higher probability than the inner curvature. The distal inner curvature is a region that is particularly spared of atherosclerosis involvement. It is by use of these quantitative statistical maps that we may begin to approach the problem of correlating the spatial pattern of the disease with local chemistry and histology, and with specific hemodynamic influences.

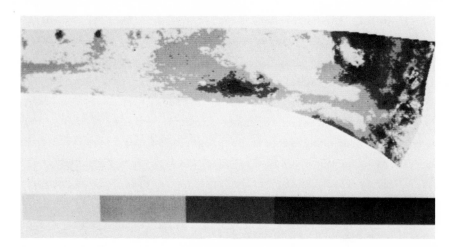

Fig. 4 Topographic map of the probability of sudanophilic lesions in the thoracic aorta of cholesterol-fed mini-pigs, generated using image analysis and computer techniques. The origin of the aorta (i.e., aortic valve) is to the right; the descending thoracic aorta at T8 is to the left. Probability bands are in 15% intervals (i.e., 0-15%, 15-30%, etc.) with the lightest colors representing low probability and the darker shades representing the highest probabilities.

ARTERIAL CROSS SECTION

Assessment of atherosclerosis severity has for many years been evaluated from histologic cross sections of arteries. Most typically, the degree of involvement has been visually estimated on the basis of relative reduction in lumen area, i.e., percent lumen stenosis. The increasing availability of instruments that are capable of accurate and efficient measurement now allow investigators the opportunity to examine quantitatively several characteristics of atherosclerotic arteries. These character-istics include linear measurements of lumen radius and diameter, circumference of lumen, internal and external elastic lamina, and mean and maximum intimal, medial and total artery wall thick-nesses. Several area measurements can also be determined including lumen, intima and media as well as internal plaque tissue charac-teristics such as fibromuscular cap, necrosis, mineralization,

etc.   In brief, the instrumentation is now available to do quantitative, morphological "dissection" of plaques and plaque components which allow investigators to express the various descriptors
of atherosclerosis severity in relative and absolute terms.

Applications of instrumentation in describing lesion severity
have been made in studies of human carotid arteries (Chapt. 13)
and in studies of atherosclerosis progression and regression using
nonhuman primate models (10-12, Chapt. 19).   Two findings that
must be taken into consideration when evaluating lesion severity
from pathology specimens have been reemphasized in these studies.
The first is that lesion severity defined as percent lumen stenosis
when estimated or measured from nonperfusion fixed vessels may not
accurately describe the effect of atherosclerosis on lumen area,
because of both configurational and size changes that potentially
occur when the artery is removed from its in vivo pressurized
state.   Secondly, there is accumulating evidence that atherosclerotic lesions can effect arteries in such a way that there may not
be an inverse relationship between plaque size and lumen caliber.

Recently, programs have been developed which not only allow
accurate and efficient measurement of lesion characteristics, but
also allow investigators to define and document more clearly the
spacial distribution of lesions and lesion components (Fig. 5).
Using the digitizer tablet, the structure of the luminal-intimal
interface, the internal elastic lamina, the medial-adventitia
border, and the adventitia may be identified.   One may calculate
numerous parameters as shown in Fig. 5.   Mean areas of the lumen,
intima, media and adventitia and the centroid of the cross section
are calculated using the inner and outer elastic lamina as a
basis.   The calculated spatial or angular polar coordinate variation of the intimal, medial, adventitial and total wall thick-
nesses may then be plotted on rectangular coordinates.   The
percent luminal stenosis and lumen-to-medial ratios may be calculated from these types of measurements.   In addition, length of
the internal elastica, areas of atheronecrosis within the plaque

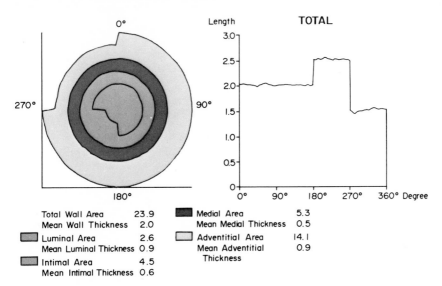

Total Wall Area	23.9		Medial Area	5.3
Mean Wall Thickness	2.0		Mean Medial Thickness	0.5
Luminal Area	2.6		Adventitial Area	14.1
Mean Luminal Thickness	0.9		Mean Adventitial	0.9
Intimal Area	4.5		Thickness	
Mean Intimal Thickness	0.6			

Fig. 5   Schematic representation of the use of polar coordinate plotting to determine the radial distribution of arterial wall morphology using the centroid, as determined by the internal elastic membrane, as the origin.   The distribution as a function of angle for the luminal, intimal, medial, and adventitial sections are shown.

or within the media, and length of destroyed internal and external elastic lamina may be determined.

QUANTITATIVE CELLULAR MEASUREMENTS

The quantitative measurement of cellular size and shape both in vivo and in vitro has recently been used extensively for the study of the cellular components of the arterial wall.   In Fig. 6, one such method for the quantification of en face endothelial cell cell morphology is presented.   The borders of this cell and its nucleus are outlined using a digitizing system; measurements of area, parameter, angle of orientation, length, width, length-to-width ratio, axis-intersection ratio, and shape index are then calculated (13).   From these data, histograms of each variable for a population may be determined, and both the average and deviating cells may be identified.   Such techniques have been employed in studies which include the effects of hemodynamics on

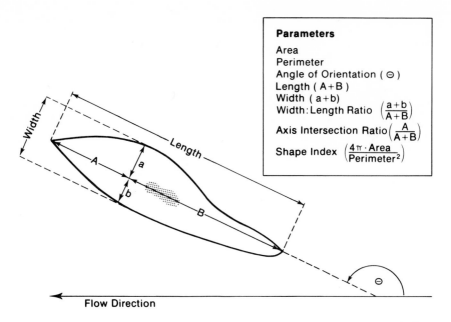

Fig. 6   Scheme of the morphometric parameters calculated for individual endothelial cells.   (From Ref. 13.)

the organization of the endothelium (14), and the identification of site of predisposition for the development of atherosclerotic lesions (15).

SUMMARY

Several quantitative methods have been developed for the evaluation of atherosclerosis from pathology specimens.   The techniques presented in this chapter are not inclusive of all those being used currently, but do provide a wide range of applicability and complexity.

Importantly, morphometric methods are not ends in themselves, but rather, provide investigators with tools that can be used to approach questions in both basic and clinical research.   Questions for instance, that seek to define subtle synergetic relationships among multiple risk factors that are operable at the level of the arterial wall, or others that are aimed at determining quantitatively the rate and direction of atherosclerosis.

Morphometric data derived from pathology specimens may also form a basis for comparing not only the biochemical and functional correlates of lesions, but also in helping establish the validity and reliability of clinical evaluations using B-mode and Doppler ultrasound images, intravenous digital subtraction angiography and nuclear magnetic residence.

REFERENCES

1. Cornhill JF, Roach MR (1974) Quantitative method for the evaluation of atherosclerotic lesions. Atherosclerosis 20:131-136
2. Cornhill JF, Roach MR (1976) A quantitative study of the localization of atherosclerotic lesions in the rabbit aorta. Atherosclerosis 23:489-501
3. Roach MR, Fletcher J, Cornhill JF (1976) The effect of the duration of the cholesterol feeding on the development of atherosclerotic lesions in the rabbit aorta. Atherosclerosis 25:1-11
4. Roach MR, Cornhill JF, Fletcher J (1978) A quantitative study of the development of sudanophilic lesions in the aorta of rabbits fed a low-cholesterol diet for up to six months. Atherosclerosis 29:259-264
5. Cornhill JF, Levesque MJ, Nerem RM (1980) Quantitative study of the localization of sudanophilic coeliac lesions in the White Carneau pigeon. Atherosclerosis 35:103-110
6. Sinzinger J, Silberbauer K, Auerwald W (1980) Quantitative investigation of sudanophilic lesions around the aortic ostia of human fetuses, newborn and children. Blood Vessels 17:44
7. Cornhill JF, Akins DE, Hutson MS, Chandler AB (1980) Localization of atherosclerotic lesions in the human basilar artery. Atherosclerosis 35:70-79
8. Cornhill JF, Barrett WA, Fry DL (1980) Quantitative topography of experimental atherosclerosis. In: Nerem RM, Guyton JR (eds) Hemodynamics and the arterial wall. Proceedings from a specialist meeting. University of Houston, pp 94-99
9. Barrett WA (1981) An iterative algorithm of multiple threshold detection. Proceedings of pattern recognition and image processing. IEEE, Computer Society, pp 273-278
10. Clarkson TB, Bond MG, Bullock BC, Marzetta CA (1981) A study of atherosclerosis regression in *Macaca mulatta*. Exp Mol Pathol 34:345-368
11. Clarkson TB, Lehner NDM, Wagner WD, St Clair RW, Bond MG, Bullock BC (1979) A study of atherosclerosis regression in *Macaca mulatta*. I. Design of experiment and lesion induction. Exp Mol Pathol 30:360-385
12. Bond MG, Adams MR, Bullock BC (1981) Complicating factors in evaluating coronary artery atherosclerosis. Artery 9:21-29

13. Cornhill JF, Levesque MJ, Herderick EE, Nerem RM, Kilman JW, Vasko JS (1980) Quantitative study of the rabbit aortic endothelium using vascular casts. Atherosclerosis 35:321-337
14. Nerem RM, Levesque MJ, Cornhill JF (1981) Vascular endothelial morphology as an indicator of the pattern of blood flow. J Biomech Eng 103:172-176
15. Lewis JC, Taylor RG, Jones ND, St Clair RW, Cornhill JF (1982) Endothelial surface characteristics in pigeon coronary artery atherosclerosis. I. Cellular alterations during the initial stages of dietary cholesterol challenge. Lab Invest 46:123-138

5

Physical Biochemistry of the Lesions of Man, Subhuman Primates, and Rabbits

DAVID A. WAUGH AND DONALD M. SMALL

Our task is to summarize briefly the biochemical constituents of the vessel walls and how these change during the progression from normal intima to an atherosclerotic plaque. The intima is made up of a variety of cellular and noncellular components, including endothelial and occasional smooth muscle cells, glycosaminoglycans, collagen, and elastin ground substances. There is evidence that all of these intimal constituents undergo some changes during the progression from normal intima to atherosclerotic lesion. The major changes in mass and therefore volume during the progression to atherosclerotic lesions in man are in the lipid constituents of the vessel wall. In the normal vessel wall at different ages the total dry weight of the intima contains only a very few percent of its total mass as lipid (1); in the discrete small lesions called fatty streaks the lipid content of the intima in that lesion has increased to approximately 20% of the total mass. However, in carefully dissected, large, raised lesions described as atherosclerotic plaques, the percent dry weight is often greater than 50% (2). Since the density of the lipids is some 30-40% less than the density of the other constituents (proteins, polysaccharides),

This research was supported by National Institutes of Health grants HL-26335 and HL-07291. We wish to thank Saul S. Katz for permission to use Fig. 2 and Irene Miller for typing the manuscript.

absolute volume occupied would be greater than the mass. Thus in
human atherosclerotic lesions lipids account for a major fraction
of the nonwater volume occupied by the lesion and therefore must
be considered in the pathogenesis. The rest of this discussion
will be directed mainly towards lipids, although other substances
which increase in mass during the development of atherosclerotic
lesions also include some cellular and connective tissue elements.

PHYSICAL CHEMISTRY OF LIPIDS OF ATHEROSCLEROTIC LESIONS

Matter can exist in a number of physical states such as gas,
liquids, solids, and some intermediate forms between liquids and
solids called liquid crystals. Thus it is possible that lipids
in the arterial wall during the progression of atherosclerosis
could be present in different states (liquids, liquid crystals,
or solids), and that the reversibility of these lesions might be
related to the state(s) of the deposited lipids. Therefore, many
years ago we undertook to understand the physical interactions
of the major lipids found in atherosclerosis (3).

The major lipids that accumulate in atherosclerosis are
phospholipids, cholesterol, and cholesterol esters. The interactions of equilibrated mixtures of these substances in aqueous
systems can be represented on a triangle, in which there are four
major zones (Fig. 1). Zone I, a lamellar liquid-crystalline
phase, contains bimolecular leaflets of phospholipid into which
free cholesterol and small amounts of cholesterol ester can be
incorporated. The maximum amount of free cholesterol incorporated
is about 33% of the amount of phospholipid by weight, or approximately 1 mol free cholesterol per mol phospholipid. The maximum
amount of cholesterol ester incorporated is about 2%, or approximately 1 mol cholesterol ester per 40 mol phospholipid. In this
phase, which is analogous to the lipid regions of many cell
membranes and cell-organelle membranes (4), the lamellar liquid
crystals may be more or less fluid, depending on the type of
phospholipid, the fatty acyl chains within it, and the other

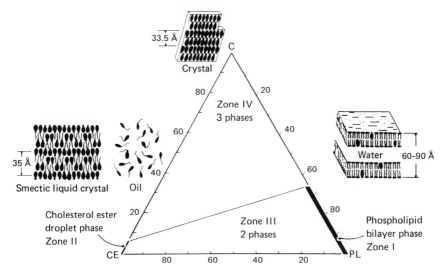

Fig. 1. Phase diagram of three-component system cholesterol (C),
phospholipid (PL), and cholesterol ester (CE) in excess water at
37°C and 1 atmosphere pressure. Zone I has a single phase of
phospholipid lamellar liquid-crystal with up to 33% cholesterol
and 2% cholesterol ester. Zone II also contains a single phase
of liquid or liquid-crystalline cholesterol ester. Zone III
contains both the cholesterol ester and phospholipid phases. Zone
IV has a third phase, cholesterol monohydrate crystals. Schematic
molecular representation of the phases are shown near each apex
of the triangle. The irregular lines denote phospholipid molecules, the solid symbols cholesterol molecules and the solid,
tailed symbols cholesterol ester.

membrane components present, such as cholesterol, glycosphingo-
lipids or proteins.

Zone II contains a single phase of cholesterol ester, which
incorporates small amounts of free cholesterol--about 4% at 37°C.
Depending on the fatty acid that is esterified to cholesterol,
this phase may be in one of four states: a liquid state, in which
the molecules are randomly associated; a cholesteric liquid-
crystal state, in which the molecules are nearly oriented along
their long axes; a smectic liquid-crystalline state, in which the
molecules form a layered structure perpendicular to the long axis
(Fig. 1); or a crystalline solid state. Equivalent amounts of
cholesterol--4% by weight--are incorporated by the liquid,

cholesteric, and smectic phases, but crystalline ester excludes free cholesterol from its lattice.

In Zone III, mixtures of these lipids separate into the cholesterol-ester phase (Zone II), which floats in water, and the lamellar liquid-crystalline phase (Zone I), which sinks. In Zone IV, three phases with fixed composition coexist: the lamellar phospholipid liquid-crystalline phase saturated with cholesterol and cholesterol ester; an oily cholesterol-ester phase saturated with free cholesterol; and a cholesterol-monohydrate-crystal phase (3,5).

Each of these phases has physical characteristics that can be identified with polarizing or electron microscopy, by colorimetry, or by x-ray diffraction. The liquid-crystalline phase in Zone I has a characteristic appearance under polarizing and electron microscopes, and its x-ray diffraction is typical of a one-dimensional lamellar lattice. The first-order lamellar spacing reflects the thickness of the bilayer and its accompanying layer of water. This thickness, determined by the lipids and the amount of water present, may vary from about 6 to 9 nm (60 Å to 90 Å), but it is characteristic for a given lipid at a given temperature.

Zone II, the cholesterol-ester phase, may be liquid, liquid crystalline, or crystalline. If liquid, it is isotropic (non-birefringent between crossed polars) and produces x-ray scattering with very diffuse maxima at approximately 0.5 nm (5 Å) and 3 nm (30 Å). The cholesteric and smectic phases have different bire-fringent textures under the polarizing microscope (6).

Furthermore, the cholesteric phase scatters x-rays like the liquid, but the smectic phase produces very sharp maxima from which the organization of ester molecules in layers has been deduced (Fig. 1) (7). Each ester has a characteristic transition temperature that can be quantitated by microscopy and colorimetry, and mixtures of esters undergo transitions in a predictable manner--for example, the more double bonds in the acyl chains of the mixture, the lower the transition temperature (6). Thus the transition temperature provides evidence of the chemical composition of the esters in Zone II.

The cholesterol-monohydrate-crystal phase in Zone IV has been characterized extensively in plaques (3,5). The crystals show characteristic x-ray spacing and appearance under the microscope; they melt at 85°C (8); and their crystal structure has been identified (9).

PHYSICAL CHEMICAL PROPERTIES OF THE NORMAL INTIMA

Katz (10) has recently shown that the normal intima of newborn children contains virtually no cholesterol ester as indicated in Fig. 2. As the person passes through the various decades of life the mean intimal lipid composition increases, a separate cholesterol ester phase is formed, which is largely extracellular and progresses down the line toward LDL composition as noted in Fig. 2. In the fifth decade this line changes its direction as the intima becomes enriched in free cholesterol and deviates from the direction of the lipid deposition in the younger intima. Lipid deposition in the intima up to 40 years looks as if lipids from low-density lipoproteins are added to the vessel wall. However, the composition at older ages, richer in cholesterol, is different and thus appears to have undergone biochemical changes. It should be stressed that the intima in all these cases would look grossly normal and be considered pathologically normal.

PHYSICAL PROPERTIES OF ATHEROSCLEROTIC LESIONS

The first grossly recognizable lesions are the fatty streaks, slightly raised yellow lesions from 1 mm up to 1 cm in size, which contain large masses of foam cells and whose composition is plotted on Fig. 3. The origin of the lipid in foam cells has stimulated great interest recently and several reviews concerning the cellular metabolism of cholesterol and lipid deposition have been worth consulting (11,12,13). Most of the lipids in fatty streaks are present in the foam cells and are present as

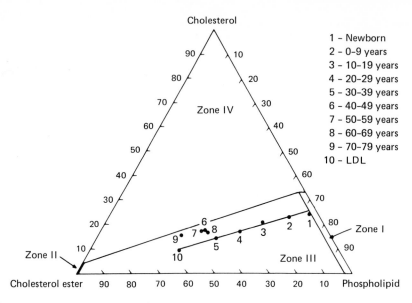

Fig. 2   Compositions of normal intima lipids of newborns and
people of subsequent decades as plotted on the cholesterol,
phospholipid, and cholesterol ester phase diagram (see Fig. 1).
Plots 1-9 represent intima lipids, whereas point 10 is the composition of human LDL.   Intima lipid compositions up to the fourth
decade fall on a straight line joining newborn to LDL (From Ref.
10, with permission.)

cholesterol ester phase, readily observable under the polarizing
microscope as shown in Fig. 4A.   The intermediate lesions appear
rather similar although perhaps slightly larger than fatty streaks,
but they fall in a region where three phases are predicted to
coexist, that is, the cholesterol ester phase, the membrane phase,
and cholesterol monohydrate crystals.   However, only a few of the
lesions in this zone actually had cholesterol monohydrate crystals
and the number of crystals is very small (5), which suggests that
these lesions contain cholesterol in a supersaturated system.

The gruel-containing plaques have a composition having much
greater free cholesterol.   Unlike fatty streaks and intermediate
lesions the plaques are necrotic and contain much dead cellular
material, and most of the lipid is extracellular (2,5).   The
predicted lipid physical state should contain large numbers of
crystals of cholesterol monohydrate and these are in fact present.

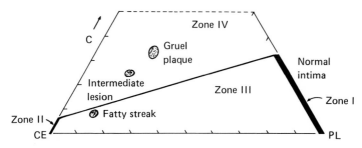

Fig. 3   Mean composition of fatty streaks, intermediate lesions, and gruel-containing plaques plotted on the phase diagram (see Fig. 1).   (From Ref. 5, with permission.)

In human lesions, the cholesterol monohydrate crystals may reach the size of 1 mm in length.   They are present as large plates as indicated in Fig. 4B.

A simplified thesis of the development of the plaque (13,14) is outlined in Fig. 5.   First, during the early period of life the intimal cells and the extracellular intima contain very little cholesterol-ester-rich lipid material.   Most of the lipid is present as membranes in cells and has a composition lying near the phospholipid zone.   With increasing age the composition of the

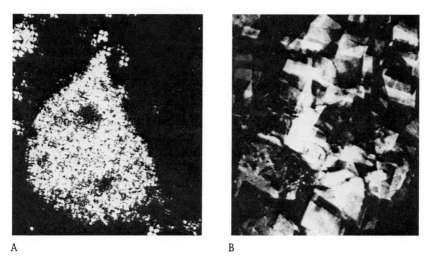

A   B

Fig. 4   A: Polarized light photomicrographs of a foam cell.
B: Cholesterol monohydrate crystals at 22°C (X100, multicrossed polarizers).

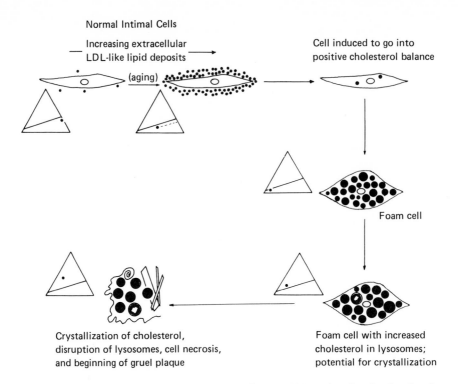

Fig. 5 Schematic representation of possible physical-chemical changes that occur during the development of gruel-containing plaques. In normal intima, lipid droplets accumulate extracellularly with age, predominantly associated with connective tissue fibrils. At some time, some cells are induced to go into positive cholesterol balance and the cell begins to accumulate cholesteryl oleate-rich storage droplets. If this process continues foam cells develop. In some cells a lysosomal defect may develop which does not allow the exit of free cholesterol or a relative deficiency of cholesterol carrier protein. Lysosomes become supersaturated with cholesterol, nucleation occurs, crystals form, the lysosomes rupture, and necrosis and cell death begin.

intima proceeds toward LDL. Thus more and more LDL-like lipid (this does not necessarily mean native LDL but could mean an altered form of LDL (see 14,15,16), accumulates in the extracellular space, but the cells apparently remain normal. At some point in time in the vessel wall some cells are induced to go into positive balance, more cholesterol enters the cell than leaves, and the cell begins to accumulate cholesteryl oleate-rich storage droplets. If cholesterol balance continues to be positive the cells become

foam cells and a group of such cells is called a fatty streak.
These lesions are obviously reversible if cholesterol balance can
be reversed. In time some of these lesions may develop a lysosomal defect that allows the continued intake of cholesterol ester
into lysosomes and the hydrolysis into free cholesterol, but blocks
exit out of lysosomes either due to cellular mechanisms being
saturated with cholesterol or a relative deficiency in cholesterol
carrier protein. This allows free cholesterol concentration to
increase within lysosomes to the point where nucleation may occur,
crystals form, the lysosomes rupture, cells autolyze, and cell
death and necrosis begin. Such a progression would lead to a
relative decrease in cholesterol ester and an increase in free
cholesterol as is seen in the atherosclerotic plaque (Fig. 3).
Furthermore, such necrosis would allow other elements such as
thrombosis, fibrobrosis, collagen deposition, and calcium precip-
itation to accompany the necrosis and give rise to the other
elements found in advanced calcified atherosclerotic plaques.

THE CORRELATION OF THE HISTOLOGICAL APPEARANCE OF LESIONS
AND THE POSITION OF THE LIPIDS IN THE LESIONS

In lesion fragments as shown in Fig. 4, it is possible to dissect
unfixed lesions and observe foam cells, lipid droplets, and cholesterol monohydrate crystals. Dissection and removal of parts of
lesions to microscopic slides were necessary because the usual
fixation techniques for vessel walls involve changes in temperature and medium, particularly organic solvents and dyes, which
alter the physical state of the lipids. However, the techniques
utilized by us to observe the native physical state does not allow
fixation of the tissue or preservation of the normal architecture
of the vascular wall. Thus we would like to know where the cellular and extracellular lipids are in respect to the vessel wall
architecture and whether the physical state varies in different
regions of the arterial wall.

     In normal histological sections of atherosclerotic lesions the
presence of lipid is either inferred from empty spaces or detected

with dyes such as oil-red-O and Sudan black (17), both of which
alter the physical properties of lipid. Polarized light microscopy (PLM) however has the advantages of not only detecting lipid
in its natural state, but also by determining some of the physical
properties of the lipid (such as birefringence, morphology and
melting) one can deduce the biochemical nature of the lipid (5).
For example, what is thought to be cholesterol in plaques as inferred from "clefts" can really be confirmed only by PLM. In
certain cases the clefts could well be artifacts.

As it has been mentioned, although PLM has been used to detect
the presence of lipid in its various phases within lesions, it has
been done in squashed tissue, thus destroying any chance of knowing the original site of the lipid. However, we have found that
by rapidly freezing tissue in hexane at -70°C excellent sections
could be obtained with good definition of the lipid and mainte-
nance of its physical properties. This allows correlations to be
made between histology and biochemistry at a level not possible
with other techniques.

An example of the technique can be seen in the micrographs of
a lesion taken from an atherosclerotic rabbit (Fig. 6). A section
stained with hematoxylin & eosin (HE) shows marked intimal thickening with smooth muscle cells and early foam cell formation deep
in the intima. A lipid stain of the adjacent section shows evidence of lipid deposition, which is confirmed by PLM. At higher
magnification it is difficult to be certain if the lipid is intra-
or extracellular, and it also appears to be in large droplets.
However, when viewed by a PLM the lipid is obviously intracellular
in small discrete droplets (Fig. 7). Thus the CE-filled cells
correspond to the foam cells seen on HE.

If the unstained section is then heated and observed under
the PLM, melting temperatures of the droplets within each cell
(or extracellular droplets as well) can be easily determined and
photographically recorded. In the absence of impurities in the
droplets the melting temperature of cholesterol ester is a
reflection of the fatty acid composition (6). Thus, biochemical

differences in cells throughout the lesion can be observed histologically. Within the early rabbit lesions the lipid appeared to
melt fairly uniformly. This uniform melting is not surprising
since it is known that cholesterol is initially deposited in foam
cells predominantly as cholesterol oleate (18). However, as lesions progress to intermediate lesions and fatty plaques, the
ester composition changes (5) and this should be observable within
certain regions of the lesion. These biochemical differences may
also be correlated with other histological changes that may be
occurring in progressive and regressive lesions. For instance,
when appropriate cellular markers are used, the changes in lipid
biochemistry in smooth muscle cells and macrophages can be followed. Furthermore, changes in lipid biochemistry may be in
certain cells of intermediate lesions which may be precursers to
cellular necrosis and development of the plaques.

Preparation of the tissue in this way also allows detection
of enzymatic activity, which can also be correlated with lipid
deposition and its physical properties. For instance, using a
substrate to detect β-galactosidase (19), a lysosomal enzyme, we
can see slight activity in normal rabbit artery within smooth
muscle cells. However, following production of atherosclerosis,
activity is greatly increased but only in regions of cholesterol
ester deposition. In areas of intimal thickening without CE deposition only minimal amounts of activity are present. It would
appear that the enhanced lysosomal activity is associated with
CE-filled cells.

At present we are using the technique to study the effects of
various diets on the biochemistry of lesions in the atherosclerotic rabbit. Obviously the technique can be used to study
lesions in any animal model, including man. However, we have
found that it is necessary to use fresh, unfixed tissue to get the
best results, which requires being present at autopsy. By concur-
rently determining biochemical, biophysical, and histological
changes on the same histological section, a greater understanding
of the mechanism of progression and regression should be possible.

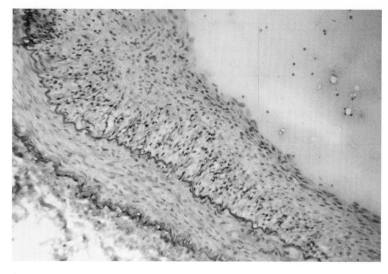

A

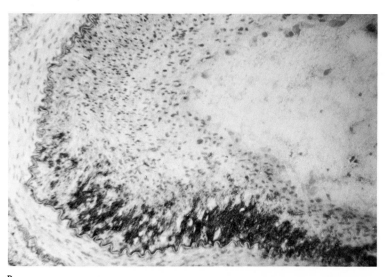

B

Fig. 6 A: Adjacent sections of rabbit artery showing intimal
thickening and foam cell formation deep in the intima. B: An
oil-red-0 stain confirms the presence of lipids. C: Photographed
under polarized light the birefringent areas correspond exactly to
the lipid seen on oil-red-0.

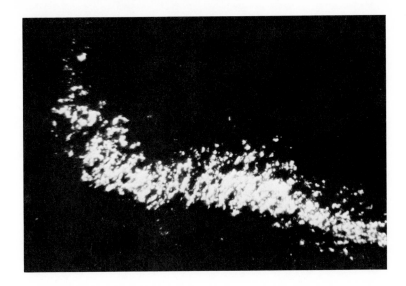

C

Fig. 6 Continued

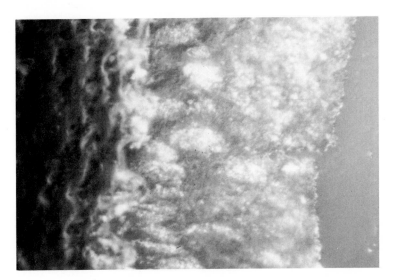

A

Fig. 7 At high magnification, (X400) photomicrographs of the same section before and after staining for lipid. Polarized light microscopy (A) gives better definition of cellular origin of the lipid than does oil-red-O (B).

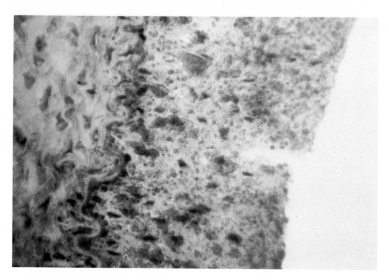

B

Fig. 7 Continued

REFERENCES

1. Smith EB, Evans PH, Downham MD (1967) The lipid in the aortic
   intima. The correlation of morphological and chemical characteristics. J Atheroscler Res 7:171-186
2. Smith EB, Slater RS (1972) The microdissection of large
   atherosclerotic plaques to give morphologically and topo-
   graphically defined fractions for analysis. Part 1. The
   lipids in the isolated fractions. Atherosclerosis 15:37-56
3. Small DM, Shipley GG (1974) Physical-chemical basis of lipid
   deposition in atherosclerosis. Science 185:222-229
4. Small DM (1977) Liquid crystals in living and dying systems.
   J Colloid Interface Sci 58:581-602
5. Katz SS, Small DM, Shipley GG (1976) Physical chemistry of
   the lipids of human atherosclerotic lesions. Demonstration
   of a lesion intermediate between fatty streaks and advanced
   plaques. J Clin Invest 58:200-211
6. Small DM (1970) The physical state of lipids of biological
   importance--cholesterol esters, cholesterol and triglyceride.
   In: Blank M (ed) Surface chemistry of biological systems.
   Plenum Press, New York, pp 55-83
7. Atkinson D, Deckelbaum RJ, Small DM, Shipley GG (1977) The
   structure of human plasma low-density lipoproteins. The
   molecular organization of the central core. Proc Natl Acad
   Sci USA 74:1042-1046
8. Loomis CR, Shipley GG, Small DM (1979) The phase behavior
   of hydrated cholesterol. J Lipid Res 20:525-535

9. Craven BM (1976)   Crystal structure of cholesterol monohydrate. Nature 160:727-729
10. Katz SS (1981) The lipids of grossly normal human aortic
    intima from birth to old age. J Biol Chem 256:12275-12280
11. Brown MS, Goldstein JL (1976) Receptor-mediated control of
    cholesterol metabolism. Science 191:150-154
12. Fredrickson DS, Brown MS, Goldstein JL (1978) The familial
    hyperlipoproteinemias. In: Stanbury JB, Wyngaarden JB,
    Fredrickson DS (eds) The metabolic basis of inherited disease.
    McGraw-Hill, New York, pp 604-655
13. Small DM (1977) Cellular mechanisms for lipid deposition in
    atherosclerosis. N Engl J Med (Seminars in Physiology)
    297:873-877, 924-929
14. Small DM (1980) Summary of concepts concerning the arterial
    wall and its atherosclerotic lesions. In: Gotto AM Jr, Smith
    LC, Allen B (eds) Atherosclerosis V. Springer-Verlag, New
    York, pp 520-524
15. Hoff HF, Heideman CL, Gaubatz JW (1980) Low-density lipopro-
    teins in the aorta: In: Gotto AM Jr, Smith LC, Allen B (eds)
    Atherosclerosis V. Springer-Verlag, New York, pp 533-536
16. Hollander W, Paddock J, Colombo M (1979) Lipoproteins in
    human atherosclerotic vessels. Exp Mol Pathol 30:144-171
17. Humason GL (1979) Staining lipids and carbohydrates. In:
    Animal Tissue Techniques. WH Freeman and Company, San
    Francisco, pp 284-293
18. St Clair RW (1976) Cholesterol ester metabolism in athero-
    sclerotic arterial tissue. Ann NY Acad Sci 275:228-237
19. Bayliss-High OB, Adams CWM (1980) The role of macrophages
    and giant cells in advanced human atherosclerosis.
    Atherosclerosis 36:441-447

DISCUSSION: RICHARD W. ST. CLAIR

Drs. Small and Waugh have already described some of the physical biochemical changes that take place in the lipids of the athero- sclerotic lesion. I would like to summarize for you in a very simplified way some of the other biochemical changes that take place in the atherosclerotic lesion and, finally, attempt to give you some perspective as to the role of the cellular components of the arterial wall responsible for some of these changes.

The following is a summary of the major biochemical changes that are found in atherosclerotic arteries:

Increased permeability to macromolecules and perhaps blood
    monocytes
Cholesterol and cholesteryl ester accumulation (intra-
    and extracellular)
Increased cholesterol esterification and fatty acid
    synthesis
Increased cell proliferation and cell death
Increased synthesis and accumulation of connective
    tissue matrix (collagen, elastin, proteoglycan)
Necrosis and mineralization.

These by no means represent a complete list, but instead are meant to include those processes that appear to be related to the basic pathogenesis of the lesion.

The first of these changes is an increase in the permeability of the arterial wall to macromolecules such as low-density lipo- protein, and other plasma proteins. In addition, if the endothe- lial surface is examined by scanning electron microscopy, one frequently sees blood cells that can be identified principally as monocytes adhering to the endothelium at the growing edge of the raised lesions. This may be the forerunner of the entry of blood monocytes into the arterial wall, where they ultimately are converted into macrophages. The hallmark of atherosclerosis is the accumulation of cholesterol and cholesteryl esters, both intra- and extracellularly. This does not represent a simple accumulation of cholesterol and cholesteryl esters from lipoproteins, but rather the arterial wall plays a significant role in remodeling the composition of the cholesteryl esters that accumulate. This is done by initial hydrolysis of lipoprotein cholesteryl esters, followed by reesterification to fatty acids either synthesized by the arterial wall or derived from the plasma. As a result, one of the earliest biochemical changes to occur in the developing lesion is an increase in cholesterol esterification. Increased cell proliferation is also a prominent early feature of the developing lesion. This is associated with an increased rate of cell death, but obviously since cells accumulate in the atherosclerotic intima cell proliferation must initially exceed cell death. As the lesion progresses there is an increased accumulation of connective tissue components, including collagen, elastin, and proteoglycans. This is then followed somewhat later in the progression of the disease by necrosis and mineralization and, ultimately, other events such as ulceration, hemorrhage within the plaque, and thrombosis. The major components of the atherosclerotic lesion that are responsible for the mass of the atheroma are the increased number of cells, connective tissue, and in particular, the massive accumulation of cholesterol and cholesteryl esters.

What cells are responsible for the above described metabolic changes? If one looks at an electron micrograph of an atherosclerotic lesion at least two types of fat-filled cells known as foam cells are seen. A number of these foam cells are clearly smooth muscle cells as evidenced by the presence of a prominent basement membrane, numerous pinocytotic vesicles, and large numbers of myofilaments. On the other hand, there are clearly other foam cells that are more difficult to identify. They do not have the above described characteristics of smooth muscle cells and, at least by morphologic and some biochemical criteria, probably represent macrophages. The proportion of foam cells derived from smooth muscle cells and of macrophages within the lesion can vary considerably, and there is little information to explain the reasons for this distribution.

Let's consider the specific biochemical roles of each of these three cell types. First of all, the endothelium plays a major role as a permeability barrier for cells and macromolecules entering the arterial wall. It now seems clear that in the developing atherosclerotic lesion one does not necessarily have to have frankly denuded endothelium in order to have alterations in endothelial permeability. Consequently, more subtle metabolic changes in the endothelium would appear to play a critical role in determining the integrity of this endothelial barrier. In addition, the endothelium serves as an antithrombogenic surface by insulating the blood components from tissue constituents such as collagen and by the production of prostacyclin that acts to inhibit platelet aggregation. Smooth muscle cells represent the major cellular component of the arterial wall. They possess receptors for the uptake of normal LDL and this uptake of LDL can result in the accumulation of cholesteryl esters within the cell. Although it is difficult to envision how such a highly regulated process might result in the pathologic accumulation of cholesteryl esters, there must be such mechanisms since smooth muscle cells with abnormal accumulations of cholesteryl esters clearly are present in the atheroma. Another important process in which smooth muscle cells participate is in the proliferation of cells within the intima. Smooth muscle cell proliferation occurs early in the pathogenesis of the developing lesion and is thought to be stimulated by a variety of factors, including platelet-derived growth factor as well as growth factors produced by both macrophages and endothelial cells. Smooth muscle cells are also thought to be the major cell type responsible for the synthesis of the connective tissue matrix of the arterial wall, although again endothelial cells have also been shown to synthesize certain types of collagen. What stimulates connective tissue synthesis is unknown. Macrophages are not a major cellular component of the normal arterial wall. As a result, their appearance in the atherosclerotic lesion is thought to result from the migration of blood monocytes into the arterial wall in response to certain unknown stimuli. Macrophages have receptors for the uptake of abnormal lipoproteins. These abnormal lipoproteins are taken up by the cell in massive amounts, since this receptor is very poorly down-regulated. Consequently, the macrophage can accumulate large amounts of cholesteryl esters and show substantial increases in cholesterol esterification. As a result, it is not clear whether the early increase in cholesterol esterification in the developing lesion can be attributed to macrophages or to smooth muscle cells or both. As mentioned previously, macrophages have also been shown to produce growth factors that can stimulate proliferation of both smooth muscle cells and endothelial cells. As a result, the effect of one cell type on another may play an important role in the pathogenesis of atherosclerosis.

In conclusion, it seems clear that the components that accumulate in the atheroma are the result of a complex interaction of plasma constituents with the cellular elements of the arterial wall. As a result, both the plasma-derived and cell-mediated processes must be understood if the pathogenesis of the disease is to be fully appreciated.

6

Angiography in Experimental Atherosclerosis
Advantages and Limitations

Ralph G. DePalma

The ability to detect atherosclerotic plaques and to document changes in their luminal intrusion *in seriatim* are important operational goals of experimental design. During the past 12 years we have evolved methods for serial arteriography in monkeys and dogs (1-3) and have performed more than 100 of these procedures. Initially, arteriography was used as a tool in experimental atherosclerosis much as it is used clinically: to detect the presence of gross atherosclerotic disease. Serial interventions in animal models, which could not be performed in humans, made it possible to monitor radiographically atherosclerotic plaque dynamics at known and characteristic sites (4,5). Angiography in combination with serial morphologic observations was found to be useful in detecting regressive lesion change in individual animals (6,7). This report presents data on sensitivity and specificity of angiography for detection of atherosclerosis. These data also provide an estimate of the degree of discrepancy between angiographic and conventional pathologic grading. Advantages of

---

This work was supported by USPHS Grant #7 R01 HL 26338-01. The author wishes to acknowledge the support from the University of California, Davis Primate Facility and the School of Veterinary Medicine. The contributions of Dr. Errol M. Bellon in angiographic grading and for contributing Figs. 4, 6, and 8 are gratefully acknowledged.

angiography, as well as its assumptions and limits, will be considered in relationship to experimental design.

METHODS AND CRITIQUE

Animal Colonies and General Methods

Angiograms, followed in a short time by autopsy or surgical morphologic observations, were obtained from three colonies of adult male rhesus monkeys (*M. mulatta*) and one colony of juvenile male cynomolgus monkeys (*M. fascicularis*). Our early developmental work with rhesus monkeys, from 1969 to 1972, evaluated the effects of atherogenic diets in inducing hypercholesterolemia of sufficient intensity and duration to yield plaques with luminal intrusion. These early experiments provided eight rhesus monkeys with either normal arteries or only minimal disease. When intrusive lesions were ultimately produced, other rhesus monkeys were investigated using sequential surgical and angiographic evaluations. We were able to demonstrate plaque development in individual animals and subsequent lesion regression in response to lowering serum cholesterol concentrations. The documentation of regression and the methods of serial angiographic and surgical evaluation have been described previously (2,3).

We later used serial angiographic and morphologic observations to assess the efficacy of intervention with a bile acid sequestrant in another colony of 10 atherosclerotic rhesus monkeys (6,7). A study of antiplatelet therapy in a third colony of 10 atherosclerotic rhesus monkeys has recently been reported (8). Angiographic and morphologic data were also available from a group of six cynomolgus monkeys with atherosclerosis studied for collagen dynamics (9). Five of these animals were sacrificed six weeks after angiography and biopsies confirmed the presence of stenotic plaques. A sixth, adult male with advanced disease was sacrificed immediately after angiography for a correlative study. Arteriograms were also done on 12 adult male atherosclerotic beagles for developmental studies of ulcerated plaques.

These experiments were not designed to obtain quantitative data relating angiographic with morphologic characteristics under physiologic conditions. Rather, these investigations focused upon disease induction and detection of regressive trends in individual animals after treatment. Fixation perfusion with glutaraldehyde at arterial pressure done in two comparably atherosclerotic rhesus monkeys confirmed the presence of anatomically intrusive lesions. However, these necropsies were done at a time and place sufficiently remote from angiograms and did not permit correlation of angiographic and anatomic stenosis. Time limitations inherent in experimental design, the need to obtain serial observations on individual animals, and chemical analyses of lipid and fibrous proteins in unfixed arterial segments did not allow sacrifice of a colony for a radiographic-pathologic correlative study.

A review of previous experimental data allowed calculation of sensitivity and specificity of angiography in detecting lesions in characteristic sites in 34 monkeys. These sites included the internal carotid and spermatic arteries, lumbar aorta, and the origin of the inferior mesenteric artery. The data also allowed comparison of angiographic grades with the more conventional morphologic estimates of plaque severity. Angiographic grades were assigned to intrusive lesions by Erroll M. Bellon. Subsequently, morphologic lesions were graded by surgical or necropsy observers: R. G. DePalma, S. Koletsky, and recently, Pacita Manalo-Sears.

Angiographic Techniques

As previously described (3,4), femoral arteries were used for angiographic access and as sites for obtaining index arterial biopsies. A fine (5F Gensini) angiographic catheter, well lubricated with sterile mineral oil, was introduced through the common femoral artery, which was exposed under local anesthesia after appropriate sedation. The mineral oil facilitated catheter passage and minimized wall friction and trauma. With the catheter

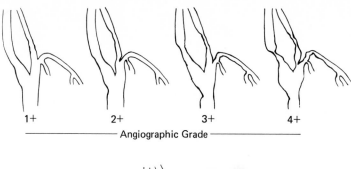

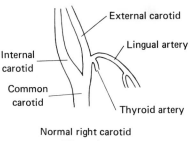

Fig. 1 Normal rhesus carotid artery bifurcation and appearances
of angiographic grades 1+ - 4+ in representative diagrams.

tip in the appropriate site, 76% Renographin was injected and films
were exposed using a Schonander rapid film changer. Repeated
lateral views of the abdominal aorta were obtained by positioning
the animal under fluoroscopic control so that the third lumbar
vertebra was positioned in the true lateral plane while the
femoral heads were superimposed. This allowed, on each occasion,
repetitive study of the origins of the inferior mesenteric artery,
aorta, and lumbar arteries in exactly comparable projections.
This technique also visualized the spermatic arteries. As the
importance of internal carotid artery lesions became apparent,
separate views of the thoracic aorta and carotid artery bifur-
cation--mainly on the right--were also obtained. Utilizing either
the brachial arteries or reentry through femoral artery sites, at
least four sequential arteriograms were done in some animals. For
sequential angiographic studies in the adult rhesus animals the
initial x-rays were inspected for closure of the proximal humeral

epiphyses. Five of the six cynomolgus monkeys were found to have open epiphyses at the time of the first angiogram.

Grading of Lesions

Angiograms were graded as follows: 1+ corresponded to a perceptible contour defect; 2+ corresponded to luminal reduction up to 20%; 3+ corresponded to luminal reduction up to 50%; and 4+ corresponded to luminal reduction greater than 50% or extensive linear involvement (Figs. 1 and 2).

Using mainly grossly visible lesions, disease severity was estimated from pathology specimens as follows:

Severity	Gross Morphology	Histology
1+	Visible yellow streaks	Minimal intimal fibrous plaque lipid deposit and foam cells
2+	Raised yellow plaque with minimal luminal encroachment	Well-developed intimal fibrous or fatty-fibrous plaque; proliferation of smooth muscle cells and lipid deposition in media
3+	Extensive plaque with luminal encroachment	Large intimal fatty-fibrous plaque with cholesterol slits; narrow lumen; proliferation of medial smooth muscle cells with lipid and collagen deposition
4+	Plaque complicated by thrombosis and/or calcification	Atheromatous plaque with necrosis and abundant lipid; deposition of collagen and calcium

The aorta and internal carotid arteries were graded at necropsy. At surgical exposures the spermatic, inferior mesenteric, and femoral arteries were scrutinized for plaques observable through their thin walls. The femoral and spermatic arteries were excised at standard sites for histologic analysis while plaques of the inferior mesenteric artery were exposed, palpated, and their appearance recorded by color photography. Generally, after a second or third angiogram and sacrifice, the contralateral femoral

and spermatic arteries were removed and the morphology of the
inferior mesenteric artery origin was evaluated grossly and
histologically at necropsy.

Data Analysis

Positive and negative angiograms were compared to morphologic
findings in the same arterial segments. A simple comparison of
positive and negative results provided estimates of sensitivity
and specificity of arteriograms in plaque detection. Sensitivity
was defined as the fraction of true angiographic positives;
specificity was defined as the fraction of true angiographic
negatives. In addition, comparison of paired gradings for each
site was used to estimate the relationship between independently
obtained angiographic and morphologic estimates of lesion severity.
Lesions were also observed at other sites including the presacral
artery, iliac and vertebral arteries, and the origin of the
superior mesenteric artery. These will be described in detail in
a future publication. For this report, sufficient numbers of

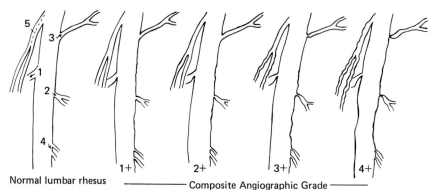

Normal lumbar rhesus
aorta and branches = lateral view ———————— Composite Angiographic Grade ————
1: Inferior mesenteric artery origin   Atherosclerosis of Aorta
2, 3, 4: Lumbar arteries;   and Associated Branches
    2 and 3 superimposed
5: Spermatics; superimposed

Fig. 2   Lateral view of normal rhesus aorta, inferior mesenteric
artery origin, lumbar and spermatic arteries. Appearance in
representative composite diagrams of angiographic grades 1+ - 4+.
Changes in all vessels may not occur synchronously.

correlated observations were available for the internal carotid artery, the inferior mesenteric artery origin, the lumbar aorta and lumbar artery origins, and the spermatic arteries.

RESULTS

Table 1 summarizes specificity and sensitivity data for the internal carotid, inferior mesenteric artery, lumbar aorta, and spermatic artery. Angiography was found to be a highly specific method for detecting the presence of atherosclerotic plaques in nonhuman primates. The incidence of false positive arteriograms was, for practical reasons, zero except in the spermatic artery, where specificity was 0.82. Here lesion grading was based also on an estimate of tortuosity not present in the other sites, which comprised origins of branched arteries. In the femoral artery, early fatty lesions were evident as yellow bulges on gross examination, but were not detected angiographically (Fig. 3).

Sensitivity for detection of lesions of the internal carotid artery was 0.45; the inferior mesenteric artery origin 0.73; the lumbar aorta 0.54; and the spermatic artery 0.58. At arterial pressure it would not be expected that minimally elevated lesions such as fatty streaks would be detected by angiography. Eliminating paired values of angiographic grade 0: pathologic grade 1 (i.e., 0.1 category) raised the angiographic sensitivity to 0.63 for the internal carotid artery; 0.88 for the inferior mesenteric artery origin; 0.78 for the lumbar aorta and lumbar arteries; and 0.73 for the spermatic arteries.

The utility of serial angiography in demonstrating atherosclerosis progression and regression is shown in Fig. 4. This individual rhesus monkey was fed from 1969-1971 a high (2-4%) cholesterol containing diet with butter and coconut oil (10). Angiography, surgical exploration, and biopsy after 24 months of feeding the atherogenic diet revealed no gross lesions. The results with this regimen in our first colony are shown in Fig. 5. Intrusive lesions detected by the combination of angiography and surgery

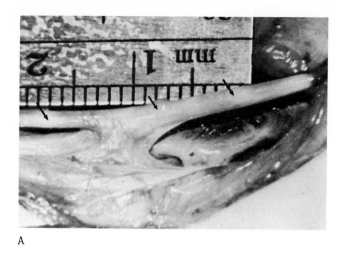

A

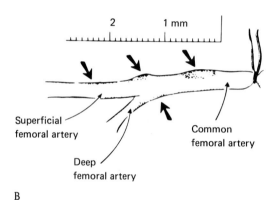

B

Fig. 3 A: Left femoral artery; B: Diagrammatic presentation; C:
Right femoral artery. Atherosclerotic involvement of femoral
arteries in rhesus monkey after 23 months of atherogenic feeding.
Note bulging of vessels at sites of plaques in this type of
lesion. (From Ref. 7,   1980 American Medical Association with
permission.)

occurred in only three instances. The presence of intrusive

lesions was, on the average, related to elevation in serum choles-

terol concentration. Overall results in lesion production on this

atherogenic diet fell short of our expectations, therefore we

began feeding the colony a diet revised after that reported by

Armstrong and coworkers (11). This new diet contained 0.5%

cholesterol and egg yolk, with sucrose as the main source of

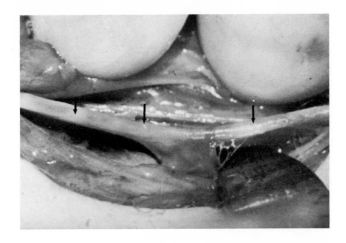

C

carbohydrate. Arteriograms and surgical exploration later showed
the development of intrusive atherosclerotic lesions. Subsequent
feeding with low-lipid monkey chow and other interventions that
lowered serum cholesterol concentration revealed regression of
luminal intrusion as early as 11 months (1,2).

In our regression experiments the angiographic observations
of lessening stenoses were accompanied by serial biopsies of
paired arteries which had compact, residual fibrous plaques that
contained scanty lipid-staining material (3,6,7). The efficacy
of feeding this atherogenic diet was confirmed by angiographic and
and morphologic observations, therefore it was adopted as our
standard method of inducing atherosclerosis in subhuman primates.
This diet produced intrusive lesions in almost all animals after
18-24 months. On the average, lesion severity was related to the
degree of elevation in serum cholesterol concentrations, although
there was, as expected, variability among animals (6). Therefore,
before intervention, animals were segregated into groups on the
basis of disease severity as determined by angiography.

Angiography also revealed, on occasion, dramatic disease
progression that might otherwise have passed undetected. Fig. 6
illustrates sequential arteriograms obtained on an individual
animal in the last colony studied for the effects of antiplatelet

R. G. DePalma

Table 1. Sensitivity and specificity of angiography in detecting atherosclerosis in animals.

Internal Carotid Artery

Morphologic Result	Positive angiogram	Negative angiogram	Sensitivity[a]
With lesion	[1·2]·2 1·3·2 1·4·1 2·3·1 3·3·1 4·4·3 n = 10	[0·1]·6 0·2·5 0·3·1 n = 12	10/22 = 0.45
			Specificity[b]
Without lesion	n = 0	[0·0]·6 n = 6	6/6 = 1.0

Inferior Mesenteric Artery Origin

Morphologic Result	Positive angiogram	Negative angiogram	Sensitivity[a]
With lesion	1·1·5 [4·2]·2 1·2·5 [4·4]·2 1·3·2 1·4·1 2·3·3 3·2·1 [3·4]·1 n = 22	[0·1]·5 [0·2]·3 n = 8	22/30 = 0.73
			Specificity[b]
Without lesion	[1·0]·1 n = 1	[0·0]·12 n = 12	12/13 = 0.92

Lumbar Aorta

Morphologic Result	Positive angiogram	Negative angiogram	Sensitivity[a]
With lesion	1·1·1 [4·4]·2 1·2·2 1·3·4 2·2·1 2·3·1 3·2·2 [3·3]·1 n = 14	[0·1]·8 0·2·3 0·3·1 n = 12	14/26 = 0.54
			Specificity[b]
Without lesion	n = 0	[0·0]·8 n = 8	8/8 = 1.0

Spermatic Artery

Morphologic Result	Positive angiogram	Negative angiogram	Sensitivity[a]
With lesion	1·1·3 1·2·3 1·3·1 2·4·1 [3·3]·2 n = 11	0·1·4 0·2·2 0·3·1 0·4·1 n = 8	11/19 = 0.58
			Specificity[b]
Without lesion	[1·0]·2 [2·0]·2 n = 4	[0·0]·18 n = 18	18/22 = 0.82

[a] Fraction of true positives.
[b] Fraction of true negatives.

Note: The angiographic grade is the first figure given in the brackets; the morphologic grade is the second.

intervention (8). During the interval between the two angiograms, a thrombosis of the left subclavian artery occurred and was detected by angiography prior to sacrifice. The morphology of this lesion is shown in Fig. 7. Overall, in a colony consisting of seven animals treated with antiplatelet agents and three control animals, atherosclerosis appeared to progress more rapidly radiographically and morphologically in the treated monkeys. This experiment to evaluate antiplatelet therapy contributed the bulk of angiographic and morphologic grades of 4+. The lesions in treated animals were mainly calcified stenotic plaques, while none of the arteries from control animals had calcified plaques. The only spontaneous thrombosis occurred in a treated animal in this colony. Serial angiograms in other animals fed atherogenic diets for up to 6 years did not demonstrate a similar event. Ulceration was not diagnosed angiographically in any artery, even those graded 4+, nor was gross ulceration ever detected at necropsy.

In contrast, the canine model of atherosclerotic beagles did develop ulcerated plaques (1) and ischemia (12,13). Recent angiograms obtained in this colony have been of interest. Fig. 8 shows the angiographic appearance of the carotid artery bifurcation in a hypercholesterolemic beagle dog after 18 months of feeding an atherogenic diet. On the basis of this advanced lesion, the animal was selected for a pilot study utilizing injection of isotopically labelled platelets to reveal possible localization in arteries that were prone to ulceration.

DISCUSSION

The ideal method of plaque detection and measurement would identify all lesions, determine severity and distribution, be repeatable, and neither provoke nor destroy lesions in the arterial segment under observation. This ideal method would yield precise quantitative relationships between luminal intrusion in vivo, plaque pathology and composition, and ultimately hemodynamic parameters. Angiography offers some, but not all of these capabilities. This

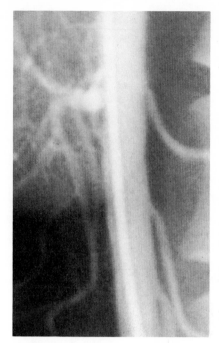

A

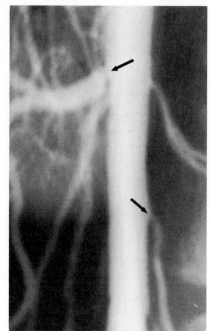

B

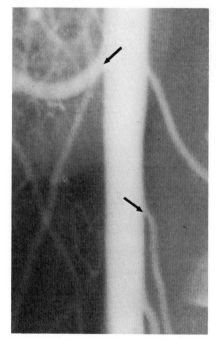

C

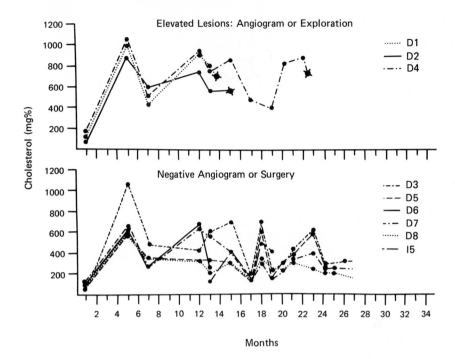

Fig. 5 Upper panel: response of first experimental colony in producing intrusive lesions detectable by angiography in two and
aortotomy in one animal. Lower panel: Negative angiograms and
explorations. Note relationship to magnitude of serum cholesterol
response.

technique, as with morphology evaluation, includes both assumptions
and intrinsic disadvantages. Clearly, angiography estimates lumen
compromise, but gives little or no information about wall thickness
unless, as in aneurysms, a rim of calcium exists. Here ultrasonography may provide useful information about wall thickness and
thrombus as well.

Fig. 4 (Opposite) Lateral views of lumbar aorta. A: 24 months:
diet 2-4% cholesterol, butter, and coconut oil (10): average cholesterol 410 mg/dl. Angiogram interpreted as negative, exploration
revealed no lesion of inferior mesenteric artery. B: Diet changed
to 0.5% cholesterol and egg yolk with sucrose (11). 22 months:
average cholesterol 620 mg/dl. Note involvement of inferior
mesenteric and lumbar arteries. C: Diet normal chow (Purina).
11 months: average cholesterol 120 mg/dl. Note regression of
luminal intrusion at inferior mesenteric and lumbar arteries.

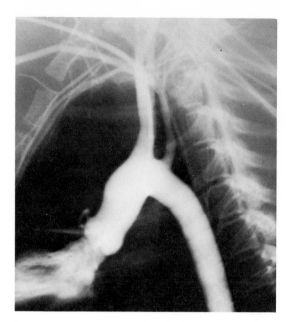

A

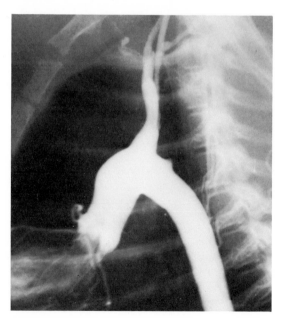

B

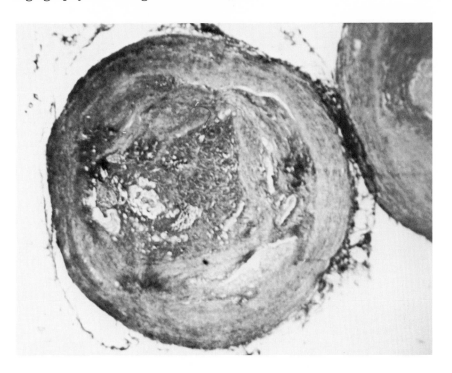

Fig. 7 Cross-sectional view of thrombosis superimposed on calcified left subclavian artery plaque corresponding to Fig. 6B.
Mallory trichome (x40).

Our experiments first intended to use angiography as it is
used clinically: to detect intrusive arterial disease similar to
that occurring in man. The limited sensitivity and high specificity of angiography were advantageous in that we wished to study
changes in more advanced plaques. Using this technique, we were
certain of the presence of intrusive lesions when interventions
were begun. Conversely, studies of the dynamics of fatty streak
or very early nonintrusive lesions would have been unreliable
without surgical interventions such as aortotomy and arterial
exploration (1,2). It is a well-recognized clinical dictum that

Fig. 6 (Opposite) A: Arch aortogram of Rhesus D-11 after atherogenic feeding 25 months. Average cholesterol 690 mg/dl. B:
Arch aortogram of Rhesus D-11 after atherogenic feeding 71 months.
Average cholesterol 692 mg/dl antiplatelet therapy for 12 months
prior to angiograph. Note thrombosis of subclavian artery.

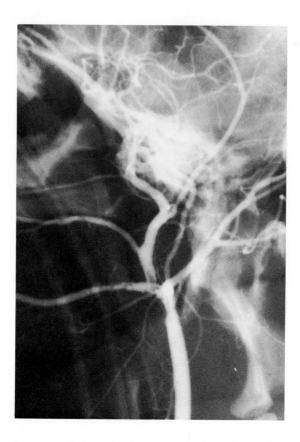

Fig. 8 Angiogram of beagle dog 25 months after thyroid ablation
and atherogenic feeding for 18 months. Note lesion at bifurcation.

angiography underestimates disease severity. Interesting site
limitations in sensitivity of angiography exist in the femoral
arteries of rhesus monkeys, where disease was never detected;
limitations in specificity also exist in the spermatic arteries,
where false positive findings occurred. However, angiographic
estimates of atherosclerotic change in these involved index
vessels were confirmed morphologically, and were found to be
effective in estimating changes in lesion type and composition
(3,6,7).
    Morphologic change correlated well with progressive and
regressive angiographic trends (i.e., lessening of stenoses) in

other involved arteries. Our morphologic and chemical observations of femoral artery segments showed lessening of plaque lipid
during angiographic regression due to lipid lowering (7) and
progression with calcification during antiplatelet treatment of
hypercholesterolemic monkeys (8). The requirement for catheter
passage via the external iliac arteries potentially initiates
trauma which might mar serial observations in these vessels and
is disadvantageous for sequential viewing of femoral arteries
distally. Thus arterial samples for chemical analyses were always
obtained distal to the site of catheter passage (3). Trauma due
to catheter passage appeared insignificant in the larger common
iliac arteries (7).

The assumption that lessened plaque luminal intrusion, detected angiographically or morphologically, represents improvement appears reasonable. This concept is supported by our own
correlated observations and those of others (11,14,15). Nonethe-
less, this general assumption must be qualified. Lessening of
luminal intrusion could result from arterial dilation during
disease progression. This, in fact is known to occur in varying
degrees in coronary arteries (16,17) of different nonhuman
primates. Apparently this effect is enhanced by growth during
atherogenesis. We controlled for this factor in our adult rhesus
experiments by ensuring that there was closure of the humeral
epiphyses before beginning feeding. This was a problem, however
in the experiment with juvenile cynomolgus monkeys (9).

Another obvious limitation of angiography is that early fatty
plaques are compressible, while the artery wall increases in bulk.
The result is an external bead-like bulge which is seen early in
the course of the disease. This is best illustrated in the femoral
and spermatic arteries. We also observed negative arteriograms in
infants fed an atherogenic diet for three years from the time of
weaning. In this circumstance, compressible fatty plaques tend to
yield false negative results, lessening sensitivity of angiography.
The converse possibility exists; certain minor lesions might also
produce segmental spasm and cause a false positive angiographic

result, thus overestimating disease severity. This event is probably rare; our data (Table 1) show overestimation of lesion severity in only 11 of 146 observations.

In the rhesus, after up to 6 years of atherogenic feeding, we observed mainly intimal stenotic plaques that correlated well with the angiographic findings in characteristic sites described here. In monkeys no aneurysms were seen, while aortic aneurysms and medial changes were seen in the atherosclerotic dog (18). Medial injury, in fact, appeared commonly in canine arteries; aneurysms were seen twice in 50 animals. Although more precise quantitative data could be obtained for each species using perfusion studies with baric fixation (19), this desirable refinement was not our intent. It did not prove to be essential in detecting progression or regression in our experimental interventions. Angiography was found to be a reliable reflection of disease severity, giving us the information we desired prior to regression interventions. Morphologic and chemical changes confirmed regressive or progressive lesion trends detected by angiography.

An important qualification requiring consideration is that angiographic stenoses might lessen while less cross-linked, and potentially unstable arterial fibrous proteins might increase in the arterial wall. Divergent chemical responses with increases in collagen accompanying decreases of lipid (7) and failure of regression attempts (12) suggest this possibility in certain circumstances. Possibly this undesirable change might occur when serum cholesterol fails to fall below a threshold for regression (6,12). While the intrusive bulk and lipid content of plaques might lessen, fibrous or necrotic lesions might become more unstable and prone to complications of intraplaque hemorrhage, dissection, or ulceration. These events can, in turn, produce sudden luminal intrusion, occlusion, or embolization. This undesirable sequence demands examination in relevant animal models. Each of these events occurs in human atherosclerosis and causes morbidity and mortality. However, when such a sudden

event occurs in an unstable arterial segment, angiography is a
most useful means of detecting dramatic lesion change.

With the exception of the single angiographically detected
thrombosis in the rhesus treated with aspirin and dipyridamole,
arterial occlusion leading to ischemic complications never occurred in our experience with this species. No angiographically
positive atherosclerotic rhesus monkeys exhibited EKG change or
distal-flow-related Doppler changes. However, these abnormalities
do occur in this species with prolonged atherogenic feeding containing peanut oil (20). In contrast, atherosclerotic dogs
developed complicated plaques and clinical ischemic events. Atherosclerotic cynomolgus monkeys and dogs, in our hands, have also
been subject to sudden death with severe coronary atherosclerosis
not detected by our current angiographic techniques. Therefore,
experimental design must take into account limitations of each
particular animal model as well as those of angiographic and
morphologic quantitative methods. The quest for a "gold standard"
might ultimately define measures of atherosclerotic disease *and*
disordered physiology sufficient to cause complications mimicking
those of human disease. Reversal of arterial pathology *and* prevention of complications caused by the disease process constitute
effective therapy. Defined in this manner, no single "gold
standard" yet exists for quantitating atherosclerosis.

In spite of conceptual and methodologic limitations in quantitative radiographic and morphologic studies, methods ensuring
standardized reproducible arteriograms in animal models and in
humans will continue to be of great value. Almost all of our clinical decisions for surgical interventions are based on arteriography combined with measurements of symptom severity and disordered
physiology. Fig. 9 shows two divergent angiographic examples of
ulcerative lesions involving the human carotid artery. Note that
the lesions may be barely perceptible, or may be present as a
dilatation in the extreme case. Either lesion is prone to produce
stroke due to embolization of plaque debris. Both patients were

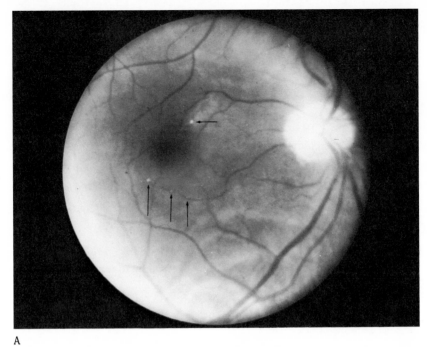

A

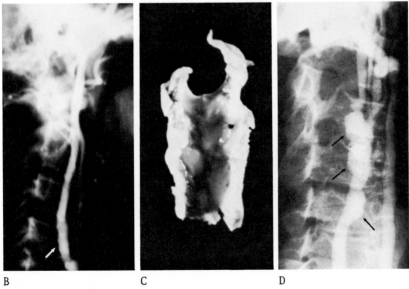

B   C   D

operated upon based on the results of angiography. However, the sensitivity of angiography in detecting dangerous ulcerated plaques in the human carotid artery has been reported to be only 60% (21). Methods combining angiography and platelet tracer studies which detect early and minor ulceration and offer the promise of enhancing sensitivity would be developed best in an animal model.

CONCLUSIONS AND RECOMMENDATIONS

For future research, angiography offers a valid assessment of efficacy of various interventions and can be used even more precisely to estimate lesion characteristics when combined with morphologic and other types of observations. Table 2 illustrates an experimental design utilizing serial angiography. This plan acknowledges a requirement for correlative angiographic and morphologic measurements that maximize information and compensate intrinsic limitations in either method of observation. Small colonies can be used, but larger colony size permits more elaborate chemical and hemodynamic studies. Wider application and further refinement of digital subtraction angiography (22) also promise more liberal use of serial angiography in man. Therefore, in man serial observations beginning at point B (Table 2) could be obtained using this less invasive and easily repeated form of angiography to estimate changes in plaque luminal intrusion. Wall dynamics and changes in wall thickness might be estimated by further refinement of commonly used ultrasound noninvasive scans. These are now increasingly capable of higher resolution. In combination with other techniques, and in spite

Fig. 9 (Opposite) A: Embolic lesion. Fundus of right eye: 47-year-old male patient. B: Carotid angiogram, lateral view, 48 h later. Note slightly irregular contour of internal carotid. No stenosis. C: Specimen removed at endarterectomy. Note ulcerations with little lumen encroachment. D: Carotid arteriogram 60-year-old male. Note extensive dilation with multiple ulcerations proximal to stenoses of internal and external carotid arteries (arrows).

Table 2. Experimental Design

Animal Colony

Baseline Angiography: Sacrifice of selected animals for
perfusion fixation at arterial pressure

Period I   Disease Induction

Angiography: Femoral and spermatic aa biopsy;
photography of inferior mesenteric artery
sacrifice of selected animals for perfusion fixation

Desired Severity of Disease Obtained

Colony Segregated
on Basis of Lesion Severity

Experimental   Controls

Hemodynamic Event
Period II
Intervention   Interval Angiography   No Intervention

Angiography: Second index aa biopsies and photography
Necropsy and selected animals for perfusion fixation

---

of its recognized limitations, angiography is a useful, if not
completely quantitative tool for estimating atherosclerotic plaque
dynamics.

SUMMARY

The ability to detect atherosclerotic plaques and to document
changes in luminal intrusion *in seriatim* are important operational
goals of experimental design. Over the past 12 years methods were
evolved for serial angiography in monkeys and dogs and over 100
arteriograms were performed. Progression of intrusive lesions
related to hypercholesterolemia and regressive effects of lowered
serum cholesterol induced by diet, internal biliary diversion,
and bile acid sequestrant were observed. A study of antiplatelet
therapy in monkeys was recently completed and developmental
studies of ulcerated canine plaques initiated.

The technique for serial angiography used controlled lateral projections for repetitive studies of carotid bifurcations, thoracic aorta, and abdominal aorta to include superior and inferior mesenteric origins, and lumbar and spermatic arteries. Estimates of radiographic lesion severity were graded blindly by the angiographer and later compared to morphologically graded lesions recorded at surgery or necropsy.

The results of a total of 146 observations at four sites showed that angiography was a highly specific method of plaque detection. There were virtually no false positives with the exception of the spermatic arteries, where specificity (i.e., fraction of true negatives) was 0.82. Sensitivity for detection of early fatty lesions was low, especially in the femoral arteries, where fatty plaques resulted in an external bulge with no luminal encroachment. Sensitivity for detection of all lesions of the internal carotid artery was 0.45; the inferior mesenteric artery origin 0.73; the lumbar aorta 0.54 and the spermatic artery 0.58.

Limitations of angiography mainly include its low sensitivity for only lesion detection due to dependence on detection of luminal intrusion. Angiography also does not give information about wall thickness or external bulging of early plaques. Its advantages include its high specificity, indicating advanced disease before beginning regression interventions; its ability to estimate arterial lesion distribution and severity in individuals, permitting segregation of colonies prior to treatment; and its repeatability, without provoking or destroying lesions under observation. When combined with morphologic and possibly ultra-sonic techniques, angiography is a useful tool for estimating atherosclerotic plaque dynamics.

REFERENCES

1. DePalma RG, Insull W Jr, Bellon EM, Roth WT, Robinson AV (1972) Animal models for study of progression and regression of atherosclerosis. Surgery 72:268-278

2. DePalma RG, Bellon EM, Insull W Jr, Roth WT, Robinson AV (1972) Studies on progression and regression of experimental atherosclerosis. Techniques and application to the rhesus monkey. In: Goldsmith EI, Moor-Jankowski J (eds) Medical Primatology. Karger, Basel III, pp 313-323

3. DePalma RG, Bellon EM, Klein L, Koletsky S, Insull W Jr (1977) Approaches to evaluating regression of experimental atherosclerosis. Adv Exp Med Biol 82:459-470

4. Bellon EM, DePalma RG, Klein L, Koletsky S, Robinson AV (1979) The utility of arteriography in the evaluation of experimental atherosclerosis: a ten-year experience with rhesus and fascicularis monkeys. Abstracts of Fifth International Symposium on Atherosclerosis, Houston, TX

5. Bellon EM, DePalma RG, Insull W, Koletsky S (1976) Sequential angiography for measurement of progression and regression of lesions of experimental atherosclerosis. Invest Radiol 11:382

6. DePalma RG, Bellon EM, Koletsky S, Schneider DL (1979) Atherosclerotic plaque regression in rhesus monkeys induced by bile acid sequestrant. Exp Mol Pathol 31:423-439

7. DePalma RG, Klein L, Bellon EM, Koletsky S (1980) Regression of atherosclerotic plaques in rhesus monkeys. Arch Surg 115:1268-1278

8. DePalma RG, Bellon EM, Manalo PM (1981) Failure of antiplatelet agents to control dietary atherosclerosis. J Cardiovasc Surg 22:445

9. Klein L, DePalma RG, Insull W Jr, Koletsky S, Bellon EM (1976) Stability of original collagen and elastin and gain of new collagen in atherosclerotic plaques. Abstracts of 30th Annual Meeting Council on Atherosclerosis, p 3

10. Wissler RW (1968) Recent progress in studies of experimental primate atherosclerosis. Prog Biochem Pharmacol 4:378-392

11. Armstrong ML, Warner ED, Connor WE (1970) Regression of coronary atheromatosis in rhesus monkeys. Circ Res 27:59-67

12. DePalma RG, Koletsky S, Bellon EM, Insull W Jr (1977) Failure of regression of atherosclerosis in dogs with moderate cholesterolemia. Atherosclerosis 27:297-310

13. DePalma RG (1981) Regression or arrest of atherosclerosis-- Does it happen? In: Greenhalgh RM (ed) Proceedings of International Symposium: Hormones and vascular disease. Pitman Publishers, Ltd, London, pp 71-92

14. Blankenhorn DH, Brooks SH, Selzer RH, Barndt R (1978) The rate of atherosclerosis change during treatment of hyperlipoproteinemia. Circulation 57:335-361

15. Bond MG, Bullock BC, Lehner NDM, Clarkson TB (1978) Regression of primate carotid artery atherosclerosis at 200 vs 300 mg/dl plasma cholesterol concentration. Stroke 9:97-98

16. Bond MG, Adams MR, Kaduck JM, Bullock BC (1981) The effects of coronary artery size: Implications for myocardial infarction. Fed Proc 40:773

17. Bond MG, Adams MR, Bullock BC (1981) Complicating factors in evaluating coronary artery atherosclerosis. Artery 9:21-29

18. DePalma RG (1981) Biochemical abnormalities and atheroscle-
    rotic aneurysm. In: Bergan JJ, Yao JST (eds) Aneurysms:
    Diagnosis and treatment. Grune and Stratton, New York,
    pp 45-59
19. Clark JM, Glagov S (1976) Evaluation and publication of
    scanning electron micrographs. Science 192:1360-1361
20. Bond MG, Bullock BC, Bellinger DA, Hamm TE (1980) Myocardial
    infarction in a large colony of nonhuman primates with
    coronary atherosclerosis. Am J Pathol 101:675-692
21. Edwards JH, Kricheff II, Riles T, Imparato A (1979) Angio-
    graphically undetected ulceration of the carotid artery as a
    cause of embolic stroke. Radiology 132:369-373
22. Mistretta CA, Crummy AB (1981) Diagnosis of cardiovascular
    disease by digital subtraction angiography. Science 214:
    761-765

DISCUSSION: ERROL M. BELLON

You have heard about the increasing sophistication of arteriography and its extension.   I think it would therefore be useful to
review some of the basic concepts that underlie the arteriographic
process.   You have also heard that we ought to take a fresh look
at our approach to atherosclerosis as if we were encountering it
for the first time today.   Let's try to do that.

In discussing these conceptual considerations in terms of
their application to arteriography, I can't emphasize too strongly
that arteriography is a two-dimensional representation of a three-
dimensional object.   The problems of interpretation are much
related to abstraction.   One must keep in mind, when viewing an
arteriogram, that one is not seeing either A or B, but rather
something else, perhaps C.

Secondly, arteriography measures what is *not* there.   It is the
hole in the donut.   Thus the arteriogram offers a two-dimensional
columnar representation of a space within the artery, the lumen.

Perspective is also important and arteriographically, the view
of the arterial tree is longitudinal and not cross-sectional.   It
is that distinction in *form* between histological cross section and
arteriogram that causes me conceptual difficulty with any comparison studies.   Matching the kind of abstraction that the in vitro
cross section is with an in vivo column seems at times like
comparing donuts to trees.   No correlation technique that I have
observed to date compensates for this difference.

One of the most difficult concepts related to understanding
arteriography concerns the dual relationship which exists between
the contrast material column on the inside and the arterial wall
on the outside.   The lumen is defined by the wall of the artery
at the intimal layer, and the contrast material column defines
the internal complement of the arterial wall, the lumen, by shape;
and in so doing, reflects, in the contrast material column edge,
the shape of the intimal layer of the wall.

   This classic wineglass/face illustration replicates exactly,
in psychologically pure form, the contrast material/intima duality:
the wineglass is the contrast material column. The face on either
side is the intimal wall surface--each equally defines the other.
Thus the contrast material column cannot be viewed as an entity
separate from the wall, nor the wall apart from the contrast
material column. Arteriography demonstrates no more than the
intimal surface of the wall. You have seen plaques demonstrated
at all locations throughout the arterial wall. For the purposes
of arteriography, those lesions are simply *not* there, i.e., the
medial and outer layers of the arterial wall are arteriographically silent.

   Finally, as we consider the increased sophistication of other
techniques and secondary derivative applications of the basic
arteriographic image, one must note that there is an assumption
here that arteriography is not a distortional process. This
assumption remains to be examined and validated.

7

Digital Intravenous Subtraction Angiography

THERON W. OVITT

The digital intravenous subtraction angiographic system utilizes modern, low-noise, video and digital electronic equipment, and high-speed image processors to provide enhanced images of major arteries after the intravenous injection of contrast media. This image system (Fig. 1) consists of five major components: (1) modern x-ray generation equipment; (2) a high-quality x-ray image intensifier; (3) precision high-signal video cameras; (4) an image processor with multiple processing algorithms; (5) and either a digital or analog storage system. Images obtained before the intravenous injection of contrast material are subtracted from subsequent images; the subtracted image is then electronically enhanced to produce the final image of arterial structure, which is viewed on a cathode ray tube display.

EQUIPMENT

X-ray Generator and Tube

Calculations indicate that a 1 mrad exposure per frame at the intensifier face is needed to detect 2% contrast levels in 1 mm structures (1). Cardiovascular exams, where multiple short exposures (5 ms) of high intensity are needed to produce an exam, require a high-flux, high-heat-capacity x-ray source. At present no 0.6-1.2 mm focal spot x-ray tubes can meet this requirement.

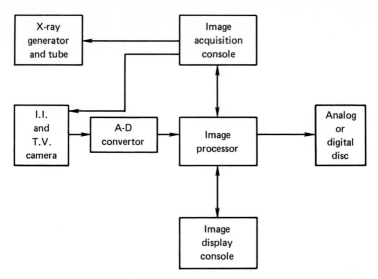

Fig. 1 General diagrammatic description of a digital video subtraction system for intravenous angiography.

The generator has to reliably produce short exposures of equal intensity over the entire series for satisfactory subtractions. Cardiac exams thus put a burden on all but the most modern CPG and three-phase generators, with moderate tube limitations.

For other procedures, examining relatively stationary peripheral vascular structures, this requirement of very high performance x-ray tubes and generators can be relaxed. Exams such as carotid and cerebral artery studies, are usually performed with longer exposures (up to 0.1 s) and slower image acquisition rates (1-2 images per sec), compatible with general angiographic equipment.

Image Intensifier

The image intensifier should be able to accept a 1 mrad exposure without loss of either resolution or contrast. Conventional intensifiers, especially those with high conversion efficiencies, suffer loss of resolution when exposed to this high flux rate, due to the repelling of electrons at the crossover point in the neck of the

intensifier. New intensifiers are being designed and tested to
meet these high-exposure requirements to further improve the
quality of images.

Many examinations are compromised by limited intensifier
field size. For example, 9-inch intensifiers do not have sufficient field size to incorporate the entire head and neck, even
though all vessels are opacified. Therefore, injections have
to be repeated for complete head and neck evaluation. Thus the
development of larger field intensifiers is needed, so that whole
arterial systems can be included with one injection. The Philips
14-inch intensifier is the first step in this direction; other
manufacturers are developing prototype 16-, 20- and 24-inch
intensifiers.

Video Tube and Camera

The video tube and camera are superior to those provided in
standard fluoroscopic systems. The video camera must have a high
signal-to-noise ratio in order not to degrade the signal ema-
nating from the image intensifier, which is approximately
200-300:1. At present most systems are using an Amperex 45XQ
frog's head plumbicon video tube incorporated into a Sierra
camera. Its most important feature is the high signal output of
up to 3 mA, with only 1-2 nA of preamplifier noise, so that a
signal-to-noise ratio in excess of 800:1, at 5 MHz, is achieved.
The camera can operate in the noninterlaced mode, so that
interfield motion differences are eliminated when performing
cardiovascular examinations. At present all systems operate in
a 512 line-interlaced or noninterlaced mode, which produces
satisfactory resolution on a 9-inch intensifier, with negligible
interfield motion differences in extrathoracic vascular examinations. However, with the incorporation of larger field
intensifiers, cameras capable of performing at 1000-2000 TV lines
will have to be used to maintain present resolution of approximately 2LP/mm.

Analog/Digital Converter

The analog/digital converter is a high-speed converter capable of
10 megawords per second with 13 bit accuracy. This allows digiti-
zation of 512 x 512 rasters at 30 frames per second. At higher
raster rates, slower video scan techniques will be used, however,
20 megaword rate A/D converters are becoming available.

Video Image Processor

The video image processor accepts the incoming digitized images
from the A/D converter and temporarily stores them in 512 x 512
memories contained within the processor. These memories serve
as a temporary holding device, so that incoming images can either
be immediately processed or stored on digital discs in raw form.
Because digital discs are limited in the rate of information they
can receive, an all-digital system, at present, can accept only
approximately three images per second in the 512 x 512 configuration. If an analog storage system is used these images can
be unloaded in real time, 30 images per second, onto the video
disc or tape with some degradation of information. Memories can
be placed in parallel so that real-time subtraction can be performed, resulting in immediate continuous display and recording
of subtracted images. By this method, the first image without
contrast is stored in a memory and serves as the mask from which
all subsequent images are immediately subtracted.

The video image processor is a high-speed digital data acquisition and processing device designed to efficiently handle large
volumes of data such as those present in digitized video images.
The rapid commercial development of these processors is recent,
and is in response to the needs of complex image analysis required
for space and satellite pictures. This technology is readily
applied to digital video x-ray imagery. Memories can also serve
to add images together to improve the signal-to-noise ratio before
being unloaded onto a disc or tape. All of these functions are
controlled by the acquisition console, which has keyboards, knobs,

and joy sticks, similar to computed tomography analysis consoles. Complex image enhancement techniques, some used in space and satellite image analysis, are being examined and new techniques are constantly being developed, so that a complete, current description of image enhancement techniques is quickly outdated.

Storage

Images can be stored either in digital form, on digital discs, or in analog form, on analog discs or tape recorders. The advantage of storing images on digital discs is that all information remains digitized and image degradation is minimized. Images are recalled from storage, sequentially manipulated and displayed very rapidly until the best subtracted, enhanced image is obtained. The final image is usually recorded on film by a multiformat camera for a permanent record.

CLINICAL APPLICATION

Because this is a subtraction technique, it is preferable to examine only cooperative patients. While patient motion may be corrected by postprocessing in some patients, motion artifacts, both voluntary and involuntary, are major degrading factors in many images, to the extent that some examinations may be non-diagnostic. Since no premedication or postexamination care is required, this is an outpatient procedure. Injection procedures vary from use of a 3-inch angiocatheter placed in an antecubital vein to the placement of pigtail catheters within the superior vena cava. Contrast injection rates vary from 12 to 30 cc per second with total dosages of about 40-50 cc per injection. There is considerable dilution of the contrast material as it traverses from the venous to the arterial circulation, thus the better the bolus, the better the images that are obtained.

The primary indications for use of digital intravenous sub-traction angiography have been major-vessel atherosclerotic disease. The most intensively studied vessel has been the carotid bifurcation (Fig. 2) with reports of 70-90% diagnostic accuracy when compared with conventional arteriography (2,3). Other arteries readily studied are the aorta, both in the thorax and in the abdomen, and the renal, iliac, and femoral arteries. Other areas that have drawn interest are postoperative evaluation of bypass grafts, renal transplants, and pulmonary arteries. Because of the newness of the technique, validation studies have not been reported in these areas.

Experimental animal work has laid the foundation for clinical cardiac exams. We have examined both normal ventricles and abnormal ventricles in the experimental model and have been able to produce excellent ventriculograms. These ventriculograms were performed at 30 frames per second and clearly demonstrate abnormal areas of ventricular contractility. We are now in the process of developing software programs to develop a semiautomated method, or interactive method, to outline the contrast filled ventricle and perform ejection fraction analysis. Future hardware development will include the incorporation of a DC-coupled video preamplifier so that video densitometry can be performed accurately. It is hoped that with the addition of this piece of equipment and with expanded dynamic range to 10 bits, volumetric studies as well as flow rate studies can be performed.

Further experiments will be performed to evaluate the ability of this procedure to visualize the coronary arteries in their entirety. We realize this is a difficult project and may not be obtainable in the near future. However, new processing techniques are being developed, and it is hoped that diagnostic coronary artery exams can be performed in the near future.

One of the major limitations of intravenous angiography is its susceptibility to motion artifacts; this includes both voluntary and involuntary motion, such as peristalsing bowel gas, involuntary swallowing, and cardiovascular pulsations. It is possible to correct some of these motion artifacts with image manipulation, such as reregistration of the subtraction mask, or rubber sheeting

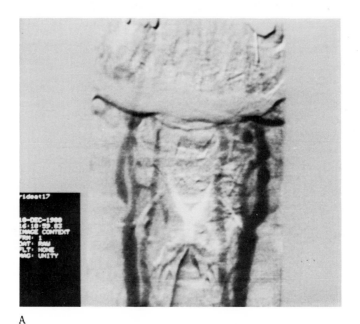

A

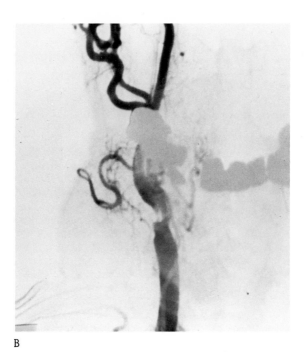

B

Fig. 2   Stenosis of origin of right carotid artery in patient with right carotid bruit and vaque symptomatology.

the contrast mask to fit the contrast image. Another major
limitation is the superimposition of vessels, especially in
intracerebral and abdominal examinations. With proper patient
positioning these shortcomings can be overcome. It is possible
that, with stereo techniques, this problem may be substantially
alleviated.

Now that major manufacturers are in the process of producing
these devices, major equipment modifications specifically adapted
to this procedure can be expected to further advance the technology. In addition, with software development advances borrowing
heavily from space image analysis techniques, and with the rapid
development of high-speed image processors, image enhancement
techniques should improve rapidly. This is a developing technology in which substantial advances can be expected over the next
several years.

REFERENCES

1. Frost MM, Fisher HD, Nudelman S, Roehrig H (1977) A digital
   video acquisition system for extraction of subvisual
   information in diagnostic medical imaging. Society for
   Photoelectronic Instrumentation Engineers 127, Optical
   Instrumentation in Medicine 6:208-215
2. Chilcote WA, Modic MT, Pavlicek WA, Little JR, Furlan AJ,
   Duchesneau PM, Weinstein MA (1981) Digital subtraction
   angiography of the carotid arteries: A comparative study in
   100 patients. Radiology 139:287-295
3. Seeger JF, Weinstein PR, Carmody RF, Ovitt TW, Fisher D III,
   Capp MP (1982) Digital video subtraction angiography of the
   cervical and cerebral vasculature. J Neurosurg 56:173-179
4. Brennecke R, Hahne HJ, Moldenhauer JH, Bürsch JH, Heintzen PH
   (1978) Improved digital real-time processing and storage
   techniques with applications to intravenous contrast
   angiography. Proceedings of conference, "Computers in
   Cardiology", Stanford, CA, September 12-14, 1978, pp 191-194
5. Meaney TF, Weinstein MA, Buonocore E, Pavlicek W, Borkowski
   GP, Gallagher JH, Sufka B, MacIntyre WJ (1980) Digital
   subtraction angiography of the human cardiovascular system.
   AJR 135:1153-1160
6. Ovitt TW, Christenson PC, Fisher HD III, Frost MM, Nudleman S,
   Roehrig H, Seeley G (1980) Intravenous angiography using
   digital video subtraction: X-ray imaging system. AJR
   135:1141-1144

7. Christenson PC, Ovitt TW, Fisher HD III, Frost MM, Nudelman S,
    Roehrig H (1980) Intravenous angiography using digital video
    subtraction: Intravenous cervicocerebrovascular angiography.
    AJR 135:1145-1152

 8. Crummy AB, Strother CM, Sackett JF, Ergun DL, Shaw CG, Kruger
    RA, Mistretta CA, Turnipseed WD, Lieberman RP, Myerowitz PD,
    Ruzicka FF (1980) Computerized fluoroscopy: Digital sub-
    traction for intravenous angiocardiography and arteriography.
    AJR 135:1131-1140

DISCUSSION: P. DAVID MYEROWITZ

For the last three years at the University of Wisconsin, there
have been two areas of interest using digital subtraction angiography, imaging capability and quantitative measurements from these
images. I will try to highlight our work on digital subtraction
angiography (DSA). Imaging of static vessels using intravenous
injections has been our first area of accomplishment, although our
equipment was originally designed to be a cardiac-imaging device.
Carotid studies using intravenous injections are able to demonstrate stenoses well. DSA also provides good qualitative resolution for aortoiliac disease. The aortic arch has been well
visualized, demonstrating congenital and acquired lesions of the
thoracic aorta, as well as postoperative studies following inter-
position grafting for coarctation. As far as clinical studies for
qualitative estimates of lesions in the vascular tree, I think our
group, as well as others, has shown that this is a reasonable
technique.

During this time we continued looking at left ventriculography
and the question of visualizing coronary arteries on intravenous
injections of contrast. The left ventricle is defined nearly as
well using intravenous DSA as by direct left ventriculography. We
feel we have achieved much better resolution of the left ventricle
than that provided by many of the nuclear radiology techniques
used for the same purpose. Coronary arteries, however, have not
yet been seen well on intravenous DSA studies. There is some
visualization of the left anterior descending and circumflex
coronary arteries on some studies, but nothing that could be
considered diagnostic. We, therefore, looked at intraarterial
injections for visualizing coronary arteries. We had already
looked at intraarterial injections for visualizing peripheral
vasculature in patients with severe proximal stenoses of the
distal arterial tree. When looking at coronary arteries in a
dog following aortic root injection of contrast, visualization
by using the subtraction process is markedly improved. Major

coronary artery obstructions can be seen by this technique. With improvement in our injection technique we showed that, using aortic root injections, coronary arteries could be visualized well in dogs. This led to our first human study of aortic root injection for coronary visualization in which we could see the left anterior descending and circumflex system and a nondominant right coronary artery. A few months prior to this study the patient had coronary arteriography which showed no major obstructive lesions. This study was done during angiography to evaluate carotid disease. This technique might be useful to reduce the morbidity and mortality of selective coronary injection as well as for screening for coronary artery disease in patients with peripheral vascular disease who are being studied by standard arteriography. Coronary artery disease is a major cause of operative and late mortality in these peripheral vascular surgery patients.

We had been interested in intravenous coronary bypass visualization and had studied 26 aortic anastomoses in 11 patients back for recatheterization with chest pain following bypass surgery. We correctly identified 11/15 patent and 11/11 occluded bypass grafts. However, although the bypass grafts can be seen, it is not possible with current technology to evaluate anastomoses or run-off. Although we could identify grafts, we did not feel that we could deduce much about the physiology of the system. Using aortic root injection, however, in a dog study, we were able to show a bypass graft, the distal anastomosis, and distal run-off well, which demonstrates that this technique might be useful in some selected patients. We also found that partial occlusions of a bypass graft could be detected by using this technique.

A strong interest in our group has been the development of quantitative studies of both ejection fraction and vessel flow. Using the technique of videodensitometry, we demonstrated a linear relationship between the volume of a balloon and the computer reading of contrast density. We then proceeded to ejection fraction calculations. The computer gives relative values of contrast density for a diastolic and systolic window over the left ventricle. By subtracting systolic from diastolic contrast values and dividing by diastolic values, ejection fractions can be calculated. However, much work needs to be done to eliminate some of the errors in the calculation. These errors include scatter and veiling glare corrections, and in this specific technique there is a large error late in the passage of contrast with the accumulation of iodine in myocardial tissue. Preliminary studies that we are doing to look at this particular error have shown that significant accumulation of iodine in heart tissue occurs late in the dye pass curve over the left ventricle. This concept may be important for further uses of this technique to actually look at flow to an area of myocardium. However, correction for this accumulation of iodine in tissue will produce much less variability in ejection fraction calculation during the entire dye pass curve than was previously obtained without it. In a series of dog studies, the correction reduced the variability from about 18% to about 2%. Using the concept of iodine accumulation in tissue, by placing a window of interest over the left ventricle during slow intracoronary injection of small volumes of contrast, it may also be possible to evaluate regional perfusion. Studies of different volumes of iodine injected directly into the circumflex coronary artery and of normalized videodensitometry values in systole and diastole over the area of distribution of the artery show that there was very good correlation between those two numbers. These errors may also be problems for nuclear techniques. Lastly, we are currently looking at vessel flows using time delay curves and phase washout studies. Early dog studies with these techniques show that there might be a way of calculating vessel flow in either the coronary system or peripheral vasculature. The exact accuracy of this technique remains to be defined, but as a cardiac surgeon, I believe it is important for us to determine the physiological importance of atherosclerotic lesions. Just determining whether or not there is an obstruction does not tell the story.

8

Quantitative Evaluation of Atherosclerosis Using Doppler Ultrasound

E. RICHARD GREENE, MARLOWE W. ELDRIDGE, WYATT F. VOYLES, FERNANDO G. MIRANDA, AND JERRY G. DAVIS

A quantitative evaluation of the effect of atherosclerosis on the blood transport capabilities of the human cardiovascular system would ideally require a method which could noninvasively, nontraumatically, and dynamically measure blood vessel morphology and intraluminal flow variables.

Recent technological developments in ultrasonic echo Doppler instruments have resulted in systems which appear more capable of exhibiting the characteristics of an ideal cardiovascular diagnostic and research tool. Many of these new technological capabilities have been sophisticated modifications of the initial, simple, inexpensive Doppler units (1,2). The impetus for the improvement of the technical capabilities of Doppler instruments has resulted from (1) the unfamiliarity of clinicians with the physiological nature of the Doppler blood velocity, (2) the uncertainty in medicine on the clinical importance of detecting multiple grades of stenotic lesions, (3) the technical difficulties in

The authors would like to thank Drs. U. C. Luft, Jack Loeppky, Neal Halpern, Jonathan Sands, Robert Jahnke, David Somerville, Robert Croke, Emmett Mathews, Pratap Avasthi, David Hoekenga, and Richard Conn for their professional expertise. John Adams, Treva Miller, Pat Reilly, Arthur Witt, Ruth Graham, Linda Bernhardt, and Isidora Miranda provided excellent technical support. The work was supported by grants from the American Heart Association and NHLBI grants 5-R01 HL 26025-02 and 1-R01 HL 27095-01.

producing accurate and reproducible measurements of the Doppler flow variables required to quantitatively correlate disturbed flow regions with atherosclerotic lesions, and (4) the requirement of reliable and precise measurements of the variables needed to calculate volumetric flow (cm^3/sec). Moreover, we still do not fully understand the epidemiology of vascular disease, the pathophysiology of occlusive changes, the natural history of arterial lesions, or the precise mechanisms of transient ischemic attacks distal to a stenotic lesion. Doppler ultrasound instruments were developed in the hope of providing techniques which would decrease this general lack of understanding.

Clinical Doppler ultrasound systems that at present are commercially available can be listed in order of their complexity and cost: (1) directional and nondirectional portable continuous wave (CW) devices, (2) continuous and pulsed wave Doppler (PD) flow imaging scanners, and (3) real-time ultrasonic sector scanners incorporating a range-gated pulsed Doppler, identified as a duplex scanner. These methods not only vary in initial cost but also in their technical capabilities, limitations, versatility, and clinical reliability. Importantly, each Doppler procedure of noninvasively evaluating atherosclerotic lesions requires different degrees of operator skill and clinical interpretation of the raw data. Presently, it appears that no best test exists, but a combination of various Doppler techniques (direct or indirect interrogation of a given vessel) produces the most effective way of diagnosis (1).

The purposes of this chapter are threefold: to briefly describe the general, theoretical, and technical aspects of current ultrasound Doppler methods; to discuss the important clinical advantages, assumptions, accuracy, reliability, and technical problems associated with each method; and to suggest future research and development that could improve the accuracy and precision of noninvasive, nonionizing Doppler ultrasound in the quantitative evaluation of the anatomy, pathophysiology, and natural history of atherosclerosis.

METHODS

General Considerations

Accurate use of any Doppler ultrasound device, whether continuous, pulsed, flow imaging, or real-time duplex, requires an appreciation of the hemodynamic phenomenon being measured as well as an understanding of the interaction of acoustic energy with biological tissues and moving blood particles. A brief summary will be presented here, and the reader is referred to the literature for a more comprehensive treatment (2-7).

The term "ultrasound" is used to describe mechanical vibrations at frequencies above the limit of human audibility. Most nontraumatic ultrasound used diagnostically operates between 1 and 20 megahertz (MHz) and produces peak energy levels at less than 5.0 W/cm^2. The acoustic waves are generated when a piezoelectric crystal, the transducer, vibrates at its resonant frequency after the application of a controlled burst of electromagnetic energy to its surface. When the vibrating transducer contacts the skin, two important changes occur as the acoustic energy propagates through the tissue. The energy will be absorbed to reduce its intensity at each point along the beam, and it will also be reflected at points along the beam where the acoustic impedance changes. The acoustic impedance depends on the mechanical properties of the biological tissue. If ultrasonic energy from the transducer is delivered in short bursts of energy, or pulsed, the same transducer can then be used to receive reflected energy.

If the location of the interface between two tissues with different values of acoustic impedances is stationary, the frequency of the reflected wave will be approximately the same as the incoming wave and can be received by the same or separate transducers for dynamic structural information, such as cardiac chamber (8) and blood vessel dimensions (9,10). In contrast, a moving interface will cause the reflected signal frequency to be frequency-shifted by a magnitude proportional to the velocity of the interface in the direction of the sound beam axis (2). In the

simplest form, this relationship is given by the classic Doppler
equation:

$$\Delta f = \frac{2\ V\ f\ \cos\ \Theta}{C}$$

where Δf represents the Doppler shift expressed in kilohertz (kHz);
V is the velocity vector of the interface, generally expressed in
cm/sec; f is the frequency of the transmitted ultrasound; C is the
velocity of sound (1500 m/sec) of the tissue media supporting the
acoustic energy; and Θ is the Doppler incident angle between the
transmitted beam and the velocity vector. Clearly, if the values
of f and C are assumed constant (a reasonable assumption in most
applications) and Θ can be measured or held constant, Δf will be
proportional to V.

When the incident sound beam traverses a blood vessel and its
energy is not absorbed or reflected by significant amounts of
calcium (11), small amounts of energy are absorbed by each moving
red cell. Since the dimensions of the red cells are small compared to the wave length of the acoustic energy, the reflected
wave is radiated in all directions (12). This phenomenon is
called backscatter and allows detection of acoustic signals with
the receiving transducer held at any angle with the backscattering
particles. If the red cell is moving relative to the transducer,
a backscattered Doppler shift can be recorded (2). Since a
distribution of blood velocities is present in each segment of
a blood vessel (6), a spectrum of Doppler shift frequencies will
be developed (13). These spectra can become quite dynamic and
complex in physiological states of blood flow and particularly
within the region of atherosclerotic lesions (14,15). Analysis
of the Doppler shift frequencies is further complicated by the
inherent pulsatile motion of the blood vessel (16).

Even if the velocity distributions of the interrogated blood
vessel are well-behaved and not influenced by a focal lesion
and/or changes in distal impedances (17), other factors which
affect the Doppler spectra must be known in order to be certain
that the Doppler spectrum genuinely reflects the various blood

velocities, (2) whether there is a uniform sound beam, which is required for uniform insonation of the vessel, and (3) whether there is distortion of the Doppler signal due to nonlinearities and overall band-pass characteristics of the device.

If the *mean* frequency shift $\overline{\Delta f}$ can be electronically extracted from the Doppler spectrum generated from a uniformly insonified velocity profile, the spatial average velocity (V) as a function of time can be measured (3). Volumetric blood flow ($\dot{Q}$) can then be determined from an independent ultrasonic measurement of lumen diameter (D) (assuming a circular cross section) by the equation:

$$\dot{Q} = \frac{\pi \ V \ D^2}{4}$$

The Doppler ultrasound methods of calculating V and $\dot{Q}$ are deceivingly simple. This has led some investigators to use simple, commercially available, noninvasive Doppler systems to arrive at quantitative measurements without appreciation of the complexities involved in making the measurements and processing the data (18-20). One must recognize that V and $\dot{Q}$ are variables that cannot be directly obtained with a singular noninvasive measurement of one physiological variable. Noninvasive Doppler methods of measuring V require the following three distinct steps: (1) location of the vessel, (2) determination of the Doppler incident angle, and (3) measurement of the spatial average Δf, which represents V. To calculate $\dot{Q}$, a measurement of the lumen diameter is also required.

The third step, determination of the value of Δf and hence V, can be quite difficult. Technological improvements have provided more control of the blood velocity sensing region known as the sample volume. Consequently, specific locations of blood velocities can be more uniformly insonated to provide Doppler spectra which accurately reflect the true mean velocity or distribution of velocities within the vessel (3,21). From these spectra, appropriate signal processing can yield a more reliable display of a normal or disturbed velocity profile or a more accurate calculation of $\dot{Q}$.

A summary of important design parameters and operational controls of either CW or PD units that influence the extraction of Doppler audio spectra from the received ultrasonic signal is given in Table 1.

In current clinical practice, only the presence, normality, and degree of abnormality of the Doppler spectral patterns generated by a Doppler unit form the basis of the noninvasive detection and quantification of atherosclerotic lesions. In spite of their clear theoretical importance (17), quantitative Doppler flow measurements ($\dot{Q}$) in diseased vessels are still of unknown clinical utility. These measurements are subject to all the physiological and technical assumptions outlined above.

Doppler Audio Signal Analysis

Although several methods of Doppler signal analysis have been developed to extract a mean Δf or to correlate Doppler spectral characteristics created by disturbed flow regions to anatomical lesions (22-24), the initial clinical analysis of the signal is generally an audible interpretation by the person performing the procedure. In the majority of cases, this audible interpretation provides the operator with reliable feedback information which governs the quality of the noninvasive examination and subsequent permanent recordings (25,26). Audio interpretation is obviously the simplest and cheapest method of detecting arterial lesions. Clearly, the observer must learn to recognize and differentiate normal and abnormal velocity signals. This skill is not obtained without extensive training. Furthermore, the method is relatively subjective, qualitative, and it does not allow for a permanent record.

The most common technique used to analyze and display the detected Doppler shift signal is the inexpensive zero-crossing frequency meter (2,3,12). This device produces a voltage output

Table 1. Relationship of Doppler design parameter and operational controls with measurement characteristics

Design Parameters or Operational Controls	Relationship	Measurement Characteristics
Transmitter frequency (all units)	Direct	Resolution, scattering power attenuation
	Inverse	Near field, longitudinal dimension
Transducer diameter (all units)	Direct	Returned power, near field dimension
	Inverse	Resolution, signal/noise ratio
Transducer $\dot{Q}$ value (all units)	Direct	Returned power
	Inverse	Bandwidth resolution
Pulse width (pulsed units)	Direct	Returned power
	Inverse	Resolution
Gate interval (pulsed units)	Direct	Returned power
	Inverse	Resolution
Pulse repetition frequency (pulsed units)	Direct	Processed power, maximum measurable frequency (Nyquist)
	Inverse	Range

that is proportional to the number of zero-crossings that occur in the Doppler audio signal. In the analysis of narrow band spectra with a good signal-to-noise ratio (>20:1), this method provides an analog signal that adequately reflects the mean frequency within the spectra (27). Furthermore, it is possible to depict forward and reverse flow velocity on a common or on separate channels. The significant disadvantages of this method, especially when applied to disturbed flow regions near lesions, are as follows (20): (1) the method requires high signal-to-noise ratios which are often difficult to achieve from the Doppler signal, (2) the output is not always linear with wide band input audio frequencies, (3) the output varies with the amplitude of the input audio signal and threshold control settings, and (4) no display of the spectra width (which is sensitive to disturbed flow regions) is obtained.

As a result of these difficulties, several generations of spectral analyzers have been developed. The most recent and versatile units are the digital fast Fourier transform (FFT) systems (28,29). These expensive devices can be obtained as multipurpose units applied to the audio output of any Doppler instrument or they can be incorporated into an integrated Doppler system. Generally, the FFT technique accurately and reliably displays normal and abnormal Doppler audio spectra and allows various spectral indices (yet to be standardized) to be calculated and correlated to anatomical lesions (22-24,30). Results from our laboratory are shown in Fig. 1 which illustrates the FFT display (kHz) of Doppler spectra obtained from angiographically normal, mild, moderate, and severe internal carotid diameter reductions (DR). Note the significant increases in peak frequencies and spectral width associated with increased stenosis. Peak frequencies are significantly dependent on the location of the sample volume (13) and will be proportional to the degree of stenosis only until the stenosis becomes hemodynamically significant. It is important to realize that gray scale or color-coded FFT devices and subsequent calculated indices derived from the spectra are also subject to the gains and dynamic range settings of the input Doppler signal and the FFT display. Fig. 2 demonstrates two spectral waveforms obtained from a normal internal carotid artery at different Doppler gain settings. An additional calculation, the mode, displays the frequency with the highest energy level at any time (an estimate of Δf and V). Even in this example of narrow band spectra associated with normal flow patterns, note the variation in gray scale presentation of the spectra. These variations may influence the calculations of various correlative

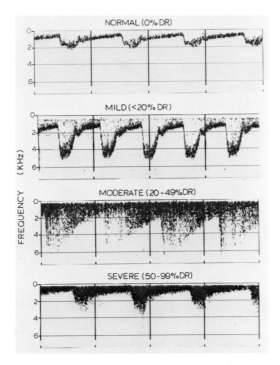

Fig. 1 Fast Fourier transform (FFT) display of image-guided
pulsed Doppler spectra obtained from angiographically normal
(>0% DR); mild (<20% DR); moderate (20-49% DR); and severe
(50-99% DR) internal carotid maximum diameter reduction (DR).
Note the significant increases in peak frequencies and spectral
width associated with increased stenosis. Waveforms are inverted
to signify flow away from transducer.

indices associated with spectral width. The effect of this and
other controls on the audio spectra display is even more pronounced
in high-energy broadband spectra generated from disturbed flow
regions. Clearly, if one is to quantitatively analyze Doppler
spectra generated from flow velocity fields created by different
degrees of arterial narrowings, careful attention to the control and
display settings of the instrument is most important. As with all
applications of noninvasive diagnostic ultrasound, optimal instrument control settings will vary with application and patient habitus.

The preceding theoretical comments and operational suggestions
have been general to all three categories of Doppler ultrasonic

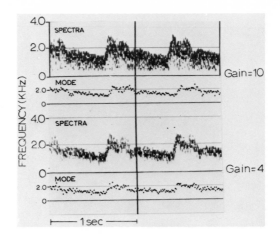

Fig. 2   FFT spectral waveform obtained from a normal internal
carotid artery at different Doppler gain settings which are
operator controlled.   Note the increased spectral width at a gain
setting of 10 db compared to 4 db, which may influence the interpretation of the spectra and hence the quantification of the
degrees of arterial stenosis.   It is also important to note that
small degrees of spectral broadening can also be present in
normal, unstenotic flow regions such as vessel branches.   An
additional waveform, the mode frequency, represents the frequency
of highest amplitude and may be used to estimate Δf and V.

instruments regardless of clinical application.   Each modality has

specific characteristics, capabilities, and limitations, which

will now be discussed.

CRITIQUE AND DISCUSSION

Continuous Wave Devices

Simple, inexpensive continuous wave (CW) devices are certainly the

most versatile and widely used Doppler instruments in clinical

practice (31,32).   Initial systems were nondirectional but more

recent versions were designed to differentiate flow directionality,

which is often of clinical importance.   The major technical

deficiency of the CW units is their lack of depth resolution.

Consequently, if two distinct flow fields (vessels) are insonated

by the relatively large sample volume (created by the three-

dimensional overlap of the beam patterns of the transmitting and receiving crystals), unspecific Doppler audio spectra will be developed. As an example, overlapping veins and arteries, a common anatomical situation, can distort the CW Doppler spectra. Directional units have helped differentiate flow fields, but they have not completely resolved this problem. Although no range resolution is possible, continuous wave units allow ultrasonic Doppler signals to be continuously sampled. Consequently, no artifactual distortion (aliasing) of the audio signal is produced by high-frequency shifts associated with elevated blood velocities and/or small Doppler angles (3). This distortion can be created by pulsed units that sample high flow rates. The distortion due to aliasing can mimic abnormal spectra created by anatomical lesions (33).

Application in Peripheral Vascular Disease. In spite of its technical limitations, the simple hand-held continuous wave device (with or without sophisticated spectral analysis) has found wide acceptance in the diagnosis of hemodynamically significant (flow and pressure reducing) lesions in the peripheral arteries during rest and exercise (23,31,32). In this application, the procedure can be undertaken by a technician without extensive training in the interpretation of Doppler spectra. Unpublished results from our laboratory with over 100 angiographic correlates support published results with an overall accuracy of 98% compared with angiography. Thus, in our institution, peripheral angiography is reserved only for surgical candidates. In addition, unique baseline physiological data (segmental pressures, qualitative flows, and vascular reserve) of significant importance to patient management are also obtained in a cost-effective manner. Few limitations are present in the application of continuous wave units to peripheral vascular disease. In advanced occlusive arterial disease, no Doppler shifts may be generated due to lack of blood velocity which will not create high enough Doppler shifts to pass the band-pass output filters of the unit. In addition, Doppler-determined cuff blood pressures may be artificially elevated (>200 mmHg) due to arterial calcification. Generally, these conditions are self-evident and do not compromise the accuracy of the noninvasive diagnosis.

The genuine success of simple, nonimaging continuous wave units in peripheral vascular disease can be attributed to the advanced state of the occlusive arterial disease (hemodynamically significant) in most patients presenting with resting or intermittent claudication. Significant flow and pressure reduction can be detected reliably and correlated to stenotic lesions demonstrated angiographically. Reliable detection of nonhemodynamically significant lesions (arbitrarily defined as <50% maximum diameter reduction in any angiographic plane) that do not significantly reduce flow and pressure clearly put unresolvable technical demands on simple continuous wave devices in peripheral and other applications.

Application in Cerebrovascular Disease Although their relative importance remains controversial, nonhemodynamically significant but emboligenic lesions in the extracranial cerebrovascular system have been implicated in cerebral ischemia (transient ischemic attacks) and infarcts (strokes) (12,34,35). Consequently, attempts to noninvasively detect hemodynamically and nonhemodynamically significant stenosis using continuous wave units were undertaken. Due to inherent physiological and anatomical complexities of the cerebral circulation, simple indirect periorbital Doppler techniques are not accurate enough to detect all hemodynamically significant and few nonhemodynamically significant lesions in the extracranial vasculature (36). Generally, total occlusion of the internal carotid gives a positive test result (particularly with compression maneuvers) and thus allows this simple indirect procedure to be a useful and commonly applied adjunct to more direct methods (1).

Direct, continuous wave Doppler interrogation of the carotid bifurcation using audio interpretation (26), zero-crossing detection (37) and FFT methods (38) have allowed useful differentiation between angiographically determined significant and insignificant lesions. One of the difficulties with these nonimaging methods is the critical problem of the proper identification of the three major vessels (common, internal, and external carotids) in a small region (39,40). Consequently, Doppler flow imaging systems with and without audio spectra analysis were developed.

Doppler Flow Imaging

Continuous Wave Flow Imaging In order to meet the need of proper vessel identification in the carotid system, Doppler flow imaging systems have been developed. The Doppler flow image is created by a video display whose spot patterns indicate a detected flow velocity. To be displayed, this velocity (frequency shift) must exceed a certain threshold value. The transducer is coupled to a a scanning arm, which can be used to create a map of the detected flow loci. Continuous wave Dopplers can be used to drive the transducer (41) and create the ultrasonic arteriogram, whose image format has been more readily acceptable to image-oriented radiologists and clinicians. One advantage (of undetermined significance) of the flow image over standard echo imaging (B-mode ultrasound scanning) is that the true flow lumen can be displayed in many planes. Unfortunately, the flow lumen image may not coincide precisely with the actual vessel wall if there are calcified plaques or other lesions in the interrogated vessel. The resolution of the flow image (which requires several minutes to produce from a stationary patient) is dependent on the lateral width of the acoustic beam pattern, whose present resolution (7) precludes the detection of plaques less than 1 mm. For the same reason, the imaged flow lumen may also be several millimeters larger than actual size. Although an image of the carotid bifurcation is generated by the Doppler, allowing identification of the vessels, the quantification of the atherosclerotic involvement generally depends on concurrent analysis of the Doppler audio spectra (22,24). CW Doppler flow imaging correlated with angiography has been promising for both nonhemodynamically significant and hemodynamically significant lesions (22,42,43). In an attempt to quantitate stenotic lesions, Spencer and Reid (24) obtained best-fit regression lines relating percent stenosis by angiography to percent stenosis by Doppler frequency ratios obtained from CW Doppler flow imaging. Unfortunately, their results showed significant scatter. Color-coded CW Doppler imaging (44,45) has also proved successful in reliably separating occlusive, significant, and insignificant lesions, but the more elaborate color technique has yet to be shown more clinically efficacious compared to earlier black and white displays. Although CW flow imaging systems have made important contributions in detection of cerebrovascular disease, their main limitation, spatial resolution, has prompted the development of pulsed Doppler flow imaging units.

Pulsed Doppler Flow Mapping Comparatively, pulsed Doppler (PD) flow imaging units are more complex and expensive than are the CW devices (46). Due to their capacity to detect flow velocity from discrete points in space independently and simultaneously (multi-gated), PD flow imaging units theoretically provide more specific flow images and Doppler spectra (47). Compared with CW imaging, increased operator skill is required with PD devices due to the problem of finding the desired vessel in three dimensions rather than two, as is done with CW Doppler techniques. Similar to CW imaging but unlike arteriography, multiplane views of the carotid bifurcation can be obtained. As with CW imaging methods, angiographic correlates using PD imaging and Doppler spectral analysis are encouraging (48) and their pitfalls can be delineated (39). Generally, imaging errors caused by calcification could be overcome by sonographic spectral analysis. It is important to note that inoperable occlusive disease can be reliably separated from operable, highly stenotic lesions. Due to the finite spatial and velocity resolution of Doppler flow imaging instruments (either CW or PD), improvements in image resolution (even at higher frequencies) seem unlikely. Consequently, improved quantitative evaluation of atherosclerotic lesions using flow imaging will probably come from improved methods of Doppler spectral analyses. This is presently a difficult matter due to the spatial distribution of various disturbed velocity patterns within and distal to lesions and their convolution with the generally ill-defined CW and PD sample volumes (33). In spite of the clinical success of static flow imaging instruments, their problems of (1) spatial resolution, (2) narrow fields of view and versatility, (3) time required from image production, and (4) relatively poor image quality were not overlooked. Predictably, the development of sophisticated and quite expensive systems which incorporate ongoing high resolution real-time echo imaging technology (10) and pulsed Doppler velocimetry was achieved (49). This instrumentation was denoted as duplex scanning.

Duplex Scanning

Available duplex scanning (DS) systems vary in their emphasis on imaging, image processing, pulsed Doppler capabilities, and audio spectra analysis (50). Units are being applied in cardiology (47, 51) and in carotid (52-56) and femoral arteries (4). In spite of the improved resolution in vessel imaging (9), quantitative evaluation of the lesion has often rested on the analysis of the range-gated Doppler audio spectra. Quantitative peak blood velocities calculated from calibrated FFT velocity spectra (43) have been used. Fig. 3 demonstrates Doppler audio spectra sampled from a normal common carotid artery examined by a 5 MHz DS in our laboratory. Note the narrow band Doppler spectrum created by undisturbed velocity profiles. Due to the ability of DS to provide measurements of the Doppler angle and vessel diameter, estimates of volume flow rate can be calculated (3,51). Doppler spectra from normal external and internal carotids are shown in Fig. 4. The high diastolic flow due to the low-impedance vascular bed supplied by the internal artery is clearly distinct from the reduced diastolic flow of the high-impedance bed of the external carotid. The shape of the spectral waveforms demonstrates an

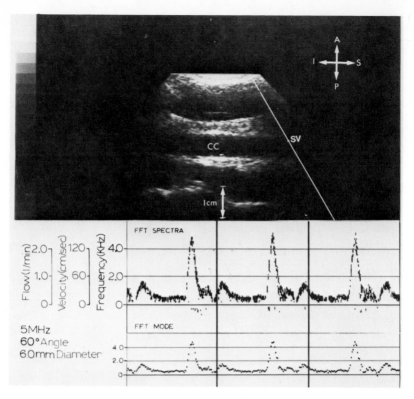

Fig. 3 A freeze frame of a DS image with the sample volume (SV)
in a normal common carotid artery (CC). Note the narrow band
spectra (velocities) created by undisturbed laminar velocity
profiles. Due to the ability of the DS to provide measurements
of Δf, Doppler angle and vessel diameter, the FFT spectra can be
calibrated in kHz, velocity (cm/sec), or flow (1/min).

important discriminatory feature of the DS method. By analyzing
the Doppler signal, vessel identity can be further defined by its
inherent flow patterns. In Fig. 4, spectral data are displayed in
kilohertz to emphasize that the velocity and/or flow calibration
requirements of angle and diameter are not always reliable in
internal and external carotids in consecutive patients in our
laboratory. This is contrary to reports of other investigators
(30,52). Fig. 5 illustrates a carotid bifurcation with Doppler
audio spectra created by a moderate stenotic lesion (10-49%
diameter reduction) in the internal carotid artery. Note the

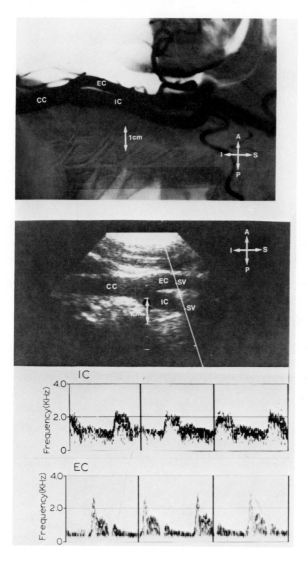

Fig. 4   Angiographic (top) and freeze-frame DS images (bottom)
with FFT spectra of a normal carotid bifurcation with the sample
volume (SV) placed in the external carotid (EC) and later in the
internal carotid (IC) distal to the common carotid (CC). Note
the high diastolic flow velocity in the IC compared to the EC.
In our experience, real-time noninvasive images of the carotid
bifurcation that are similar to angiographic presentation are
not easily obtained. Often the far walls of the EC and IC are
not visualized, hence calibration of the spectra into V and $\dot{Q}$ is
not always feasible.

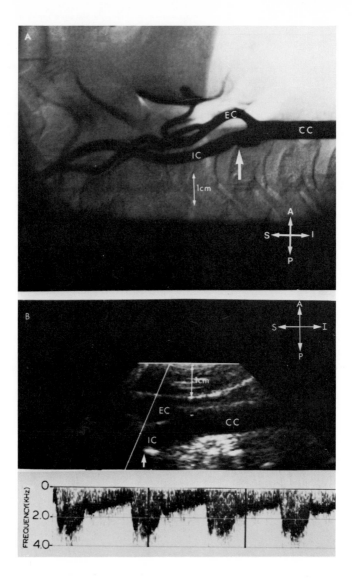

Fig. 5 Angiographic (top) and freeze-frame images (bottom) of an
abnormal carotid bifurcation with abnormal FFT spectra created by
a moderate stenotic lesion in the IC. Note the imaged vessel
calcification (white arrow). Abbreviations are the same as in
Fig. 4. The spectral waveform can be electronically inverted if
desired, but is displayed here in the downward direction to
demonstrate flow away from the transducer. It is most important
to note that calculations of Δf and V are unreliable in the
distinct regions of disturbed flow.

imaged vessel calcification, which provides morphological information along with the Doppler physiological data. As suggested by
Fell et al. (56), implementation of the FFT spectra analysis with
the expensive DS has provided new, refined capabilities of lesion
categorization. These noninvasive capabilities appear to stress
the quantitative limits of biplane angiographic interpretations.
By careful separation of external and internal blood velocity
signals and by noting the lack of diastolic flow velocity in the
proximal common carotid (55), total occlusions can be reliably
differentiated for highly stenotic lesions in the internal carotid.
Other calculated spectral indices obtained from the DS have been
proposed and prospectively studied with favorable angiographic
correlates in the internal carotid (3). As previously demonstrated
by Fig. 2, careful attention must be made to gain and other control
settings to obtain reliable results.

   Serial clinical results using different Doppler methods which
demonstrated the ability of our laboratory to noninvasively identify angiographically demonstrated lesions that obstructed $\geq$20% of
the internal carotid lumen in different patient groups are given
in Fig. 6. Results using the DS with FFT spectral analysis
obtained in 1980 are compared to results using simple nonimaging
CW audio spectral analysis in 1979 and results using oculoplethysmography (OPG) in 1978. These results suggest that relatively
inexpensive CW methods with careful operator training and Doppler
audio spectral analysis can significantly increase the diagnostic
efficacy of the noninvasive cerebrovascular laboratory with OPG
only. More costly, yet more versatile imaging DS methods can
further improve (but not significantly) the overall accuracy of
the noninvasive detection of lesions of $\geq$20% diameter reduction
in the extracranial vasculature. Importantly, the percentage of
negative angiographic procedures decreased significantly with
implementation of either CW or DS methods. These results suggest
that only patients with a high probability of carotid disease are
subjected to the risks and costs of angiography.

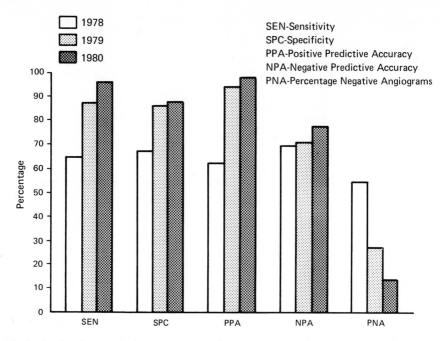

Fig. 6 Serial clinical results in our laboratory using different Doppler methods to identify angiographically demonstrated IC lesions of >20% diameter reduction and occlusions. See text for details.

Upon consideration of the good clinical results published by others and results from our laboratory using the DS in carotid disease, an important question arises (37). If adequate noninvasive diagnostic procedures that lessen the need for angiography and provide unique qualitative physiological information can be done with simple Doppler equipment, why develop expensive DS systems that should not and will not be competitive with standard arterial injection or intravenous digital angiography (57) in the appropriate workup of patients presenting with symptoms of vascular insufficiency? In the experience of this laboratory, the answer to this question is twofold. First, due to its unique imaging and range-gating Doppler capabilities, a DS system with variable transmit frequencies can be used noninvasively to detect and quantitate anatomical lesions not only in the carotids and femorals, but also in other segments of the cardiovascular system

which are not surrounded by bone or air. The same DS unit can
be used to examine intracardiac DS as well as systemic vascular
lesions. As shown in Fig. 7, application of the DS to the renal
arteries has been reported (58). Attempts to noninvasively detect flow characteristics of the left main coronary artery using
tracking devices (16) are presently being undertaken in our
laboratory (Fig. 8). Fig. 9 illustrates the various applications

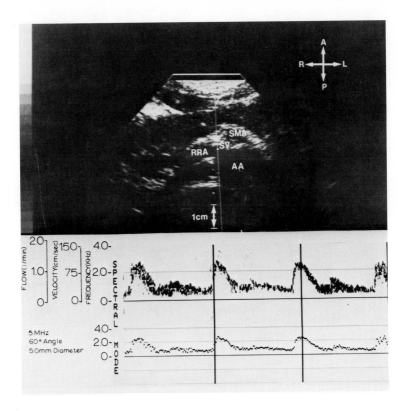

Fig. 7 A freeze-frame DS image with the sample volume (SV) placed
in a normal right renal artery (RRA). Anatomical landmarks include a cross section of the superior mesenteric artery (SMA) and
the abdominal aorta (AA). Note the narrow band spectra with
significant diastolic flow associated with the low impedance renal
bed. Vessel diameter and Dopper angle can be estimated to allow
calibration in V and Q̇. These spectra patterns will change with
the region of a stenotic lesion. Significant increases in distal
vascular impedance will reduce the diastolic flow component.

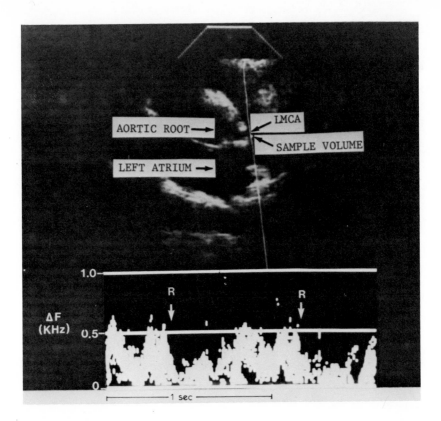

Fig. 8 A freeze-frame DS image of the left main coronary artery
at its origin with the aortic root. In these preliminary studies,
the sample volume (SV) is tracked in the left main coronary artery
(LMCA), thus allowing only blood velocity spectra and not wall
reflections to be recorded throughout the cardiac motion. Note
the predominant diastolic flow velocity (R is the R-wave of the
EKG). It is hoped that lesions of the LMCA can be detected and
noninvasive estimates of LMCA flow variables can be made.

of DS to obtain vessel images and calibrated blood velocity

signals (and subsequent flow rates) throughout the cardiovascular

system. Spectral analysis techniques to identify arterial lesions

can be applied to any of the vessels. Gray scale (59) and color-

coded, real-time, multigated, echo-Doppler images (60) have also

been developed from DS technology to demonstrate the immense

amount of physiological information and display formats that can

be obtained from pulsed Doppler ultrasound.

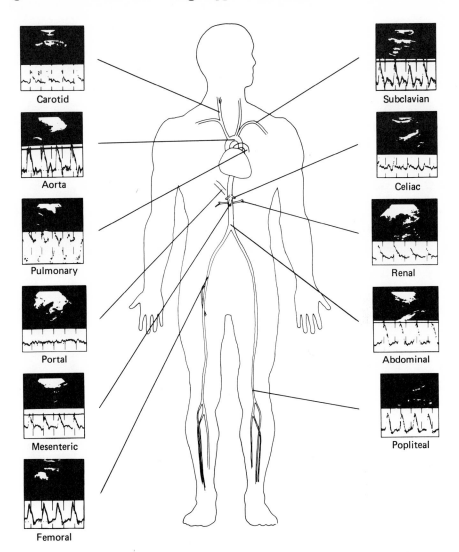

Fig. 9 A schematic representation of the various cardiovascular applications of a single, multifrequency DS. Not shown here are its additional intracardiac applications and its ability to measure cardiac output. Note the variations of the blood velocity waveforms, depending on the input impedance to different vascular beds. These results suggest that image-guided Doppler spectra and calculated hemodynamic variables obtained from the DS can be used to detect anatomical lesions and to quantify the true hemodynamic significance of these lesions throughout the cardiovascular system.

Secondly, it is the opinion of this laboratory that technological innovations associated with the DS have allowed reliable noninvasive estimates of cardiac output (61) and regional blood flow rates (51). These measurements will become increasingly important for the following reasons. The hemodynamic severity and clinical consequences of reduced oxygen transport due to an anatomical lesion depend on many physiological factors (17). Unfortunately, these factors have not been quantitatively related to the ischemic symptoms or metabolic disorders (62). In our view, a uniplane or biplane anatomical description of an atherosclerotic lesion is important but does not supply sufficient information to the understanding and quantitative evaluation of atherosclerosis. Hopefully, the development of a computer-controlled videodensitometry method will allow quantitative blood flow data to be obtained during angiography. Until then, more specific anatomical and dynamic physiological information may be obtained noninvasively (and without radiation exposure) in the human from the DS.

CONCLUSIONS AND SUGGESTIONS

Clearly, the simple continuous wave velocity detector with or without sophisticated audio spectral analysis will retain and increase its role as an important noninvasive tool in the qualitative evaluation of cerebral and peripheral vascular disease. No significant modifications of these devices and methods that would not decrease their favorable cost-effectiveness seem warranted.

The diagnostic efficacy of CW and PD flow imaging devices is generally determined by the capability of Doppler spectral analysis to reflect flow disorders secondary to anatomical lesions. These relatively inexpensive imaging units are quite specialized only to carotid examinations, but they appear able to adequately separate occlusive, less than 50% diameter reduction and greater than 50% diameter reduction in lesions of the internal carotid artery. Compared to other modalities, relatively little operator training and expertise is required for reliable results. Standardization

of the examination procedure and the interpretation of results
will further enhance the utility of these modalities.

In the extracranial vascular system, duplex scanning methods
appear equally precise as angiographic interpretations in the
quantification of atherosclerotic lesions. This capability should
extend to applications in other superficial and deep-lying vessels.
Due to pure technical constraints of resolution, fields of view,
and penetration, ultrasonic images (63) will unlikely provide the
extensive anatomical detail of either standard or digital angiography. With improved transducer design, sample volume control
(33), digital coding, adequate vessel images, and Doppler spectra
can be recorded to provide the acquisition of unique blood velocity
and flow data. Consequently, a better clinical and pathophysio-
logical understanding of the true hemodynamic severity of an
atherosclerotic lesion can be obtained.

SUMMARY

During the last two decades, various Doppler methods have been
successfully used to screen patients with significant cerebral
and peripheral vascular disease. In general terms, the principal
advantages of Doppler ultrasound techniques in the evaluation of
atherosclerotic lesions are that they (1) are noninvasive, (2)
are nontraumatic, (3) are relatively inexpensive, (4) provide
anatomical and physiological data, and (5) provide direct and
dynamic measurements. Nevertheless, the general limitations of
the techniques are of equal importance: (1) the techniques are
difficult in some subjects due to obesity and anatomical variations; (2) the technique cannot examine tissues surrounded by air
or bone; (3) the techniques require operator skill and a thorough
knowledge of human anatomy and cardiovascular dynamics; (4) the
techniques have finite spatial resolutions that may compromise
the important measurement of vessel diameter, ulceration, and
percent stenosis; and (5) the techniques have finite velocity
measuring capabilities which may compromise some measurements

of highly disturbed blood velocities outside the range of 2-200 cm/sec.

As clinical demands for the early diagnosis and quantification of vascular lesions increased, improvements in Doppler ultrasonics and spectral analysis significantly increased the technical and clinical capabilities of existing simple, inexpensive instruments. Presently, both anatomical and physiological images along with quantitative Doppler spectra from superficial and deep-lying vessels can be obtained. Consequently, the ability of new, expensive imaging equipment to quantitate atherosclerotic lesions using spectral analysis techniques compares favorably with the interpretational precision of standard invasive or intravenous digital angiography. New data suggest that unique hemodynamic information, which reflects the effects of cardiac output and vascular input impedance on the hemodynamic consequences of an anatomical lesion, can also be obtained.

REFERENCES

1. Franklin DL, Schlegel WA, Rushmer RF (1961) Blood flow measured by Doppler frequency shift of backscattered ultrasound. Science 132:564-565
2. Baker DW (1970) Pulsed ultrasonic Doppler blood flow sensing. IEEE Trans Ultrasonics 17:170-185
3. Baker DW, Daigle RE (1977) Noninvasive ultrasonic flowmetry. In: Hwang NH, Norman N (eds) Cardiovascular flow dynamics and measurements. University Park Press, Baltimore, pp 151-189
4. Blackshear WM Jr, Phillips DJ, Strandness DE Jr (1979) Pulsed Doppler assessment of normal human femoral artery velocity patterns. J Surg Res 27:73-83
5. Jorgensen JE, Campau D, Baker DW (1973) Physical characteristics and mathematical modelling of the pulsed ultrasonic flowmeter. Med Biol Eng Comput 2:404-421
6. McDonald DA (1974) Blood flow in arteries, 2nd edn. William and Wilkins, Baltimore
7. Wells PNT (1977) Biomedical ultrasonics. Academic Press, New York
8. Feigenbaum H (1981) Echocardiography, 3rd edn. Lea and Febiger, Philadelphia
9. Comerota AJ, Cranley JJ, Cook SE (1981) Real-time B-mode carotid imaging in diagnosis of cerebrovascular disease. Surgery 89:718-719

10. Cooperberg PL, Robertson WD, Fry P, Sweeney V (1979) High-resolution real-time ultrasound of the carotid bifurcation. JCU 7:13-17
11. Hartley CJ, Strandness DE (1969) The effects of atherosclerosis on transmission of ultrasound. J Surg Res 9:575-582
12. Flax SW, Webster JG, Updike SJ (1970) Statistical evaluation of the Doppler ultrasonic blood flowmeter. Biomed Sci Instrum 7:201-222
13. Reneman RS, Spencer MP (1979) Local Doppler audio spectra in normal and stenosed carotid arteries in man. Ultrasound Med Biol 5:1-11
14. Gidden DO, Mabon RF, Cassanova RA (1976) Measurement of disordered flows distal to subtotal vascular stenoses in the thoracic aortas of dogs. Circ Res 39:112-119
15. Greene ER, Histand MB (1979) Ultrasonic assessment of simulated atherosclerosis: in vitro and in vivo comparisons. J Biomech Eng 101:73-81
16. Davis JG, Richards KL, Greene ER (1979) A sample volume tracking unit for pulsed Doppler echocardiography. IEEE Trans Biomed Eng 26:285-288
17. Young DF (1979) Fluid mechanics of arterial stenoses. J Biomech Eng 101:157-175
18. Baker DW, Johnson SL, Strandness DE (1974) Prospects for quantitation of transcutaneous pulsed Doppler techniques in cardiology and peripheral vascular disease. In: Reneman RS (ed) Cardiovascular applications of ultrasound. North Holland, Amsterdam, pp 108-124
19. Gill RW (1979) Pulsed Doppler with B-mode imaging for quantitative blood flow measurement. Ultrasound Med Biol 5:223-235
20. Reneman RS, Spencer MP (1974) Difficulties in processing of an analogue Doppler flow signal; with special reference to zero-crossing meter and quantification. In: Reneman RS (ed) Cardiovascular applications of ultrasound. North Holland, Amsterdam, pp 32-42
21. Nowicki A, Reid JM (1981) An infinite gate pulse Doppler. Ultrasound Med Biol 7:41-50
22. Barnes RW, Rittgers SE, Putney WW (1982) Real-time Doppler spectrum analysis. Arch Surg 117:52-57
23. Gosling RG, King DH (1974) Continuous wave ultrasound as an alternative and complement to x-rays in vascular examinations. In: Reneman RS (ed) Cardiovascular application of ultrasound. Elsevier, Amsterdam, pp 266-282
24. Spencer MP, Reid JM (1979) Quantitation of carotid stenosis with continuous-wave (C-W) Doppler ultrasound. Stroke 10: 326-330
25. Standness DE Jr (1978) The use of ultrasound in the evaluation of peripheral vascular disease. Prog Cardiovasc Dis 20:403-422
26. Weaver RG Jr, Howard G, McKinney WM, Ball MR, Jones ASM, Toole JF (1980) Comparison of Doppler ultrasonography with arteriography of the carotid artery bifurcation. Stroke 22:402-404

27. Lunt MH (1975) Accuracy and limitations of the ultrasonic Doppler velocimeter and zero-crossing detector. Ultrasound Med Biol 2:1-10
28. Greene ER, Hoekenga DE, Richards KL, Davis JG (1980) Pulsed Doppler echocardiographic audio spectrum analysis: time interval histogram versus multifilters spectrogram and fast Fourier transform. Biomed Sci Instrum 16:134-144
29. Rittgers SE, Putney WW, Barnes RW (1980) Real-time spectrum analysis and display of directional Doppler ultrasound blood velocity signals. IEEE Trans Biomed Eng 27:723-728
30. Keagy BA, Pharr WF, Thomas D, Bowes DE (to be published Ultrasound Med Biol) A quantitation method for the evaluation of spectral analysis patterns in carotid artery stenosis.
31. Barnes RW (1981) Office Doppler techniques in vascular disease. J Fam Pract 13:711-720
32. Marinelli MR, Beach KW, Glass MJ, Primozich JF, Strandness DE Jr (1979) Noninvasive testing vs clinical evaluation of arterial disease. JAMA 241:2031-2034
33. Walker AR, Phillips DJ, Powers JE (1982) Evaluating Doppler devices using a moving string test target. JCU 10:25-30
34. Bartynski WS, Darbouze P P, Nemir P Jr (1981) Significance of ulcerated plaque in transient cerebral ischemia. Am J Surg 141:353-357
35. Pessin MS, Duncan GW, Mohr JP, Poskanzer DC (1977) Clinical and angiographic features of carotid transient ischemic attacks. N Engl J Med 296:358-362
36. Bone GE, Barnes RW (1976) Limitation of the Doppler cerebro-vascular examination in hemispheric cerebral ischemia. Surgery 79:577
37. Rutherford RB, Hiatt WR, Kreutzer EW (1977) The use of velocity waveform analysis in the diagnosis of carotid artery occlusive disease. Surgery 82:695-702
38. Barnes RW, Nix L, Rittgers SE (1981) Audible interpretation of carotid Doppler signals. Arch Surg 116:1185-1189
39. Berry SM, O'Donnell JA, Hobson RW (1980) Capabilities and limitations of pulsed Doppler sonography in carotid imaging. JCU 8:405-412
40. Prendes JL, McKinney WM, Buonanno FS, Jones AN (1980) Ana-tomic variations of the carotid bifurcation affecting Doppler scan interpretation. JCU 8:147-150
41. Reid JM, Spencer MP (1972) Ultrasonic Doppler technique for imaging blood vessels. Science 176:1235-1236
42. Shoumaker RD, Bloch S (1977) Cerebrovascular evaluation: assessment of Doppler scanning of carotid arteries, ophthalmic Doppler flow and cervical bruits. Stroke 9:563-566
43. Lewis RR, Beasley MG, Hyams DE, Gosling RG (1978) Imaging the carotid bifurcation using continuous-wave Doppler-shift ultrasound and spectral analysis. Stroke 9:465-471
44. O'Leary OH, Clouse ME, Persson AV, Edwards SA (1982) Nonin-vasive testing for carotid artery stenosis. II: Clinical applications of accuracy assessments. AJR 138:109-111

45. White D, Curry G (1978) Color-coded differential Doppler ultrasonic scanning system for the carotid bifurcation: Results in 486 bifurcations angiographically confirmed. In: Kurjak A (ed) Recent advances in ultrasound diagnosis. Excerpta Medica, Amsterdam, pp 239-249
46. Hokanson DE, Mozersky DJ, Sumner DS, McLeod FD, Strandness DE (1972) Ultrasonic arteriography: a noninvasive method for arterial visualization. Radiology 102:435-436
47. Baker DW (1980) Applications of pulsed Doppler techniques. Radiol Clin North Am 18:79-103
48. Hobson RW, Berry SM, Katocs AS Jr, O'Donnell JA, Jamil Z, Savitsky JP (1980) Comparison of pulsed Doppler and real-time B-mode echo arteriography for noninvasive imaging of the extracranial carotid arteries. Surgery 87:286-293
49. Barber FE, Baker DW, Nation AWC, Strandness DE Jr, Reid JM (1974) Ultrasonic duplex echo-Doppler scanner. IEEE Trans Biomed Eng 21:109-113
50. Phillips DJ, Powers JE, Eyer WM, Blackshear WM Jr, Bodily KC, Strandness DE Jr, Baker DW (1980) Detection of peripheral vascular disease using the duplex scanner III. Ultrasound Med Biol 6:205-218
51. Greene ER (1982) Noninvasive measurement of blood flow using pulsed Doppler ultrasound. In: Loeppky JA and Riedesel ML (eds) Oxygen transport to human tissues. Elsevier, New York, pp 135-150
52. Blackshear WM, Phillips DJ, Chikos PM, Harley JD, Thiele BL, Strandness DE (1980) Carotid artery velocity patterns in normal and stenotic vessels. Stroke 11:67-71
53. Blackshear WM Jr, Phillips DJ, Thiele BL, Hirsch JH, Chikos PM, Marinelli MR, Hard KJ, Strandness DE Jr (1979) Detection of carotid occlusive disease by ultrasonic imaging and pulsed Doppler spectrum analysis. Surgery 86:698-706
54. Bodily KC, Zierler RE, Marinelli MR, Thiele BL, Greene FM Jr, Strandness DE Jr (1980) Flow disturbances following carotid endarterectomy. Surg Gynecol Obstet 151:77-80
55. Breslau PJ, Fell G, Phillips DJ, Thiele BL, Strandness DE Jr (1982) Evaluation of carotid bifurcation disease. Arch Surg 117:58-60
56. Fell G, Phillips DJ, Chikos PM, Harley JD, Thiele BL, Strandness DE Jr (1981) Ultrasonic duplex scanning for disease of the carotid artery. Circulation 64:1191-1195
57. Ducos de Lahitte M, Marc-Vergnes J-P, Rascol A, Guiraud B, Manelfe C (1980) Intravenous angiography of the extracranial cerebral arteries. Radiology 137:705-711
58. Greene ER, Venters MD, Avasthi PS, Conn RL, Jahnke RW (1981) Noninvasive characterization of renal artery blood flow. Kidney Int 20:523-529
59. Burch DJ, Taenger JC (1981) Real-time quantitative blood flow measurements using Doppler ultrasound. Proceedings 26th AINM, San Francisco, CA, p 17
60. Eyer MK, Brandestini MA, Phillips DJ, Baker DW (1981) Color

measurements using Doppler ultrasound. Proceedings 26th AINM, San Francisco, CA, p 17

60. Eyer MK, Brandestini MA, Phillips DJ, Baker DW (1981) Color digital echo/Doppler image presentation. Ultrasound Med Biol Biol 7:21-31

61. Loeppky JA, Greene ER, Hoekenga DE, Caprihan A, Luft UC (1981) Beat-by-beat stroke volume assessment by pulsed Doppler in upright and supine exercise. J Appl Physiol 50:1173-1182

62. Sundt TM, Sharbrough FW, Piepgras DG, Kearns TP, Messick JM, O'Fallen WM (1981) Correlation of cerebral blood flow and electrocephalographic changes during carotid endarterectomy. Mayo Clin Proc 56:533-543

63. Goldstein A (1981) Range ambiguities in real-time ultrasound. JCU 9:83-90

DISCUSSION: JOHN M. REID

I want first to give you a little background on my view of the
development of this progressively expensive technology. We are
dealing with a progressive disease. No matter how much we can
help the patient, we don't seem to be able to extend life, because
we do not know very much about the disease itself, and in my view,
the future belongs to the people who can figure out what is
causing it so that we can turn it around. Otherwise, the costs
to society will continue to escalate.

We seem to be hit with a large number of degenerative diseases
in our society and we are not doing a very effective job of get-
ting at the fundamentals. The systems that Dr. Greene described
so well have been quite useful in clinical practice, using relative
information effectively to assess the cardiovascular and particularly the cerebrovascular system. I think they offer perhaps the
greatest potential in population surveys in large scale studies.
We are like the archaeologists, we have to take what data we can
find to analyze our problem. We cannot demand that the physical
world be changed for our convenience, and set criteria on the only
kind of data we can accept. We have to take the "bone" where we
find it and use our skills and our brains to figure out what the
story is.

The imaging system, which requires less operator training,
gives some guidance by mechanical arms. I would like to point out
that this makes the data reproducible on the same patient from one
examination to the next. The probe is held to provide a fixed
Doppler angle. As Merrill Spencer has shown, the operator can,
by imaging down, get the vertebral artery, as well as the carotid
system including the carotid bifurcation and internal carotid artery. It allows the operator for the first time to see where the
Doppler data are coming from. The location of the sound within
the blood vesse is shown by the cursor. The operator is no longer
holding a hand-held Doppler probe "blind" to the vessel anatomy.

We would like to have a camera, so that we will not have to
scan back and forth in excruciating detail, although it does not

take more than perhaps 10 min to make these image pictures. We did some experiments with a scanning continuous wave (CW) array, under NIH sponsorship. This would do the scanning in one dimension, at least, automatically. The images are fraught with noise but the general approach does seem to work, and perhaps at some time in the future we may be able to make these pictures more rapidly.

To make Doppler images much more complete, we have used a multiple gated system like the Branddestini system. This system puts a Doppler gate at every position along the range axis. We rather modestly called this the infinite gate pulse Doppler, at the start, but now we have a finite number of gates, too. It measures in depth; you can read the sound-beam-blood-vessel angle off longitudinal scan pictures. We thought it and the CW image would make a nice biplane pair for the carotid system. We found that this system has some other advantages. In a preliminary study by looking at flow in aorto-coronary bypass grafts, we found that it helped considerably. Instead of searching blind in range, with one or a few gates, one can examine this rather complicated region, and pick out the flow in the bypass graft. We record proper waveform and diastolic timing. We believe that it offers considerable promise in going into this more difficult site.

There are other difficult sites that we would like to examine. These are deep, moving, and very small vessels, down to the microcirculation, where the final action is. All the systems that have been built so far have attempted to separate the Doppler signal from the stationary echo signals. The systems operate in the frequency domain, and try to separate low-amplitude, Doppler shifted information from the almost stationary structure, very high-amplitude signals with a low-frequency Doppler shift; this is extremely difficult. There are other approaches. The tracking device that Dr. Greene mentioned is one of them. One could also track in the phase domain by making a correction similar to the ones that are used on fast-moving aircraft to correct for their radar platform motion; multiple-frequency systems can extract signals from only the small Rayleigh scatterers, such as red cells.

The most extreme suggestion would be that, since we are dealing with an incoherent signal and our noise is coherent, we need to design frequency filters backward to maximize what to us is the signal-to-noise ratio, but what to everybody else is the noise-to-signal ratio!

The application of Doppler devices in early disease detection is the subject of current research work. Following the detection of disturbance in the center-line flow velocity by Dr. Giddens, it was proposed to use a Doppler transducer at right angles to the flow to detect these disturbances. Such a recording position is maximally sensitive to radial flows, which do not exist in normal straight arteries. Detection of characteristic patterns due to vortex shedding has been accomplished by Dr. Newhouse. One can combine the pulse system to do this with spectrum analysis of vessel-wall echo spectra, which we have demonstrated in our laboratory to be sensitive to changes in surface roughness.

9

B-Mode Ultrasound Interrogation of Arteries

WILLIAM M. MCKINNEY AND GARY J. HARPOLD

The development of atherosclerosis in the area of the carotid bifurcation results in arterial wall abnormalities that produce emboli and hemodynamic changes of turbulence, stenosis, and occlusion. A number of techniques have been reported in the literature to evaluate these changes by direct or indirect measurement. Clinical evaluation and correlative techniques have primarily depended upon validation by the "gold standard" of arteriography for a number of years. However, the introduction of B-mode ultrasound techniques has added a unique scientific standard for direct observation and measurement of wall characteristics, lumen diameter and dynamic pulsatile characteristics of wall motion.

LITERATURE REVIEW

Initial B-mode studies (1,2) were performed with handheld transducers, and a compound scan was recorded on a storage oscilloscope. These studies demonstrated wall abnormality and lumen

The authors express appreciation to Dr. James F. Toole, Dr. M. G. Bond, Miss Catherine Nunn, Mrs. Anne Jones, Ms. Donna Lucas, Mr. Larry Myers, and Mr. Bryan Smith for their contributions, and special appreciation to Mrs. Judy Hardy in the preparation of the manuscript. The work reflects the unified effort of the cerebrovascular/neurosonology laboratory of the Department of Neurology.

information. They were limited by the technical inability to obtain satisfactory multiple-plane scans of the bifurcation and the inability to separate the external and internal carotid arteries at the bifurcation in many cases. This was primarily related to the time-consuming effort of compound scanning as well as anatomic restrictions of the anterior/posterior scanning position.

The development of real-time B-mode imaging offers a new, rapid multiplane capability in the determination of lumen and arterial wall characteristics and dynamics. When combined with Doppler flow information (3), new parameters of measurement result with an increased ability to diagnose anatomic and hemodynamic changes. Recent reports in the literature have revealed high correlation with arteriography and other methods (4-9). New terms and concepts are being developed based on acoustical pathology.

It is essential to understand the anatomic relationship of the carotid bifurcation and branches. There is a variability in the level of the bifurcation. It may lie low in the neck, at the level of the superior thyroid cartilage, or as high as the angle of the mandible. There may be variability with the relationship of the external and internal carotid arteries. In general, the external carotid artery is most anterior to the internal carotid, however, the Prendes anomaly (10) with a reversal of this position may cause difficulty in identification. The superior thyroidal artery may be identified as well as other branches of the external carotid superior to the bifurcation, which will aid in proper identification. There may be wide variations in the bifurcation angle, from 90° to a very narrow angle resulting in parallel courses of the external and internal carotid arteries. These variations have offered difficulties in Doppler imaging; however, with real-time scanning, multiplanes of examination are possible, making identification more exact. Kinks, coils, and other ana-tomic variables, including a congenitally narrowed lumen, may be easily identified. The dynamic relationship of wall pulsation

will be dependent upon the size of the vessel, wall characteristics, and pressure relationships.

METHODS

The examination is performed in the sitting or supine position.
The sitting position offers additional accessibility to the neck
for multiplaner scanning. A coupling gel is applied to the neck.
High resolution is obtained by using frequencies of 7 MHz to
10 MHz. Transducers may be coupled with a mechanically driven
sector scan or modified by the use of a mirror system to increase
the examination area. Resolution is dependent upon frequency,
transducer design, depth of field, and echogenicity of the issue.
The figures illustrated were made with a 7 MHz transducer, a
mechanically-driven mirror, a depth of field of 4 cm and approximately 0.3 mm in axial resolution. Systematic scanning for
interrogation of the vessel begins caudad and extends cephalad
with a sweeping motion to identify the parallel vessel walls.
Multiple positions may be used; however, the anteroposterior,
lateral and posterior oblique positions are the most common.
Cross-sectional views may also be obtained by rotating the transducer 90°. These may be very useful in areas of pathology which
have been identified on the longitudinal scans. The patient's
head position is adjusted to allow proper examination. The common
carotid artery may be identified at the area of the clavicle
extending to the bifurcation. Two parallel vessel walls may be
noted with dynamic radial pulsation. A coil or kink may be
identified and result in localized longitudinal motion due to
the dynamics of the pulse wave. Gain settings are very important.
Echos extending from the near luminal wall may be created by
reverberations within the wall producing artifact. The far
luminal wall of the vessel offers a more clearly defined area
without evidence of this artifact. The identification of the more
distal portions of the far wall may produce artifact in a similar
manner as the near luminal wall. The recent use of the more

posterior position has greatly aided in the identification of the
internal carotid artery. This position allows visualization of
the internal carotid above the bifurcation without interference
of the mandible. With careful movement of the transducer, a small
linear echo may be obtained along the far luminal wall of the common carotid artery approximately 1 mm within the lumen. There has
been debate as to whether this represents an anatomic structure or
separation of the serum from cellular content of the blood. This
area may be markedly thickened in cases following radiation therapy, or in patients with diabetes, collagen vascular disease, or
diffuse arteriosclerosis. Wall abnormalities may consist of "soft
plaque" or plaque containing calcification with high echogenic
features. If calcification is sufficiently present, an acoustic
shadow may be formed. Thrombus formation may also be identified
with higher gain settings presenting a speckled appearance. The
identification of ulceration may be implied with marked irregularities of the plaque and its relationship to the wall. Measurements of the luminal diameter may be made in multiple sections.

A shearing effect has been observed in areas of plaque formation producing a mechanical stress at the boundary zone between
plaque and the underlying arterial wall. The dynamics of the
vessel wall may be studied in detail. The movement of the wall
may be radial, longitudinal, or complex. The systolic pulse wave
in the normal vessel will produce primarily radial movement unless
there is a kink or coil where longitudinal movement may be superimposed. When the vessel wall becomes thickened and develops
plaque formation, the dynamics change. Some plaques have been
observed to have a primarily longitudinal movement in relation to
the remaining vessel wall radial movement. On occasion a "dancing
flutter" may be observed at the plaque area due to the effect of
systole and diastole. A valve effect may occur with diffuse
disease when the vessel opens only during systole and allows no
flow during diastole. The effects of valvular abnormalities of
the heart may also be noted, particularly with wide pulse

pressure. Cardiac irregularities affect the dynamic motion of vessel walls.

CRITIQUE

The indications for carotid B-mode are:

Asymptomatic bruit
TIA
Stroke
Pre- and postoperative endarterectomy
Diabetes with vascular disease
Hypertension
Hyperlipidemia
In response to medical and/or surgical therapy
To follow the natural course of disease

The advantages of B-mode ultrasound are:

Noninvasive
No special patient preparation
Outpatient or inpatient procedure
Repeatable, safe, and inexpensive
Direct vessel wall and lumen visualization in
    planes of examination
Dynamic data
May be portable

Problems may be encountered with B-mode carotid scanning:

Poor patient condition or cooperation
Lack of specific knowledge of acoustical properties
    of plaque components
Marked obesity and/or short neck
Severe disease with shadow defects
Artifacts, thrombus and fresh clot
Instrument calibration and sensitivity
Inter- and intraobserver variability in obtaining
    an interpretation

RESULTS

The results are summarized in Figs 1-5, which illustrate normal and abnormal findings. The illustrations are arranged to demonstrate the common carotid, bifurcation, internal and external carotid arteries. There is loss of detail due to the dynamic range of the film. Proper interpretation requires viewing on the oscilloscope or TV presentation.

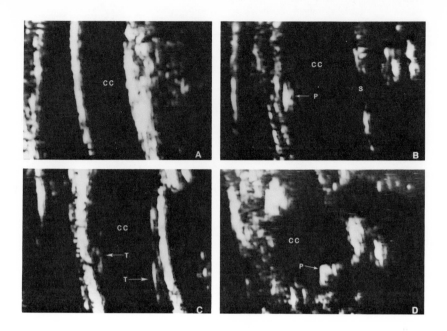

Fig. 1 A: Normal common carotid (CC). B: Common carotid (CC) with plaque (P) containing calcium producing shadow (S). C: Common carotid (CC) with thickened (T) wall from early plaque formation, diabetes, collagen vascular disease, or postradiation therapy. D: Transverse cross section of common carotid (CC) with small plaque (P). Note the poor resolution of this view due to the reflecting interfaces. Multiplanar views are necessary for proper interpretation by TV presentation.

DISCUSSION

Validation of real-time B-scanning of the carotid arteries has raised serious problems and offered new opportunities for scientific study.   Initial studies of validation with pathologic anatomy are limited by acoustical changes that occur following death, loss of dynamic information, and potential shrinkage artifact. Pathologic correlation at the time of surgery is limited by the field of view and the surgical requirements. The specimens are generally cored out and do not reflect the total vessel wall and measurements of dynamics are not evaluated. Correlation with Doppler flow studies, electroencephalography

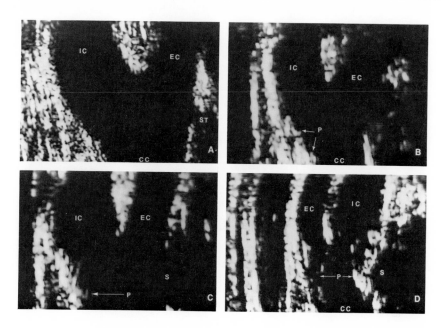

Fig. 2 A: Normal carotid bifurcation. Common carotid (CC), internal carotid (IC), external carotid (EC), and superior thyroidal artery (ST). B: Common carotid plaque (P) extending into the bifurcation without significant shadow. C: Common carotid plaque (P) extending into the bifurcation with shadow (S). D: Extensive plaque in the carotid bifurcation extending into the origins of the external and internal carotids.

(EEG), carotid phonoangiography (CPA), oculoplethyomography (OPG) and other tests are complicated by the many variables of collateral circulation and other factors. The arteriogram has been used by the clinician as the "gold standard" for clinical application and validation. The detection of wall abnormalities in the early phases of disease, however, is limited and only selected arteriogram views may be correlated. It is very important to recognize that the ultrasound examination view will be 90° from the position of the x-ray view for correlation. The ultrasound examination reveals wall abnormality directly visualized rather than a superimposed shadow. In spite of many difficulties, and the fact that they measure separate but related data, the early reports of statistical analysis of B-mode and angiogram have

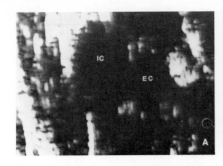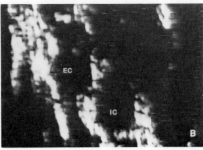

Fig. 3 A: Transverse cross section of the internal carotid (IC) and external carotid (EC) at the bifurcation. B: Transverse cross section of the internal carotid (IC) and external carotid (EC) above the bifurcation.

revealed a high correlation. The multiplaner B-mode approach, however, allows careful examination of variable anatomic plaques that may not be interpreted on angiography.

CONCLUSIONS

In conclusion, B-mode carotid artery scanning is a rapidly developing technique which may, with further definition of acoustical anatomy and pathology, be of importance in:

1. Diagnosing noninvasively, atherosclerosis in the high
    risk asymptomatic person
2. Establishing the natural course of disease in the
    individual patient with predictive value based on
    long-term follow-up studies of patients
3. Potentially tracking of atherosclerosis and progression
4. Monitoring response to medical and/or surgical therapy
5. Developing a new understanding of luminal diameter as
    it may be related to distal flow resistance
6. Evaluating the concept of mechanical stress factors in
    the development of ulceration and plaque formation

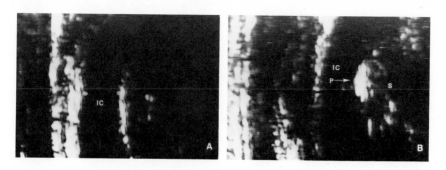

Fig. 4 A: Normal internal carotid (IC). B: Plaque (P) with shadow in the internal carotid (IC).

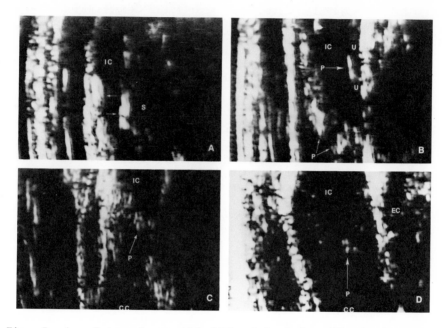

Fig. 5 A: Internal carotid (IC) with shadow (S) showing valve effect due to diffuse plaque formation on opposite walls allowing flow only during systole. B: Multiple plaque formation (P) in the internal carotid with possible ulceration at the inferior margin of the cephalad plaque. C: Total occlusion at the origin of the internal carotid (IC). D: Thrombus and plaque (P) formation at the origin of the internal carotid (IC) with a speckled pattern.

REFERENCES

1. Olinger CP (1969) Ultrasonic carotid echoarteriography.
    Am J Roentgenol Radium Ther Nucl Med 106:282-295
2. Blue SK, McKinney WM, Barnes RW, Toole JF (1972) Ultrasonic
    B-mode scanning for study of extracranial vascular disease.
    Neurology 22:1079-1085
3. Hobson RW, Berry SM, Katocs AS Jr, O'Donnell JA, Jamil Z,
    Savitsky JP (1980) Comparison of pulsed Doppler and real-
    time B-mode echo arteriography for noninvasive imaging of
    the extracranial carotid arteries. Surgery 87:286-293
4. Comerota AJ, Cranley JJ, Cooke SE (1981) Real-time B-mode
    carotid imaging in diagnosis of cerebrovascular disease.
    Surgery 89:718-729
5. Coelho JCU, Sigel B, Flanigan DP, Schuler JJ, Spigos DG,
    Nyhus LM (1981) Detection of arterial defects by real-time
    ultrasound scanning during vascular surgery: An experimental
    study. J Surg Res 30:535-543
6. Lewis RR, Beasley MG, Gosling RG (1980) Detection of disease
    at the carotid bifurcation using ultrasound - including an
    imaging system. J Royal Soc of Med 74:172-179
7. Texas Heart Institute (1980) Real-time ultrasonic imaging
    of the peripheral arteries: Technique, normal anatomy, and
    pathology. In: Cardiovascular diseases, Vol 7, No 3
    Vascular Laboratory of the Miami Heart Institute, Miami
    Beach, FL
8. Green PS (1978) Real time, high resolution ultrasonic
    carotid angiography system. In: Bernstein EF ed Nonin-
    vasive diagnostic techniques in vascular disease. Mosby,
    St. Louis, pp. 29-39
9. Cooperberg PL, Robertson WD, Fry P, Sweeney V (1979) High-
    resolution real-time ultrasound of the carotid bifurcation.
    JCU 7:13
10. Prendes JL, McKinney WM, Buonanno FS, Jones AM (1980)
    Anatomic variations of the carotid bifurcation affecting
    Doppler scan interpretation. JCU 8:147-150

DISCUSSION: TITUS C. EVANS JR.

Dr. McKinney has nicely summarized the practical features of
B-mode imaging in carotid arteries. I was impressed with his
rational approach to the use of the B-mode scanning technique.
He noted the important and good features, as well as the bad
features. I think that most of us would be in basic agreement
with his ideas, and I have no major disagreements to express.

I would like to cover four basic areas, touching on other
features that Dr. McKinney has not had time to mention. I will
discuss the techniques of B-mode imaging, some good features,
some important limitations that must not be neglected, and some
general comments for all of us, which may be a little bit
provocative.

Carotid B-mode images are relatively new, and are not yet
widespread in usage or acceptance, as is angiography. The
instruments and techniques still vary, as has been mentioned.
Differences include the frequency of the ultrasound, the resolution of the display, the stability of the image on the monitor,
and the type of transducer and whether it is supported by a
mechanically stable device or is held by the hand. In addition,
viewers have had relatively fewer years of experience than
angiographers have had.

The techniques of obtaining B-mode images are important.
They are technically easier to perform than angiography, but
still require an expert to interact with the patient, and they
are far more difficult to interpret than angiograms. In certain
cases, they require subjective overreading, as opposed to objective measurements, if lesions are long or shadowed, if anterior
and posterior portions of lesions are close together, or if
serial lesions or sequential enlargements of the same lesion are
adjacent to each other.

In carotid arteries, B-mode images are better for the detection of small lesions, such as between 1 and 25% transverse
luminal stenosis, than are angiograms. In this range, the

angiograms suffer considerably from superposition of dye and
lesions in the projection image on two-dimensional film. Small
lesions noted on B-mode images are often invisible or obscure on
angiograms, even in retrospect.

B-mode images and angiograms are about the same in terms of
ability to show middle-sized lesions from 25-50% transverse
stenosis and perhaps up to 75% stenosis. The interpreted values
by the two methods are approximately similar. Neither technique
provides much difficulty to the average observer in identifying
lesions in this range. Some shadowing may be present, but it is
generally not troublesome.

From 50-75% transverse stenosis the two techniques are also
roughly comparable, with angiograms showing good profiles if the
lesions are in silhouette against one of the arterial margins.

For 75-100% transverse linear stenosis B-mode images sometimes suffer severely from shadowing, with blank gaps covering
portions of the displayed lesions. These gaps may occur in the
center of a large lesion on either anterior or posterior surface
of the carotid artery, and especially in that part of a posterior
lesion directly behind a large or calcific anterior lesion. Here
quantitation is very difficult. Experience is needed to perform
mental extrapolation to determine where the surface of the lesion
really is and to make the appropriate estimation of the amount of
stenosis present. Objectively measured values of stenosis are
not always reliable, and when compared with angiography, they
sometimes tend to be lower than the corresponding angiogram
values. Thus it is necessary to introduce an expert's subjective
input and mentally boost the estimate of stenosis. Factors such
as lesion density and length, adjacent lesions, extent of shadowing, and disappearance of the lumen of the artery cephalad to
the lesion with very-high-grade stenosis all enter into the
subjective impression of the interpreter in grading lesions. I
feel that an experienced echo technician would not be able to do
this as well as a qualified physician. It is likely that

angiography and ultrasonography both underestimate the actual disease in many cases in this range of high-grade lesions.

Both techniques significantly underestimate the extent of apparent surface ulceration as well. Correlations between B-mode images and angiograms suffer from the lack of a unified viewing angle. B-mode images are usually taken from a slightly different to a grossly different angle from the angiogram. The optimal viewing angle to demonstrate an ulcer crater should be different for the two techniques for longitudinal views. In our experience at the Mayo Clinic ulcers seen on angiograms often do not correlate with those seen on B-mode and vice versa. This is probably due to different viewing angles and to technical limitations. Ultrasound shadows, ulcers, areas of poor reflectivity, or other conditions, may appear similar to each other and confuse the observer.

B-mode evaluation has several advantages. I will not reiterate most of them. B-mode images are easy procedures to perform once the observer becomes experienced. Patients accept them. We have had no complications at the Mayo Clinic.

The disadvantages of carotid B-mode imaging, however, are significant, and should not be neglected. Only the neck region can be studied. As most of the major lesions are in the imagable portion of the carotid artery, however, this is not usually a major problem. Intracranial disease is undetected. The more cephalad portion of the internal carotid artery is deeper in the neck and yields poorer images than does the common carotid artery. Shadowing causes more problems for the novice than the expert. Precise measurements of lesions and arteries are not always easy to make and it is difficult to standardize where to make these measurements. Intra- and interobserver variability are also potential problems, as have been mentioned.

B-mode techniques usually cannot be used to distinguish between very-high-grade and complete obstruction of internal carotid arteries with certainty. However we have noted some scans of lesions where the lumens were completely obliterated in a very short distance, and these cases were correlated with 100% obstruction on the angiograms. Multiple additional reflections in what appeared to be the lumens cephalad to the lesions have also been correlated with 100% obstruction on the angiograms.

All carotid arteries and their lesions are unique in appearance on B-mode images, and the interpretations may not contain sufficient information to determine the need for angiography. Additional noninvasive methods such as cervical Doppler, supraorbital Doppler, oculoplethysmography, and retinal artery pressures may be needed to determine the need for angiography.

Since lesions tend to occur in skip-and-hit sequences, it is not unusual to see additional lesions above and below the main carotid bifurcation location already mentioned. We have encountered two cases where significant lesions were demonstrated on the angiogram just above the field of view of the B-mode image; one of these was due to fibromuscular dysplasia and one of these was due to atherosclerosis. A normal B-mode image or a small lesion seen by B-mode imaging does not exclude significant disease beyond the field of view. Therefore, a patient with clinical symptoms probably should be considered for other additional studies, and may also need an angiogram.

The branching orientation of the carotid artery is quite variable, as has been mentioned, and even the expert has occasional trouble in determining which branches are internal and which are external. Patients with ectasia of the thoracic or carotid arteries, connective tissue laxity, or kyphosis of the spine may have the carotid arteries physically displaced higher into the neck, showing buckling or high branching. The tortuosity and increased motion are easily recognized on B-mode images.

Pulsations of the arterial walls in a radial direction or in a longitudinal direction also occur. Many factors influence this motion, however, and it does not appear that much great practical use can be made from specific measurements of wall motion.

Smearing of bright portions of the images in a posterior direction due to transducer ringing and multiple reflections are minor problems.

There is a potential risk of increased carotid sinus tone when the transducer or coupling bag is placed against the neck. Bradycardia or orthostatism after imaging may be temporary in patients of all ages, including healthy young people. It is especially important to prevent these effects in persons with carotid disease. After a carotid B-scan it is wise to allow the patient several seconds to readjust with the transducer off of the neck before resuming an upright posture. Raising the arms on standing also aids venous filling of the heart. The fact that theoretical risk of compression of the carotid artery itself by the transducer or coupling bag has not materialized can be attributed to extreme care on the part of the physician. This remains a potential problem, however. The inclusion of a pressure compensation system in the coupling bag is recommended.

Correlation studies with angiography are also easy to do. One should use a population that has about an equal number of patients with and without lesions. Many noninvasive techniques appear more sensitive than they really are when used in populations with a high percentage of disease.

Now, for the controversial part. Dr. Reid asked us what causes this disease. No one has yet spoken for the patient's care or for the physician's responsibilities. If atherosclerosis is detected in the carotid arteries of a patient, it is not sufficient to quantitate only these lesions and treat the patient with surgery or drug therapy. Atherosclerosis is likely to be widespread in the body of such a patient. One should arrange for a complete history and physical examination and pay particular attention to all areas of the body where arterial pulses are accessible. The history should include the complaints of the patient and an assessment of the major risk factors for premature or accelerated atherosclerosis. The average patient has no concept of the relative importance of the various risk factors, and many physicians and scientists do not either.   If you ask a diabetes doctor, he will say that mostly diabetics get the disease.   A hypertension doctor will say that hypertension is the main risk factor.   A lipidologist will tell you that lipids are all-important.   However, as a cardiovascular internist who studies all types of atherosclerosis without preselection of patients by risk factors I have found that it is not any of these.   Most of the patients I see with premature or excessive carotid atherosclerosis have the common history of cigarette smoking, whether it is ancient or current.   Therefore, I would make a plea for clinicians to assess risk factors along with evaluation of atherosclerosis throughout the body and to educate their peers and patients alike.

10

Radionuclide and Nuclear Magnetic Resonance Methods of Evaluating Atherosclerosis

Thomas F. Budinger, Edward Ganz, David C. Price, Martin Lipton, Brian R. Moyer, and Yukio Yano

Radionuclide techniques devoted to the evaluation of the atherosclerotic process have focused on measurements of function and metabolism of the heart and brain that might be affected by atherosclerosis, as well as on detection of thrombus formation in major arteries within and leading to these organs. This approach has more recently been joined by efforts to study the biochemical behavior of the arterial wall itself as well as the interaction of blood constituents with the components of the arteries. There is now sufficient basis to predict that we will be able to study facets of the atherosclerotic process in man using not only labeled platelets, labeled fibrin, and labeled lipoproteins, but labeled monoclonal antibodies to arterial wall constituents, fibrin, and lipoprotein receptor sites.

Nuclear magnetic resonance (NMR) promises to play an equally important but somewhat different role than radionuclide techniques. At a resolution less than 1 mm, NMR can measure the local chemical environment, including oxygen saturation, as reflected by the relaxation rate of protons. At very coarse resolutions NMR can measure tissue pH and the chemical state of some nuclear species. Of

This work was supported by the National Institutes of Heart, Lung, and Blood NIH grant No. P014L25840-02 and the U.S. Department of Energy contract No. DE-AC03-76SF00098. We appreciate Diana Morris assisting with this manuscript.

great interest is the fact that proton NMR can detect the presence of fatty deposits and calcified areas in the arterial wall.

The modes of application of radionuclide and NMR techniques for noninvasive studies are summarized in Fig. 1. This paper focuses on the status of radionuclide and NMR methods relative to noninvasive studies of atherosclerosis.

RADIONUCLIDE TECHNIQUES

Conventional Scintigraphy

Current clinical nuclear medicine is heavily devoted to nuclear cardiology because ejection fraction, segmental wall motion, and relative myocardial perfusion can be measured noninvasively. EKG-gated images of the blood pool are obtained using red cells labeled with ^{99m}Tc and relative perfusion is measured by the degree of accumulation of $^{201}Tl^+$, a cation which behaves like K^+ and Rb^+. The ejection fraction measurements by first-pass or gated blood pool methods are very reliable (1-5). Wall motion, ejection fraction, and myocardial perfusion imaging are important adjuncts to the evaluation of the patient with coronary artery disease, however, they fall short of answering questions of tissue metabolism or the mechanism of the atherosclerotic process. Even methods of positive labeling of the ischemic heart muscle (6) give limited assistance to our quest for disease mechanisms and early methods of diagnosis. Three new areas of radiopharmaceutical imaging have great potential for substantial progress in both understanding and treating atherosclerosis: (1) labeled platelet kinetic studies in man; (2) tissue specific labeled antibodies; and (3) positron and single photon tomography.

Indium-Labeled Platelet Kinetics

Almost all of the clinical complications of atherosclerosis leading to patient morbidity and mortality involve intraarterial thrombus formation (7,8). Previous attempts to image thrombi have focused on the use of radio-iodinated fibrinogen, which converts to

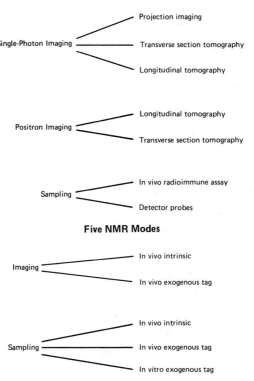

Radionuclide Methods

Single-Photon Imaging
- Projection imaging
- Transverse section tomography
- Longitudinal tomography

Positron Imaging
- Longitudinal tomography
- Transverse section tomography

Sampling
- In vivo radioimmune assay
- Detector probes

Five NMR Modes

Imaging
- In vivo intrinsic
- In vivo exogenous tag

Sampling
- In vivo intrinsic
- In vivo exogenous tag
- In vitro exogenous tag

Fig. 1 Modes of application of radionuclide and NMR techniques for noninvasive studies.

fibrin and is actively incorporated in a new thrombus. The commercially available fibrinogen is labeled with ^{125}I which, because of its low energy, limits the examination to the superficial vessels only. ^{123}I-fibrinogen has been prepared and used successfully in a study of peripheral vein thrombosis (9). ^{125}I- and ^{131}I-labeled fibrinogen have been shown to accumulate in new and old thrombi (10). The limited availability of pure ^{123}I, the variability in active uptake, and lack of quantitative methods are three factors that might account for the paucity of general enthusiasm for this technique. Furthermore, the major sites for fibrin deposition are venous thrombi, while our interest is in arterial thrombi.

Human and animal platelets have been labeled with radionuclides that are appropriate for imaging (11,12). ^{111}In-labeled autologous platelets demonstrate all of the normal functional characteristics of the more traditional ^{51}Cr-labeled platelets in terms of survival and clotting ability. Because the radionuclide ^{111}In has now been shown to bind to cytoplasmic contents that are not affected by the platelet release reaction, the label accumulates and stays in the newly formed clot as long as the platelet remains at the thrombus site. The patterns of platelet accumulation and discharge from thrombi have been studied recently in an animal model using a poly-ethylene catheter planted in one carotid via the femoral artery (13). Platelet uptake as imaged and quantitated noninvasively corresponds to the thrombus mass. In the catheter model the up-take reaches a peak within an hour after insertion of the catheter and thereafter decreases, corresponding to the loss of platelets from the clot. A similar pattern of clot formation occurs after denuding the endothelium by a balloon catheter (Fig. 2).

The value of being able to detect the presence of labeled platelet accumulation is that the clinical complications of arteriosclerosis can be detected before the onset of a cata-strophic event such as embolization or occlusion or both.

Price and coworkers (13) demonstrated that preformed thrombus does not accumulate a platelet mass significant enough for reli-able detection of a thrombus after that thrombus has formed. Approximately 0.2 μCi is required in the region of the thrombus for detection using [111]In. This means that approximately 0.1% of the circulating platelet mass (approximately 1.5×10^9 platelets) must be deposited in the thrombus to be visualized if the radia-tion dose to the spleen is to be kept below 5-8 rads.

Platelet accumulation can be quantitated during a period of a few days following endarterectomy (13). However, in three patients who had endarterectomies one week before injection of labeled platelets, there was no accumulation shown.

In the study by Price and coworkers (13) carotid arteries with significant atherosclerotic disease did not reveal any platelet

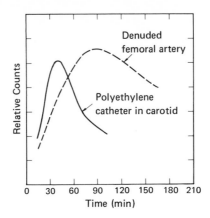

Fig. 2   Patterns of platelet accumulation and discharge from thrombi in vivo.

accumulation.   However, Davis et al. (14) demonstrated platelet accumulation in over half the patients with angiographically defined atherosclerosis at the common carotid bifurcation.   The difference between these two studies probably has to do with the use of antithrombosis medication and the pathological state of the atherosclerotic lesions.

Imaging labeled platelets is a method whereby the kinetics of platelet accumulation and discharge can be followed noninvasively in the body.   This method should be distinguished from the dynamic study of the aging thrombus, wherein the exchange of fibrin can be detected using labeled fibrinogen (10).   The studies thus far have not progressed to the point of comparative work between platelet accumulation and fibrin formation using these two techniques.

A major limitation in the ^{111}In-platelet-labeling method is the fact that a dose of only 300 µCi is acceptable due to the long half-life of ^{111}In.   The second limitation is that the ^{111}In activity from platelets in the general circulation causes some superposition of activity in normal projection imaging.   A solution to both of these problems might lie in the use of ^{68}Ga-labeled platelets. ^{68}Ga is a positron emitter with a half-life of 68 min. Using the proper instrumentation the sensitivity for detection of

[68]Ga-labeled platelets can be 10 or more times greater than that
for single photon imaging. Of equal importance is the fact that
due to the short half-life over ten times the dose can be injected.
Thus, ^{68}Ga-labeled platelets should provide a sensitivity of one
hundred times or more than that of the ^{111}In platelet procedure.

In contrast to the partial success of indium-labeled platelets
for studying some cases of carotid artery atherosclerosis, no uptake has been found in studies of the coronary arteries performed
before and after transluminal angioplasty, though active uptake is
detected at insertion sites for the arterial catheters in these
human patient studies.

The enthusiasm for platelet accumulation studies is based on
substantial evidence that platelet deposition at sites of arterial
injury plays a central role in arteriothrombosis and atherogenesis
(15,16). In the past, the only means of evaluating the process
of platelet accumulation has been through measurements of platelet
turnover (12) or of the plasma concentration of platelet specific
proteins that have been released (18). The technique of platelet
labeling and imaging, particularly using positron tomographic
approaches may permit the evaluation of localized platelet deposition on individual vascular lesions.

Labeled Lipoproteins and Monoclonal Antibodies

Human lipoproteins labeled with ^{125}I have been shown to accumulate
in the previously injured rabbit aorta (19). Based on these
observations, pioneering studies were performed in four patients
with carotid artery disease with imaging 24 hours after injection
of 100 μCi of ^{125}I-radiolabeled low-density lipoproteins (20).
Lesions were detected in the carotid arteries of three of the four
patients. The potential for studying lipoprotein kinetics in
normal and diseased arteries is high based on these early experiments, which were done under nonoptimal conditions. [125]I has a
very low-energy photon and a long half-life, so that only a
limited dose can be given to the patient. Lipoproteins can be

labeled with other tracers, including ^{123}I for single photon emission work and ^{122}I for positron tomography if the labeling procedures are sufficiently rapid. In addition to activity accumulation at arterial sites of damage or repair from damage, lipoprotein receptor concentration can be measured noninvasively by tracer techniques. Recent investigations of the lipoprotein transport system suggest that the lipoprotein receptors in both liver and extrahepatic tissues mediate the uptake and degradation of cholesterol-carrying lipoproteins and thus play a crucial role in the regulation of plasma cholesterol in man (21). There is great potential for measuring the number or concentration of lipo-protein receptors on membranes if substances specific for these receptors can be purified and labeled. One approach is to make monoclonal antibodies to lipoproteins and evaluate the distribution of those antibodies by noninvasive imaging techniques. Isolation of monoclonal antibodies that are specific for vascular smooth muscle cells of the arterial wall has been accomplished at the laboratories of Russell Ross at the University of Washington. These antibodies do not appear to cross-react with endothelial cells or fibroblasts (22,23). Distribution studies using these monoclonal antibodies have not as yet been done.

Problems With Labeled-Protein Distribution Methods

The major limitation to these suggested noninvasive imaging tech-niques is the long persistence of radiolabel in the intravascular space. Thus, if a short half-life radionuclide is used, more tracer can be given per unit radiation dose; however, the imaging must be done at a shorter time interval after injection than is required with longer half-life tracers. Because of these consid-erations, ^{121}I (4-day half-life) might be an appropriate positron emitter if labeling procedures required for radionuclides other than iodine are not available. The enthusiasm for evaluating the distribution of biologically active proteins such as antibodies to arterial smooth muscle, endothelial cells, and lipoproteins is

tempered by the fact that the labeling must be sufficiently
intense to avoid saturation of the receptors with radiolabeled
material.   In addition, for quantitative studies, emission
tomographic techniques are needed to complement the biological and
medical technological advances associated with monoclonal antibody
and protein labeling technology.

Intravascularly injected large proteins remain in the blood
and tissue surrounding the organ or membrane of interest for long
periods of time.   Thus, imaging is done hours after the injected
tracer is given, whereas the accumulation in the tissue of interest is probably very rapid.   Subtraction techniques (24), using
labeled nonspecific proteins, are effective in removing this
background.

SINGLE PHOTON EMISSION TOMOGRAPHY

Emission computed tomography involves the determination of the
three-dimensional volume distribution of a radionuclide by external
measurement of the photon emission from multiple angles.   Isotopes
that emit single photons (e.g., ^{99}Tc, ^{123}I, ^{133}Xe, ^{201}Tl) are used
in the single photon tomography mode, and those which emit posi-
trons (e.g., ^{11}C, ^{15}O, ^{13}N, ^{68}Ga, ^{82}Rb, etc.) are used in positron
emission tomography discussed in the next section.

There are two general categories of single photon emission
tomography.   They are first, longitudinal or limited angular-
range tomography, and second, transverse-section tomography or
complete angular-range sampling.   The limited angular-range
tomographic approaches have focused on the use of the seven
pinhole collimator (25), the time-coded aperture (26,27), the
rotating slant-hole collimator (28) and the rotating quadrant
slant-hole collimator (29).   Limited angle tomography using
these apertures has a questionable future because the angular
range of data acquisition is inadequate.   This conclusion is
based on theoretical and physical analyses of limited angular
viewing (30-34).   In comparison to other imaging systems, limited

angular-range tomography with the seven pinhole collimator is not as specific as transverse-section tomography for the detection of myocardial infarcts.

There has been a revival of interest in single photon tomography of the head due to the realization that the sensitivity of devices for imaging the brain is adequate for imaging blood flow using the ^{133}Xe washout method (35,36) or using the relative accumulation method with lipophylic radiopharmaceuticals such as the labeled phenylalkylanines (37,38). Commercial devices, however, lack important design features which could optimize and make practical tomography with single photon transducers (30,39).

A basic limitation of single photon tomography is the fact that particularly for the chest, the sensitivity of detection is low. This problem can be overcome to some extent if appropriate single photon radiopharmaceuticals are developed which localize specifically in the viable myocardium or alternatively in ischemic zones as hot spots. Using transverse section devices or limited angular range tomographic systems with at least 120° of angular range, studies of ejection fraction, wall motion, and infarct sizing will be far more reliable if ^{99}Tc or ^{123}I labels can be used on compounds which actively accumulate in the viable myocardium (40). Thus, although the studies with seven-hole pinhole and slant-hole tomography have been disappointing, improvements in instruments and radiopharmaceuticals can be anticipated and continued development of this mode of imaging is warranted. The poor sensitivity of single photon systems will severely limit their potential if resolution of 10 mm or less is required.

POSITRON EMISSION TOMOGRAPHY

Basic Principles

Isotopes can be accelerator-produced; these have nuclei deficient in neutrons compared to the number of protons. For example, ^{11}C has six protons and only five neutrons. There is a natural tendency for nuclei to have more neutrons than protons. Thus, for

neutron-deficient isotopes, a proton is converted to a neutron by
expulsion of a positive electron (positron) from the nucleus. This
positive electron encounters a negative electon within a few millimeters of the nucleus. Annihilation of the two particles results
in the formation of two 511 keV, which fly off back-to-back, 180
degrees from one another (Fig. 3). The photons can be detected by
scintillation crystals that surround the subject. The annihilation
photons travel with the speed of light and arrive in near time
coincidence at the scintillators. Thus, if two events occur within
a few nanoseconds, the electronic circuits accept the pair as
having come from the same positron annihilation. The position of
the source is somewhere along a line connecting the two crystals
that detected the event. If, as in Fig. 3A, the source is in a
single position, then after multiple annihilation events are
recorded the source is found at the intersection of the lines.
For multiple sources, the thousands of coincidence events are
treated by mathematical algorithms in a way similar to x-ray
computed tomography.

Positron Emission Tomography of the Heart

Positron emission tomography (PET) of the heart can measure blood
perfusion, metabolism of fatty acids, metabolism of sugars, uptake
of amino acids, and can also quantitate infarction volume. Positron tomography can also measure perfusion and metabolism of the
brain. Previous reviews of principles basic to PET instrumentation and of procedures for quantitative studies of the heart
muscle with examples of measurements of myocardial flow and metabolism are given by Budinger, Brownell et al. and Ter-Pogossian
et al. (39,41,42).

Myocardial Perfusion

For tracers such as ^{82}Rb, ^{52}Mn, and ^{13}NH$_3$, which have high extraction coefficients and low tissue clearance, flow can be deduced
from the quotient of the amount accumulated in the myocardium
at any time and the amount that has been available to the myocar-

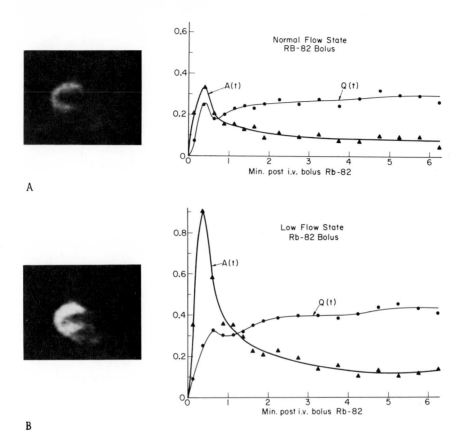

Fig. 3   Source at which positron annihilation occurs can be detected by scintillation crystals that surround the subject.

dium (4,43).   The latter can be deduced from the concentration in the left ventricular blood pool measured tomographically.

$$F \times E = \frac{Q(T)e^{\lambda T}}{\int^{T} A(t)e^{\lambda t}dt} \tag{1}$$

where Q(T) is the amount in the myocardium, at time T, F is flow, E is the tissue extraction, A is the arterial concentration, and λ is the physical decay constant.   A major asset of dynamic positron tomography is the fact that both Q(t) and A(t) can be measured simultaneously, as shown in Fig. 3.   The PET system used for our studies has a resolution of 9 mm full width at half maximum (FWHM) and can acquire complete angular sampling without motion of the detectors (44). A limitation of this procedure is the fact that extraction is a decreasing function of flow for a diffusion-limited tracer such as rubidium; however, over the flow range 0 - 2 times normal flow, the F x E values from equation (1) can be related to specific volume flow. This general model allows measurement of specific volume flow using bolus injection or constant infusion of ^{82}Rb ($t_{1/2}$ = 76 sec) from a ^{82}Sr/^{82}Rb generator (45).

Infarction detection and sizing can be accomplished by static imaging of the accumulation of a number of positron emitters (e.g., ^{13}NH$_3$ (46), ^{82}Rb (4), ^{11}C-palmitic acid (47,48), and ^{18}F-deoxyglucose (49).

Fatty Acid Metabolism

The major fuel for metabolism of the non-ischemic myocardium is fatty acids, although glucose plays a significant role when glucose and insulin are present. Palmitic acid labeled with ^{11}C in the carboxyl position has been used to evaluate the rate of β-oxidation by examination of the rate of disappearance of the activity as a function of time (48,50). Under ischemic conditions, the rate of clearance is decreased. In the normal myocardium the rate of clearance is proportional to cardiac work. The residue function (uptake-washout curve) contains unique information about the β-oxidation of free fatty acids (FFA) for the production of high-energy phosphates. However, the shape of the residue function will depend very much on the input function as well as on the β-oxidation rate determined using the model of Fig. 4. Generally, the input function can be fitted by a biexponential and the parameters of the model determined by an iterative least squares fit to the residue function. This method provides a quantitative technique for evaluation of myocardial metabolism, but requires a dynamic PET system for the acquisition of gated images, which must be collected at 5-sec intervals during the early part of the study in order to accurately describe the residue function.

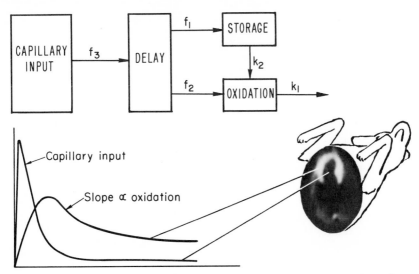

Fig. 4 Schematic representation of palmitic acid model for evaluation of the residue function (uptake-washout curve).

Glucose Metabolism of the Myocardium

The accumulation of ^{18}F-deoxyglucose in the heart makes this agent well suited for imaging the distribution of functional muscle, as well as for metabolic studies. High-resolution static images of the myocardium can be obtained with good statistics in a 5-min data accumulation interval, 40 min after injection of 4-8 mCi of ^{18}F-deoxyglucose. Deoxyglucose is transported between blood and the myocyte by the same saturable carrier that transports glucose. Deoxyglucose-6-phosphate is not further metabolized and accumulates in the myocardium without significant loss for as long as 90 min. The rate of glycolysis is determined using the moment-to-moment concentration changes in the myocardium and a compartment model similar to that employed for brain studies (51). The first studies of the myocardium using ^{18}F-deoxyglucose showed that the rate constants for myocyte glycolysis are similar to those for the brain (49,52). However, unlike the brain, the membrane transport of glucose in the myocardium is mediated by insulin, and perhaps by nonspecific permeability changes during ischemia. Thus, it appears that the assumption of average values for the rate constants will lead to serious errors. A dramatic example of the effects of insulin on glucose transport into skeletal muscle is shown in Fig. 5, wherein glucose uptake at low and high insulin levels is shown. If the moment-to-moment data from the blood pool in the left ventricle and the myocardium are observed, it is possible to experimentally derive the transport and phosphorylation rate constants for each subject rather than rely on assumed values.

The observation that there is increased glycolysis during ischemia has been thought to explain the observation that there is a less marked decrease in deoxyglucose uptake than there is a decrease in flow using $^{13}NH_3$ accumulation (52). Glycolytic flux is increased only during a short period (53), and depends upon the the glucose-insulin state of the subject. Furthermore, it is still not clear to what extent $^{13}NH_3$ ammonia extraction and accumulation in the heart is dependent on the state of myocardial protein metabolism (54,55). Should glucose uptake actually increase relative to flow as a reliable indicator of myocardial ischemia, then it is possible to use ^{82}Rb from a generator system and ^{18}F-deoxyglucose delivered from an off-site cyclotron to examine the state of the myocardium.

Amino Acid Metabolism

Amino acid kinetics of human myocardium can be studied using ^{13}N- or ^{11}C-labeled amino acids. The amino acid with the highest demonstrated uptake in the myocardium is asparagine (56). Its uptake of 13.7% of the injected dose in the dog is about four times higher than that of potassium, rubidium, glucose, and fatty acids; the uptake in man is low (57). Glutamate has a higher extraction in the ischemic myocardium than in the normal myocardium according to measurements made during coronary catheterization in man (58). A high extraction of 5.6% of the injected dose has been observed in patient studies (59). ^{13}N-alanine is also known

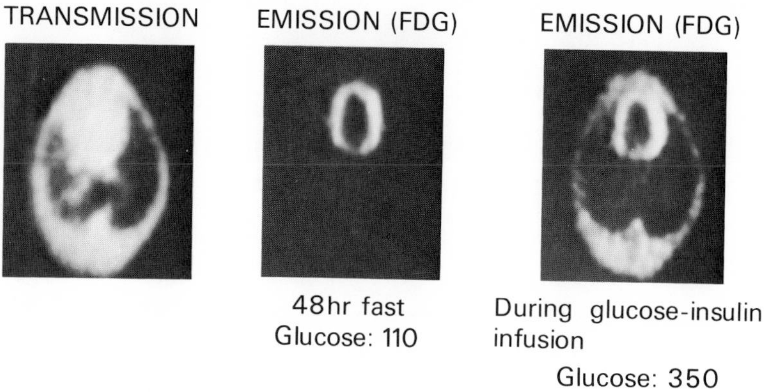

TRANSMISSION   EMISSION (FDG)   EMISSION (FDG)

                              48hr fast   During glucose-insulin
                           Glucose: 110   infusion
                                                 Glucose: 350

Fig. 5   Effects of insulin on glucose transport into skeletal
muscle shown by positron emission tomography.

to localize in the heart, but the possibility exists that after
peripheral injection the $^{13}NH_3$ from metabolized alanine is the
actual tracer in the heart. Our studies of amino acid metabolism
focused initially on ^{11}C-valine, one of the branched-chain amino
acids oxidized by muscle (60). We observed less than 1% of the
injected dose in the myocardium and no significant increase in
accumulation during fatty acid infusion. Studies on methionine
and taurine accumulation are now underway. In man and dogs about
1% of the injected dose of these compounds goes to the myocardium
with the concentration in the heart twice that of skeletal muscle.
Experience has shown that quantitative studies of myocardial
perfusion and metabolism can be made by measurement of the input
function and residue function from the sequential PET images.
Practical clinical applications require a tomograph capable of
taking data from three planes simultaneously with a resolution
less than 8 mm FWHM. Gating of the transverse section data and
measurement of the input function are the two additional requirements for quantitative studies of perfusion and metabolism.
Gating is necessary during acquisition of the residue curve
because the high activity of the adjacent ventricular blood pool
will seriously distort the information from the region of interest
over the myocardium.

NUCLEAR MAGNETIC RESONANCE

Basic Principles

The basic principles of NMR and a historical introduction to the
uses of NMR in medical imaging has been recently presented (41,61).
The nuclei of elements such as ^{1}H, ^{19}F, ^{23}Na, ^{31}P, have an odd
number of protons and neutrons and are magnetic. Each nucleus can
be thought of as a small magnet, which can assume a low energy
state when aligned with a field or a higher energy state when
aligned against the field. A weak but rapidly alternating magnetic
field applied by a coil near the subject or specimen stimulates
changes in the orientation of the nuclei relative to the direction
of a strong static magnetic field. This can be thought of as
"flipping" the direction of the nuclear spins. The energy absorbed
by the "flipped" nuclei is reemitted when the nuclei return to the
equilibrium state. The absorption and emission of energy take
place at a resonant frequency given by the formula: $\omega = \gamma H$, where
γ is the characteristic gyromagnetic ratio and H is the static
magnetic field. The γ differs for different elements and even
different isotopes of the same element, thus the resonant frequency
will differ from element to element. For example, at 0.1 Tesla
(1000 gauss) the resonant frequency for hydrogen is 4 MHz and that
of phosphorus is 1.7 MHz. Spatial distribution information can
be obtained by using the fact that the resonant frequency depends
on the magnetic field. Thus, by varying the field in a known
manner through the specimen volume, it is possible to select the
region of the specimen from which the information is derived by
using the frequency of the return signals.

In addition to being able to measure the concentration of nuclei of a particular species at a particular point in the specimen,
two other parameters of the returned NMR signal are of biological
importance: the T_1 spin-lattice relaxation time and the T_2 spin-
spin relaxation time. These parameters depend on the motion of
the nuclei, the regional temperature, the viscosity of the tissue,
and the magnetic effects of nearby nuclei and electrons.

The NMR signal is slightly (few parts in one million) shifted from the resonant frequency by electronically induced magnetic field perturbations associated with the chemical bonds near the nuclei of interest. Thus, the fine structure pattern of the return signal gives information about the chemical structure of the nuclei. This is used to evaluate high-energy phosphorous metabolism. In addition, volume flow information can be gleaned from a change in signal intensity due to the movement of nuclei through the resonance region. NMR techniques for acquiring the above information do not have equal sensitivity for all elements, NMR cannot image with the same high resolution the state of phosphorus or carbon bonds, or the tissue concentration of ^{23}Na or ^{31}P, as well as it can measure the concentration of protons or the proton T_1 relaxation parameter. This is due to the difference in sensitivity of NMR for the different elements as well as the very low concentration of the elements of interest relative to the concentration of protons in tissue (Table 1). For example, the concentration of hydrogen in tissue is approximately 90 mmol/gm while ^{23}Na concentration in blood and extracellular fluid is 1400 μmol/gm and ATP phosphorus in the brain is only a few μmol/gm. It is now well known that NMR has the potential for measurement of tissue bioenergetics such as ATP versus creatine phosphate ratios as well as pH changes using chemical shifts of the signal from orthophosphates (62-65). Though these measurements involve relatively large tissue volumes because the phosphorous concentration is low relative to protons (Table 1), regional measurements in humans can be accomplished using focused fields and surface probes (rf coil). However, a magnetic field of 1 T or more is required in a magnet with a bore diameter of at least 40 cm.

NMR Heart Studies

Five facets of NMR heart imaging discussed below are in early stages of investigation and need more theoretical and experimental work for effective implementation in the study of ischemic heart disease associated with atherosclerosis.

Table 1. Difference in sensitivity of NMR for the different elements

Element	Frequency at 0.1 T	Relative Sensitivity Varian Tables (1965)	Frequency at 0.3 T	Tissue Concentration (mM/gm)	Detection Sensitivity
^{1}H	4.3	1.0	12.9	90	1[a]
^{19}F	4.0	0.83	12.0	2.6[b]	2.7×10^{-2}
^{23}Na	1.1	0.09	3.4	0.14[c]	1.4×10^{-3}
^{31}P	1.7	0.07	5.2	0.002[d]	1.6×10^{-5}

[a] Hydrogen from 80% water in tissues.
[b] Blood concentration after injection of 500 cc of fluorocarbon.
[c] Blood and extracellular fluid.
[d] Concentration of tissue phosphorous associated with ATP or creatine phosphate.

1.   Ischemia is accompanied by an increase in longitudinal relaxation time of about 10% (66,67).

2. O_2 in the blood can change its T_1 relaxation time. Changes between the right and left ventricular cavities have been noted in ungated NMR human thorax transverse sections (68).

The influence of hemoglobin on the T_1 of blood was first demonstrated by Crooks and Singer (69) who showed a decrease due to hemoglobin. T_1 was not affected by the oxygen state of the hemoglobin; however, it is decreased by the presence of the paramagnetic O_2. T_2 is also decreased (70). It is still not clear whether T-parameter changes noted in vivo or in vitro can be related to O_2 content of blood and tissue and how these changes are related to the state of the hemoglobin.

3.   Infusion of a paramagnetic ion such as Mn^{++} will lower the proton T_1 relaxation time in proportion to the amount of Mn^{++} that reaches the tissue. The concentration of Mn^{++} in heart muscle a few minutes after injection is proportional to flow. The evidence for the effects of Mn^{++} on T_1 reduction were first reported in 1978 (63,71).

4.   Heart muscle can be distinguished from blood in high resolution images with or without gating. Ungated heart imaging studies also give results of seemingly good resolution. These early results (68,72,73) are a complex result of wall velocity as well as the intrinsic T_1 and T_2 of pericardial fat and muscle. Images can be misleading due to paradoxical T_1 as explained below.

If the pulse duration is varied appropriately with respect to T_1 and the linear velocity of the muscle (protons) in and out of the imaging plane, an apparent T_1 can be observed which is different from that of muscle not in motion. Protons outside the plane can move into the sensitive plane during a particular pulse sequence; conversely, a portion of the myocardium, or for that moving fluid volume, can leave the sensitive or resonant region during the time period between an exciting pulse and the received signal. In the latter case the signal will be lost. In the former

case the signal might be enhanced or decreased depending on the
pulse duration and movement velocity. Thus, paradoxical enhancement (positive or negative) of the T_1 rate can occur depending on
the imaging method and pulse sequence. If this paradoxical
enhancement is well understood then it should be possible to image
wall motion using varying pulse durations in ungated studies.

5. Ejection fraction and regional wall thickening can be
measured by imaging natural ^{23}Na of biological tissue. ^{23}Na acts
as a natural contrast material because its concentration in the
blood and extracellular fluid is 15 times greater than the intracellular concentration, i.e., 140 mM outside and 7-10 mM inside
the cell. The Harvard group has demonstrated the feasibility of
performing gated imaging studies using an isolated perfused rat
heart in a high field (9.45 T; 95.25 MHz) (74). The sensitivity
of ^{23}Na is 0.09 times less than that for protons at the same
magnetic field strength and the concentration in body fluids is
642 times less than that of water protons. Thus, the overall
sensitivity for ^{23}Na imaging is expected to be 7000 times less
than that for protons (Table 1).

Noninvasive Evaluation of Arterial Blood Flow

NMR provides two new approaches to measurement of blood flow and
characterization of the tissue constituents of the diseased vessel
wall. Several approaches to flow measurement are possible:
time-of-flight of tagged nuclei (75,76); magnetohydrodynamic
effect for pulsatile flow (77,78); a phase dispersion technique
(76); and examination of the relation of T_1 to the pulse timing
of the NMR instrument. From early results which compared proton
density to proton T_1 images in the human body (72) and the rat
(79) it became clear that flow information could be derived from
NMR data. In addition, tissue flow can be inferred from the
changes in the T_1 rate due to injection of a paramagnetic ion such
as Mn^{++} for those organs wherein the accumulation is proportional
to flow.

Noninvasive Measurement of Arterial Vessel Wall Composition

Because the T_1 and T_2 parameters vary with tissue type, we would
expect NMR to, be able to detect the early processes of atherosclerosis even before intraluminal protrusion of the atheromatous
plaque (Fig. 6). Fat deposits have been demonstrated in autopsy
specimens (Kaufman and Crooks, personal communication, 1982).
High-spatial-resolution NMR would be able to detect and monitor
fatty deposits in the aorta, carotid, iliac, and femoral arteries.
Unfortunately, the coronary arteries are usually embedded in a
fatty sheath so that fat deposits in coronary arteries will not
be easy to quantitate. In addition, the T_1 and T_2 parameters of
fibrinous material are also expected to vary from those of smooth
muscle.

SUMMARY

The major point made and conclusions presented in this paper on
the role of radionuclide tracer studies and NMR imaging techniques
for the noninvasive evaluation of atherosclerosis are:

1. Present methods of first-pass ungated blood pool studies
    provide effective and accurate noninvasive techniques for
    the measurement of ejection fraction and wall motion.
2. Myocardial perfusion studies using single-photon-emitting
    perfusion indicators are effective and sensitive diagnostic
    methods for evaluating the presence of ischemic heart disease
    but at a time very long after establishment of arterial wall
    pathology, except for prinzmetal angina.
3. Single photon tomographic methods for heart imaging have been
    disappointing because the limited angle systems frequently
    give unacceptable artifacts, and the transverse section
    systems commercially available have marginal resolution.
    Possible improvements in limited angle tomography can be
    realized by the development of instrumentation that gives
    more than the presently available angular distribution, and
    by the development of short half-life radiopharmaceuticals
    that accumulate in the heart, which allow the injection of
    sufficient activity for quantitative transverse section
    imaging.
4. Platelet accumulation at the arterial sites can currently
    be followed noninvasively using nuclear medicine techniques.
    There is a potential for improvement in sensitivity by a
    factor of 100, using positron emission tomography.

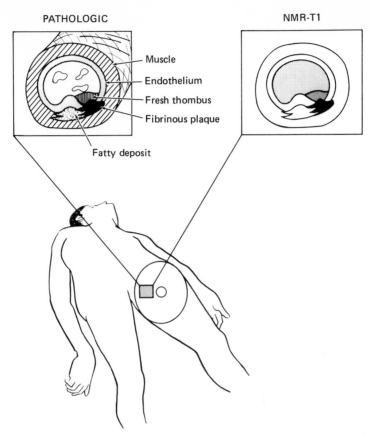

Fig. 6   Schematic representation of the prospects for imaging the
composition of arterial walls using proton NMR relaxation parameters.

5. Methods for rapid labeling of lipoproteins and monoclonal
    antibodies can be used to perfect tracers that show promise
    of describing arterial abnormalities and the distribution of
    receptor sites for lipoprotein transport.
6. Positron emission tomography will be able to measure the
    metabolism, oxygen utilization, transport of amino acids, and
    perfusion of the myocardium with a resolution of 6 mm FWHM
    in the near future.
7. Positron emission tomography offers a method of imaging the
    kinetics of antibodies and platelets in atherosclerotic
    disease, and instruments can be built with a resolution in
    the range of 2 mm FWHM.
8. Nuclear magnetic resonance imaging offers a method for the
    evaluation of the presence and degree of fatty deposition
    in the walls of large arteries.

9. Nuclear magnetic resonance methods can be used to evaluate the degree of ischemia of organs and has the potential for measuring the state of oxygen tension and pH of tissues.

REFERENCES

1. Freeman LM, Blaufox MD (eds) (1979) Cardiovascular nuclear medicine. I. Semin Nucl Med 9(4)
2. Freeman LM, Blaufox MD (eds) (1980) Cardiovascular nuclear medicine. II. Semin Nucl Med 10(1)
3. Freeman LM, Blaufox MD (eds) (1980) Cardiovascular nuclear medicine. III. Semin Nucl Med 10(2)
4. Budinger TF (1979) Physiology and physics of nuclear cardiology. In: Willerson JT (ed) Nuclear cardiology. FA Davis Company, Philadelphia, pp 9-78
5. Strauss W (1982) Nuclear medicine methods for noninvasive studies of atherosclerosis. In: Budinger TF, Berson AS, Ringqvist I, Mock MB, Watson JT, Powell RS (eds) Noninvasive techniques for assessment of atherosclerosis in peripheral, carotid, and coronary arteries. Raven Press, New York
6. Willerson JT, Parkey RW, Bonte FJ, Lewis SE, Corbett J, Buja LM (1980) Pathophysiologic considerations and clinico-pathological correlates of technetium-99m stannous pyro-phosphate myocardial scintigraphy. Semin Nucl Med 10:54-69
7. Kinlough-Rathbone RL, Mustard JF (1981) Atherosclerosis. Current concepts. Am J Surg 141:638-643
8. Fuster V, Chesebro JH (1981) Antithrombotic therapy: role of platelet-inhibitor drugs. I. Current concepts of thrombo-genesis: role of platelets. III. Management of arterial thromboembolic and atherosclerotic disease. Mayo Clinic Proc 56:102-112, 265-273
9. DeNardo SJ, DeNardo GL (1977) Iodine-123-fibronogen scintig-raphy. Semin Nucl Med 7:245-251
10. Coleman RE, Harwig SL, Harwig JF, Siegel BA, Welch MJ (1975) Fibrinogen uptake by thrombi: Effect of thrombus age. J Nucl Med 16:370-373
11. Thakur ML, Welch MJ, Joist JH, Coleman RE (1976) Indium-111 labeled platelets: Studies on preparation and evaluation of in vitro and in vivo functions. Thromb Res 9:345-357
12. Scheffel U, McIntyre PA, Evatt B, Dvornicky JA Jr, Natarajan TK, Bolling DR, Murphy EA (1977) Evaluation of indium-111 as a new high photon yield gamma-emitting "physiological" plate-let label. The Johns Hopkins Med J 140:285-293
13. Price DC, Hartmeyer JA, Prager RJ, Lipton MJ (1980) Evalua-tion of in vivo thrombus formation in dogs, using indium-111-oxide labeled autologous platelets. In: Thakur ML, Gottschalk A (eds) Indium-111 labeled neutrophils, platelets, and lymphocytes. Trivirum Publishing Company, New York, pp 183-186

14. Davis HH II, Siegel BA, Sherman LA, Heaton WA, Naidich TP, Joist JH, Welch MJ (1980) Scintigraphic detection of carotid atherosclerosis with indium-111-labeled autologous platelets. Circulation 61:982-988
15. Mustard JF (1979) Thrombosis and arterial disease. In: Joist JH, Sherman LA (ed) Venous and arterial thrombosis. Grune and Stratton, New York, pp 205-221
16. Harker LA, Ross R, Glomset JA (1978) The role of endothelial cell injury and platelet response in atherogenesis. Thromb Haemost 39:312-321
17. Harker LA (1978) Platelet survival time: its measurement and use. In: Spaet TH (ed) Progress in hemostasis and thrombosis, vol 4. Grune and Stratton, New York, pp 321-347
18. Kaplan KL (1978) Proteins secreted by platelets. Significance in detecting thrombosis. Adv Exp Med Biol 102:105-120
19. Roberts AB, Lees AM, Fallon JT, Strauss HW, Lees RS (1982) Determinants of O-density (LDL) accumulation in the healing arterial wall. Circulation IV-45
20. Lees RS, Lees AM, Strauss HW (1982) Extracorporeal imaging of human atherosclerosis. Clin Res 30:398A (abstr)
21. Brown MS, Kovanen PT, Goldstein JL (1981) Regulation of plasma cholesterol by lipoprotein receptors. Science 212: 628-635
22. DiCorleto PE, McAuliffe JB, Ross R (1982) Isolation of monoclonal antibodies that are specific for vascular smooth muscle cells. FASEB Mini-symposium No. 4013.
23. Ross R, Whight TN, Strandness E, Thiele BL (1982) Human atherosclerosis. I. Fine structure and cell culture. Circulation IV-45 (abstr)
24. DeLand FH, Kim EE, Simmons G, Goldenberg DM (1980) Imaging approach in radioimmunodetection. Cancer Res 40:3046-3049
25. Vogel RA, Kirch D, LeFree M, Steele P (1978) A new method of multiplanar emission tomography using a seven pinhole collimator and an Anger scintillation camera. J Nucl Med 19:648-654
26. Koral KF, Rogers WL, Knoll GF (1975) Digital tomographic imaging with time-modulated pseudorandum coded aperture and an Anger camera. J Nucl Med 16:402-413
27. Koral KF, Rogers WL (1979) Application of ART to time-coded emission tomography. Phys Med Biol 24:879-894
28. Gottschalk SC, Smith KA, Wake RH (1980) Comparison of seven pinhole and rotating slant tomography of a cardiac phantom. J Nucl Med 21:P27 (abstr)
29. Chang W, Lin SL, Henkin RE (1980) A rotatable quadrant slant hole collimator for tomography (QSH): a stationary scintillation camera based SPECT system. In: Sorenson JA (ed) Single photon emission computed tomography and other selected computer topics. Society of Nuclear Medicine, New York, pp 81-94
30. Budinger TF (1980) Physical attributes of single-photon tomography. J Nucl Med 21:579-592

31. Williams DL, Ritchie JL, Harp GD, Caldwell JH, Hamilton GW (1980) In vivo simulation of thallium-201 myocardial scintigraphy by seven-pinhole emission tomography. J Nucl Med 21:821-828

32. Rizi HR, Kline RC, Thrall JH, Besozzi MC, Keyes JW Jr, Rogers WL, Clare J, Pitt B (1981) Thallium-201 myocardial scintigraphy: A critical comparison of seven-pinhole tomography and conventional planar imaging. J Nucl Med 22:493-499

33. Stokely EM, Tipton DM, Buja LM, Lewis SE, DeVous MD Sr, Bonte FJ, Parkey RW, Willerson JT (1981) Quantitation of experimental canine infarct size using multipinhole single-photon tomography. J Nucl Med 22:55-61

34. Tamaki N, Mukai T, Ishii Y, Yonekura Y, Kambara H, Kawai C, Torizuka K (1981) Clinical evaluation of thallium-201 emission myocardial tomography using a rotating gamma camera: Comparison with seven-pinhole tomography. J Nucl Med 22: 849-855

35. Lassen NA, Henriksen L, Paulson O (1981) Regional cerebral blood flow in stroke by 133-Xenon inhalation and emission tomography. Stroke 12:284-288

36. Bonte FJ, Stokely EM (1981) Single-photon tomographic study of regional cerebral blood flow in stroke. J Nucl Med 22: 1049-1053

37. Kuhl DE, Barrio JR, Huang SC, Selin C, Ackermann RF, Lear JL, Wu JL, Lin TH, Phelps ME (1982) Quantifying local cerebral blood flow by n-isopropyl-p-^{123}I-iodoamphetamine (IMP) tomography. J Nucl Med 23:196-203

38. Hill TC, Holman BL, Lovett R, O'Leary DH, Front D, Magistretti P, Zimmerman RE, Moore S, Clouse ME, Wu JL, Lin TH, Baldwin RM (1982) Initial experience with SPECT (single photon computerized tomography) of the brain using n-isopropyl I-123-p-iodoamphetamine. J Nucl Med 23:191-195

39. Budinger TF (1982) Positron emission tomography: Limitation and potentials for studying atherosclerosis. In: Budinger TF, Berson AS, Ringqvist I, Mock MB, Watson JT, Powell RS (eds) Noninvasive techniques for assessment of atherosclerosis in peripheral, carotid, and coronary arteries. Raven Press, New York

40. Deutsch E, Bushong W, Glavan KA, Elder RC, Sodd VJ, Scholz KL, Fortman DL, Lukes SJ (1981) Heart imaging with cationic complexes of technetium. Science 214:85-86

41. Brownell GL, Budinger TF, Lauterbur PC, McGeer PL (1982) Positron tomography and nuclear magnetic resonance imaging. Science 215:619

42. Ter-Pogossian MM, Klein MS, Markham J, Roberts R, Sobel BE (1980) Regional assessment of myocardial metabolic integrity in vivo by positron-emission tomography with ^{11}C-labeled palmitate. Circulation 61:242-255

43. Bassingthwaighte JB (1977) Physiology and theory of tracer washout techniques for the estimation of myocardial blood

flow: Flow estimation from tracer washout. Cardiovasc Dis 20:165-189

44. Derenzo SE, Budinger TF, Huesman RH, Cahoon JL, Vuletich T (1981) Imaging properties of a positron tomograph with 280 BGO crystals. IEEE Trans Nucl Sci NS-28:81-89

45. Yano Y, Budinger TF, Chiang G, O'Brien HA, Grant PM (1979) Evaluation and application of alumina-based ^{82}Rb generators charged with high levels of Sr-82/85. J Nucl Med 20:961-966

46 Gould KL, Schelbert HR, Phelps ME, Hoffman EJ (1979) Non-invasive assessment of coronary stenoses with myocardial perfusion imaging during pharmacologic coronary vasodilation. V. Detection of 47 percent diameter coronary stenosis with intravenous nitrogen-13 ammonia and emission-computed tomography in intact dogs. Am J Cardiol 43:200-208

47. Sobel BE, Weiss ES, Welch MJ, Siegel BA, Ter-Pogossian MM (1977) Detection of remote myocardial infarction in patients with positron emission transaxial tomography and intravenous ^{11}C-palmitate. Circulation 55:853-857

48. Ter-Pogossian MM, Klein MS, Markham J, Roberts R, Sobel B (1980) Regional assessment of myocardial metabolic integrity in vivo by positron-emission tomography with ^{11}C-labeled palmitate. Circulation 61:242-255

49. Phelps ME, Hoffman EJ, Selin C, Huang SC, Robinson G, MacDonald N, Schelbert H, Kuhl DE (1978) Investigation of [^{18}F] 2-fluoro-2-deoxyglucose for the measure of myocardial glucose metabolism. J Nucl Med 19:1311-1319

50. Goldstein RA, Klein MS, Welch MJ, Sobel BE (1980) External assessment of myocardial metabolism with C-11 palmitate in vivo. J Nucl Med 21:342-348

51. Ratib O, Phelps ME, Huang SC, Henze E, Selin CE, Schelbert HR (1982) Positron tomography with deoxyglucose for estimating local myocardial glucose metabolism. J Nucl Med 23:577-586

52. Schelbert HR, Henze E, Phelps ME (1980) Emission tomography of the heart. Semin Nucl Med 10:355-375

53. Kobayashi K, Neely JR (1979) Control of maximum rates of glycolysis in rat cardiac muscle. Circ Res 44:166-179

54. Bergmann SR, Hack S, Tweson T, Welch MJ, Sobel BE (1980) The dependence of accumulation of ^{13}NH$_3$ by myocardium on metabolic factors and its implications for quantitative assessment of perfusion. Circulation 61:34-43

55. Schelbert HR, Phelps ME, Huang SC, MacDonald NS, Hansen H, Selin C, Kuhl DE (1981) N-13 ammonia as an indicator of myocardial blood flow. Circulation 63:1259-1272

56. Gelbard AS, Clarke LP, Laughlin JS (1974) Enzymatic synthesis and use of ^{13}N-labeled L-asparagine for myocardial imaging. J Nucl Med 15:1223-1225

57. Majumdar C, Stark V, Lathrop K, Harper PV (1978) Species differences in the myocardial localization of N-13-L-asparagine. J Nucl Med 19:701 (abstr)

58. Mudge GH, Mills RM, Taegtmeyer H, Gorlin R, Lesch M (1976)

Alterations of myocardial amino acid metabolism in chronic ischemic heart disease. J Clin Invest 58:1185-1192

59. Gelbard AS, Benua RS, Reiman RE, McDonald JM, Vomero JJ, Laughlin JS (1980) Imaging of the human heart after administration of L-(N-13)glutamate. J Nucl Med 21:988-991

60. Buse MG, Biggers JF, Friderici KH, Buse JF (1972) Oxidation of branched-chain amino acids by isolated hearts and diaphragms of the rat. J Biol Chem 247:8085-8096

61. Kaufman L, Crooks LE, Margulis AR (eds) (1982) Nuclear magnetic resonance imaging in medicine, Igaku-Shoin, New York

62. Hoult DI, Busby SJW, Gadian DG, Richard RE, Seeley PJ (1974) Observation of tissue metabolites using ^{31}P nuclear magnetic resonance. Nature 252:285-287

63. Hollis DP, Bulkley BH, Nunnally RL, Jacobus WE, Weisfeldt ML (1978) Effect of manganese ion on the phosphorus nuclear magnetic resonance spectra of the perfused rabbit heart. Clin Res 26:240A (abstr)

64. Garlick PB, Radda GK, Seeley PF, Chance B (1977) Phosphorus NMR studies on perfused heart. Biochem Biophys Res Commun 74:1256-1267

65. Nunnally RJ, Bottomley PA (1980) Assessment of pharmacological treatment of myocardial infarction by phosphorus-31 NMR with surface coils. Science 211:177-180

66. Williams DL, Ritchie JL, Harp GD, Caldwell JH, Hamilton GW (1980) In vivo simulation of thallium-201 myocardial scintigraphy by seven-pinhole emission tomography. J Nucl Med 21:821-828

67. Frank JA, Feiler MA, House WV, Lauterbur PC, Jacobson MT (1976) Measurement of proton nuclear magnetic longitudinal relaxation times and water content in infarcted canine myocardium and induced pulmonary injury. Clin Res 24:217A (abstr)

68. Young IR, Bailes DR, Burl M, Collins AG, Smith DT, McDonnell MJ, Orr JS, Banks LM, Bydder GM, Greenspan RH, Steiner RE (1982) Initial clinical evaluation of a whole body nuclear magnetic resonance (NMR) tomograph. J Comput Assist Tomogr 6:1-18

69. Crooks L, Singer J (1978) Some magnetic study of biological material. J Clin Engr 3:237

70. Thulborn KR, Waterton JC, Radda GK (1981) Proton imaging for in vivo blood flow and oxygen consumption measurements. J Magn Reson 45:188-191

71. Lauterbur PC, Dias MIIM, Rudin AM (1978) Augmentation of tissue water proton spin-lattice relaxation ratio by in vivo addition of paramagnetic ions. In: Dutton PL, Leigh JS, Scarpa A (eds) Electrons to tissue. Frontiers of biological energetics. Academic Press, New York, pp 752-759

72. Edelstein WA, Hutchison JMS, Johnson G, Redpath T (1980) Spin warp NMR imaging and applications to human whole body imaging. Phys Med Biol 24:751-756

73. Hawkes RC, Holland GN, Moore W, Roebuck EJ, Worthington BS
    (1981) Nuclear magnetic resonance (NMR) tomography of the
    normal heart. J Comput Assist Tomogr 5:605-612
74. Delayre JL, Ingwall JS, Malloy C, Fassell ET (1981) Gates
    sodium-23 magnetic resonance images of an isolated perfused
    working rat heart. Science 212:935-939
75. Battocletti JH, Halbach RE, Salles-Cunha SX, Sances A Jr
    (1980) NMR blood flow meter--theory and history. Med Phys
    8:435-443
76. Singer JR (1981) Blood flow measurements by NMR. In:
    Kaufman L, Crooks LE, Margulis AR (eds) Nuclear magnetic
    resonance imaging in medicine. Igaku-shoin, pp 128-144
77. Battocletti JH, Halbach RE, Sances A Jr, Larson SJ, Bowman RI,
    Kudravcev V (1979) Flat crossed-coil detector for blood-flow
    measurement using nuclear magnetic resonance. Med Biol Eng
    Comput 17:183-191
78. Gaffey CT, Tenforde TS, Budinger TF, Moyer BR (to be published
    Bioelectromagnetics) Electrocardiogram and blood pressure
    measurements on monkeys during exposure to stationary magnetic
    fields.
79. Crooks L, Hoenninger J, Arakawa M (1979) Tomography of
    hydrogen with NMR and the potential of imaging other body
    constituents. SPIE 106:120

DISCUSSION: JAMES B. BASSINGTHWAIGHTE

My comments on Dr. Budinger's presentation are directed from the point of view that what we are trying to develop are methods for quantitating the delivery of material to the cells of functioning organs. The processes involved are: (1) intravascular transport, governed by blood flow to the organ and its various regions; (2) exchange across vessel walls, mainly at the capillary level; (3) diffusion through the interstitial space, which is rapid for small solutes; and (4) transport across cell walls to sites within cells.

Most of the discussion thus far today has centered on the flow, but now Dr. Budinger has introduced the topic of adherence at the endothelial surface. Let us consider in some detail the processes involved. First, there is the flow-- not only the actual delivery, but also more minute rheological events, the cross-stream convection and molecular diffusion inside the vessel lumen, which carry the material (platelet or VLDL or monoclonal antibody or metabolic substrate) from the intravascular stream to the side of attachment on the wall. For platelets this site might be a leaky part of the wall where an endothelial cell has been damaged or lost, and for other substances it may be a receptor site on the luminal surface of the endothelial cell. In either case the likelihood of adherence is reduced by high shear rates and increased with more rapid reactions at the surface. While the effect of an increase in flow will be to reduce the fractional extraction of the solute during transorgan passage, more or less as described for capillary-tissue exchange by Renkin (1) and Bassingthwaighte (2), the total amount of solute deposited in a vascular bed is increased when flow is increased. This means that the initial distribution of any substance deposited in tissues is dominated by flow; if the extraction is complete during first passage and the substance escapes only slowly from the tissue, then the relationship between local flows and observable local concentrations remains for a long time. This means that the influences of the other processes-- exchange, diffusion and cellular uptake-- are strictly secondary in this situation. As a corollary to this principle, any tracer-labeled or externally detectable substance that is highly extracted (90-100%) and strongly retained, giving time for detection and reconstructive imaging, can be used to estimate regional blood flows within an organ.

A second corollary is that if one desires to elucidate the kinetics and the mechanisms of binding exchange or uptake of a solute by an organ, then this can only be accomplished if the first-pass extraction is *incomplete*. For metabolic substrates, escape from the blood stream is partially limited by transport across the capillary wall, and then partially again by transport across the cell membranes; this means that one can develop techniques for measuring the transport rates, e.g., as done by Rose et al. (3). It also means that by changing the conditions of the study, for example changing blood glucose concentration while doing a series of determinations of glucose uptake rate, one can obtain data on functional dependencies and then try to interpret these data in terms of an underlying transport mechanism.

This brings us back to the question of choice of technique. All three techniques, gamma, positron, and NMR imaging, offer detectability from outside the body; of these, positron imaging alone is limited to the detection of one substance at a time. This limits its utility for examining rapid uptake processes for which the tracer substrate and an intravascular nonexchanging reference tracer must be injected simultaneously in order to estimate the rate of uptake. For this purpose external scintillation detection of sets of gamma emittors having different energy peaks is the method of choice, offering detection of different substances, with good temporal resolution, but at some sacrifice in spatial resolution compared to positron tomography. NMR reconstructive imaging is still at an early stage. The ability to examine such events as the cyclic changes with the heartbeat of the several forms of phosphorus (ATP, ADP, AMP, creatine phosphate) has been demonstrated in an isolated rat heart, but the methodology is far from allowing this to be done in small regions of the myocardium of human patients.

When events are slow, the use of simultaneous reference tracers that do not participate in a transport process is less important. For example, the time course of deposition of ^{111}indium-labeled platelets on the wall of damaged coronary vessels can be well observed using single photon imaging--comparison with the time course of transport of an intravascular tracer through the organ would provide very little additional accuracy.

In summary, new imaging techniques have great potential for elucidating cellular and metabolic functions, but careful assessment of the strengths and weaknesses of a technique will be essential to making it useful in practical situations.

REFERENCES

1. Renkin EM (1959) Transport of potassium-42 from blood to tissue in isolated mammalian skeletal muscles. Am J Physiol 197:1205-1210
2. Bassingthwaighte JB (1974) A concurrent model for extraction during transcapillary passage. Circ Res 35: 483-503
3. Rose CP, Goresky CA, Bach GG (1977) The capillary and sarcolemmal barriers in the heart--An exploration of labeled water permeability. Circ Res 41:515-533

Part 2

Critical Review of Correlation and Validation Studies for Evaluating Atherosclerosis

Introduction

WILLIAM INSULL, JR. AND C. RICHARD MINICK

The purpose of the second session of the workshop is to systematically review the current status of correlations among the
various techniques for evaluating atherosclerotic lesions in man.
The ultimate goal of the review is to find rigorous validation
studies of the most advanced, clinically applicable techniques
for diagnosing and measuring atherosclerotic lesions including
contrast angiography, Doppler ultrasound, and B-mode ultrasound.
Validation is defined as a study, the goal of which is to prove
that a technique gives measurements of one or more properties of
atherosclerotic lesions, which truly represent the lesions'
properties as they exist in vivo. All the validation studies have
taken the form of quantitative studies seeking statistically
significant correlations, or associations, between measurements
of a single lesion characteristic by two different techniques.
These validation studies have been difficult to perform because
of problems inherent in obtaining clinical materials.

The overall result of these reviews is that although the
number of validation studies is limited and rigorous validation of
none of the techniques has been achieved, significant progress has
been made in developing concepts and procedures for validation
studies, and in identifying a broad range of emerging, crucial
technical problems. Two types of examination techniques dominate
as they have provided the most information and have been the most

widely used, pathology and arteriography techniques. Pathology
techniques are used most frequently as the reference methods.
The fewest correlative studies with pathology techniques have
been with Doppler ultrasound for lesser grades of stenosis and
with B-mode ultrasound. In addition, these studies are provoking reexamination and reevaluation of many concepts and data
on the pathogenesis and regression of atherosclerotic lesions.

The first review, by Dr. David S. Sumner, examines the basis
in hemodynamic theory for the relationship between a lesion's
configuration and its functional significance. This review
emphasizes that a lesion becomes significant for local hemodynamics and clinical manifestations when it causes a lumen
reduction, or stenosis of 70% or more, that some hemodynamic
effects occur with lesser grades of stenosis, but that the overall hemodynamic effects may be modulated by the occurrence of
parallel arterial channels.

Two subsequent reviews examine the studies correlating pathology examinations with antemortem arteriography and postmortem
arteriography. Dr. C. M. Fisher describes progress in correlating lesion specimens from carotid endarterectomy with clinical
angiography, and notes that angiography tends to underestimate
the extent of the lesions. Dr. C. Zarins describes the systematic study to correlate pathology examination with postmortem
arteriography, using this latter as the ideally performed arteriography. These studies emphasize the essential need to examine
arterial tissues only after distension by diastolic pressure, and
potential confounding of arteriographic estimation of stenosis
via lesions by simultaneous, localized dilatation of the artery.
The fundamental limitation of contrast arteriography for characterizing lesions remains the lack of data on the dimension and
nature of the arterial wall.

Doppler ultrasound measurements, reviewed by Dr. C. P. L.
Wood, have correlated well with arteriography when applied to
advanced stenotic lesions using instrumentation that is

well-advanced.   Its application to lesions with low grades of stenosis remains to be developed.

B-mode ultrasound measurements, reviewed by Dr. A. Comerota, have shown good correlation of stenosis evaluation with arteriographic estimation of stenosis in clinical use.   Its clinical evaluation of stenosis and other lesion characteristics is currently being studied in the U.S. Multicenter Trial for Assessment of the B-Mode Ultrasound, whose design, procedures, and progress are reviewed by Dr. J. F. Toole.

Correlations between morphological and biochemical pathology studies, reviewed by Dr. R. C. Minick, are the least developed correlation studied.   These studies promise great potential for exploiting the recent advances in biochemistry of arterial tissues in the diagnoses of lesions, as outlined by examples in the review.

Correlation studies, when systematically performed along the outline described in these reviews, will provide the basis for determining which techniques will be most useful for diagnosis of lesions and for evaluating their progression and regression.

11

Correlation of Lesion Configuration with Functional Significance

DAVID S. SUMNER

Arteriosclerotic lesions display an infinite variety of configurations. They vary in degree of narrowing and length of stenosis; their orifices may be abrupt or tapering; and the interface that they present to the bloodstream may be smooth, rough, or ulcerated. Their functional significance is manifested in two ways: by a global reduction of flow to the peripheral tissues, and by shedding emboli that obliterate terminal arteries. When the resulting flow deficit is severe, the tissues become hypoxic, nutritionally deprived, and lack the protection afforded by host defense mechanisms. Mild degrees of narrowing and even total occlusions may be well compensated by the development of an efficient collateral network and by vasodilation of the microvascular bed. In such cases, the obstruction may be asymptomatic or may cause symptoms only when the system is stressed by exercise, trauma, or infection. Severe, uncompensated obstructions, on the other hand, compromise the viability of the tissues even at rest or in the absence of extraneous trauma--leading to ischemic rest pain, nonhealing ulcers, tissue destruction by unchecked infection, and eventual gangrene. Although lesions capable of throwing emboli may not produce discernable physiologic changes; they may be functionally highly significant, particularly when the vessel involved supplies a sensitive area, such as the brain.

The challenge faced by both the scientist and clinician is to detect the presence of arteriosclerosis, to assess its functional significance, to characterize its morphology, to follow its regression or progression, and to evaluate the efficacy of any therapeutic measures that are employed.

HEMODYNAMIC EFFECTS OF ARTERIAL OBSTRUCTION

Under normal conditions, the diameter of an artery is large enough to provide adequate blood flow to the tissues that it serves without requiring an undue expenditure of energy. Some reserve is built in to maintain increased flow under conditions of stress. The imposition of a plaque that encroaches on the arterial lumen contributes additional energy losses. These occur whenever the lumen is narrowed or whenever flow vectors are required to change direction. Basically, the dissipation of energy in the arterial circulation is related to the viscosity of blood and to its inertia.

Viscous energy "losses" are described by Poiseuille's law:

$$P_1 - P_2 = Q \frac{8L\eta}{\pi r^4} \tag{1}$$

where $P_1 - P_2$ represents the drop in potential energy (pressure) between two points separated by the distance, L, in a cylindrical vessel with an inside radius, r, at a flow rate of Q. The coefficient of viscosity, η, is determined by "friction" between the molecules and formed elements of the blood.

Energy "losses" related to inertia occur whenever blood is accelerated or decelerated, as in pulsatile flow, or at the entrance to or exit from a stenosis. Since velocity is a vector quantity, any change in direction of flow will result in further dissipation of energy. Direction changes occur not only at bends or bifurcations in the arterial tree, but also at the entrance and exit of a stenosis. Because disturbed or turbulent flow creates an infinite variety of velocity vectors, energy losses are greatly increased when these conditions prevail.

Inertial losses depend on the mass or density of the blood, ρ and on the square of the velocity, V:

$$\Delta P = k \; \tfrac{1}{2} \; \rho V^2 \tag{2}$$

In the arterial tree, inertial losses generally exceed those due to viscosity, especially in the vicinity of a stenosis. The relative magnitude of these effects is illustrated graphically in Fig. 1. As blood is accelerated within the stenosis, much of the potential energy is converted into kinetic energy according to the Bernouilli principle; but, at the exit where the velocity falls to its prestenotic value, relatively little of the kinetic energy is transformed back into pressure--most of it has been dissipated in the form of heat, largely as a result of inertial factors.

Unless some mechanism is present to maintain a constant total resistance of the system, the presence of a stenosis will affect the flow rate as well as the pressure. As the degree of stenosis increases, the magnitude of the decrease in flow is equivalent to the increase in the pressure gradient across the stenosis (Fig. 2). Because energy dissipation--both viscous and inertial--is inversely related to the fourth power of the radius, little change occurs until the radius is reduced by about 50% (area reduced 75%); but beyond this point, minor decreases in radius cause major changes in both pressure and flow (1,2). Although decreasing the peripheral resistance shifts the curves to the left, the break point is still in the same approximate region. This gives rise to the concept of "critical stenosis," a concept that is of value in interpreting the potential significance of stenoses seen on roentgenographic studies and in analyzing the results of noninvasive pressure studies.

In a high-flow (low resistance) system, the drop in pressure and flow at any degree of narrowing beyond the "critical stenosis" point is much greater than it is in a low-flow (high resistance) system (Fig. 2). This observation is of importance clinically, since it explains why a lesion that has little significance at rest, when the peripheral resistance is high, may severely

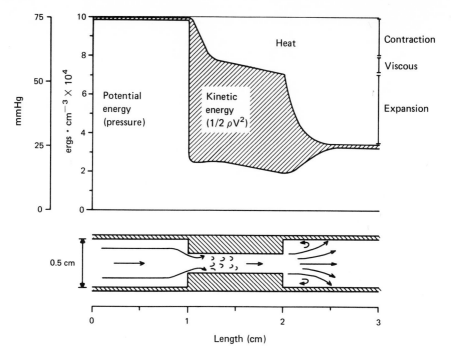

Fig. 1   Effect of a stenosis on conversion of potential and
kinetic energy to heat. Note that energy "losses" due to viscosity are much less than those related to inertia. (From Ref. 23.)

restrict blood flow during exercise, when the peripheral resistance is low.

Although the length of a stenosis affects its hemodynamic
resistance, length is far less important than radius (3). Entrance
and exit effects are modified but little by increasing the length
of a stenosis. Consequently, the length of a stenosis principally
affects energy losses related to viscosity; and viscous losses are
much more sensitive to changes in radius, which enters Poiseuille's
equation in the fourth power, than they are to length, which enters
the equation in the first power (Formula 1).

In contrast, the resistances of stenoses in series are roughly
additive, especially when there are few stenoses and the degree of
narrowing is not great. However, the cumulative effect of multiple
severe stenoses is usually somewhat less than would be anticipated

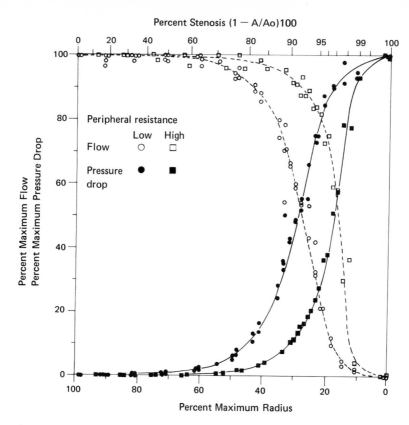

Fig. 2   Relationship of pressure gradient and flow to degree of stenosis in a canine femoral artery.

based on the sum of the individual resistances (4). Again this disparity can be attributed to inertial factors: the decreased mean flow and decreased pulsatility of flow through the entire system causes less energy dissipation at the entrance and exit of each stenosis than would have occurred had the stenosis existed in isolation.

In summary, doubling the length of a stenosis without changing its diameter would not double its resistance, but placing two stenoses of equal length in series would essentially double the resistance.

Local Effects of Stenoses

When blood passes from a vessel with a large cross-sectional area (A_1) to one with a smaller cross-sectional area (A_2), its velocity is increased.

$$V_1 A_1 = V_2 A_2$$

$$V_1 r_1^2 = V_2 r_2^2$$

(3)

Thus, the velocity of flow within a stenosis is proportional to the degree of narrowing as long as the flow through the arterial segment remains constant. However, as the artery is narrowed beyond the "critical stenosis," flow begins to decrease and velocity also decreases (Fig. 3) (5). Even when flow decreases, the ratio of the mean velocity in the stenotic region to that in the vessel of normal calibre (V_2/V_1) will always equal the area ratio, A_1/A_2 (6).

As blood approaches a stenosis, the flow stream narrows; within the stenosis there is a breakdown of orderly flow vectors, which may persist throughout the narrowed area; and at the exit, the jet emerging into the wider lumen produces areas of flow separation, eddy currents, and disturbed or turbulent flow. The magnitude of the flow disturbance is determined by Reynolds number $(Re = 2 \rho vr/\eta)$, the shape of the entrance and exit (abrupt or tapering), the degree of narrowing, surface irregularities (smooth or ulcerated), and the pulsatility of the blood. Even minor stenoses and wall irregularities produce flow disturbances that can be appreciated by analysis of the Doppler frequency spectrum (7,8). In addition, the turbulent jet tends to generate wall vibrations that are audible as bruits. The degree of stenosis and the frequency at the peak amplitude of the bruit have been shown to be closely related (9).

Changes in the arterial wall occurring in the vicinity of arterial stenoses have been attributed to flow disturbances. Vibrations weaken the arterial wall distal to the stenosis,

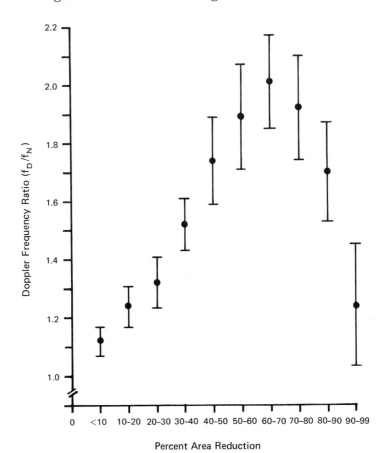

Fig. 3 Effect of increasing stenosis on the ratio of the frequency of the Doppler signal measured just beyond the site of
narrowing (F_D) to that obtained prior to the creation of the
stenosis (F_N). Frequency of the signal is proportional to the
velocity of blood flow. (From Ref. 24.)

causing poststenotic dilatation; reflected waves proximal to a

stenosis may play a role in creating aneurysms; and abnormal shear

stresses damage the endothelium, perpetuating the atherosclerotic

process. Of more immediate significance, however, is the tendency

for platelets to aggregate and clots to form in areas of relative

stasis, such as in the regions proximal to the entrance and just

distal to the exit of a stenosis or in pocket-like irregularities

in the plaque, which are commonly referred to as ulcerations.

These clots can obstruct the lumen, converting a stenosis into a total occlusion, or be carried downstream, ultimately coming to rest in a smaller artery. Small portions of the plaque itself can also break off under the influence of the flow disturbance or as a result of hemorrhage into the plaque (cholesterol emboli). It is worth emphasizing that these devastating effects can occur even in the absence of any recognizable alteration in mean pressure and flow distal to the stenosis.

Effect of Stenoses on Pulsatile Pressure and Flow

As a pulse of blood passes through a stenosis, its high-frequency harmonics are attenuated and the phase relationships between the harmonics are altered. Inertial energy losses are greater during the systolic phase of the pulse cycle than they are during diastole; thus, downstream from a stenosis, the peak velocity of flow is reduced, thereby decreasing the excursion of the flow pulse but maintaining the mean flow at its prestenotic level. The compliance of the arterial wall and that of any collateral channels constitute hydraulic capacitors, which, together with the stenosis, create a situation analagous to a low-pass filter (Fig. 4). Similar changes occur in the pressure waveform, but the mean pressure distal to a stenosis will also be reduced (Fig. 4).

Although experimentally it appears that most parenchymal organs (e.g., the kidney) function better with pulsatile flow rather than continuous flow, it is uncertain how prominent this effect is. Transcapillary exchange, critical closing pressure, arteriolar and venular tone, and lymphatic flow are all known to be responsive to pulsatile pressure. However, in most clinical situations, it is difficult to divorce changes in pulse wave configuration from the simultaneously occurring changes in mean arterial pressure and flow.

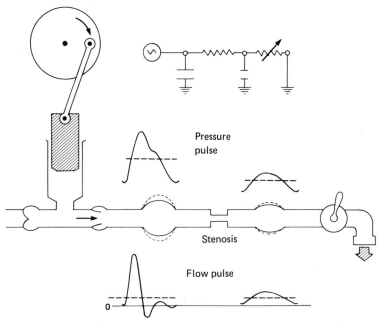

Pressure
pulse

Stenosis

Flow pulse

0

Fig. 4 Effect of stenosis on arterial pressure and flow pulse.
Dashed lines indicate mean pressure and flow values. Faucet
represents variable but high peripheral resistance. The vessels
are considered to be compliant.

PHYSIOLOGY OF ARTERIAL OBSTRUCTION

Arterial stenoses rarely, if ever, exist in isolation. As the
arterial lumen becomes more restricted by atherosclerosis,
preexisting arteries that bridge the obstructing site expand into
collateral channels (Fig. 5). The resistances of the collaterals
(R_c) are in parallel with the resistance of the obstructed or
stenotic major artery (R_s), forming a "segmental resistance," R_{cs}.
Similar to an electrical circuit, resistances in series are
roughly additive; but the total resistance offered by two or more
vessels in parallel is always less than that of the vessel with
the least resistance. Thus, the magnitude of the segmental
resistance is given by:

$$\frac{1}{R_{cs}} = \frac{1}{R_s} + \frac{1}{R_{c1}} + \frac{1}{R_{c2}} + \ldots + \frac{1}{R_{c_n}} \tag{4}$$

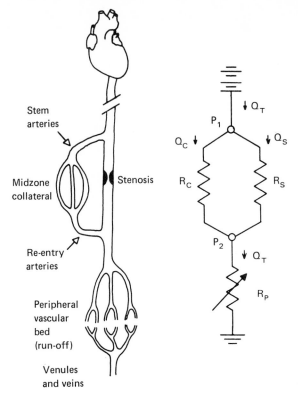

Fig. 5 Electrical analog of a typical arterial circuit containing a stenosis, collateral arteries, and a peripheral vascular bed with a variable resistance. Venous pressure is represented by ground potential. (From Ref. 23.)

Even when collaterals are well developed, the segmental resistance is seldom, if ever, as low as that offered by the major artery prior to its becoming diseased. For example, based on Poiseuille's law, it would take 256 collaterals each with a diameter of 2.5 mm or 10,000 collaterals with a diameter of 1.0 mm to reduce the segmental resistance to that of an unobstructed artery with a diameter of 10 mm.

Because segmental resistance is almost always increased in cases of arterial obstruction, most of the burden for sustaining blood flow to the tissues is assumed by the peripheral arterioles, which dilate to compensate for the increased proximal resistance.

The peripheral resistance (R_p) offered by the microvasculature is in series with the segmental resistance (R_{cs}); therefore, the total resistance of the arterial circuit (R_T) is the sum of the two resistances. Consequently, flow to the tissues (Q_T) will remain adequate as long as the peripheral arterioles retain the ability to dilate. Once maximum vasodilatation is reached, further increases in segmental resistance will result in a rapid decrease in peripheral blood flow, and the tissues will become ischemic (Fig. 6).

$$Q_T = \frac{P_1 - P_v}{R_T} + \frac{P_1 - P_v}{R_{cs} + R_p} \tag{5}$$

Although the pressure gradient ($P_1 - P_v$) across the entire arterial circuit, from the inflow arteries (P_1) to the central veins (P_v) may vary from time to time, this seldom has much effect on total blood flow. Under normal flow conditions, a rise in arterial pressure is usually offset by an increase in arteriolar resistance; and a rise in venous pressure, by a decrease in arteriolar resistance (autoregulation). However, under ischemic conditions when the peripheral vasculature is maximally dilated, an increase or decrease in perfusion pressure will lead to a corresponding increase or decrease in flow.

The pressure gradient across the diseased artery and its parallel collaterals ($P_1 - P_2$) increases as the segmental resistance increases.

$$P_1 - P_2 = Q_t R_{cs} \tag{6}$$

$$P_2 = P_1 - Q_T R_{cs}$$

Provided that the peripheral flow remains unchanged, the pressure distal to a stenosis will fall commensurate with an increase in segmental resistance (Fig. 6). When maximum peripheral vasodilatation is achieved, flow across the diseased segment rapidly decreases; and although pressure continues to fall as the segmental resistance increases, it does so at a reduced rate (Fig. 6). Collaterals developing around a stenosis often keep the

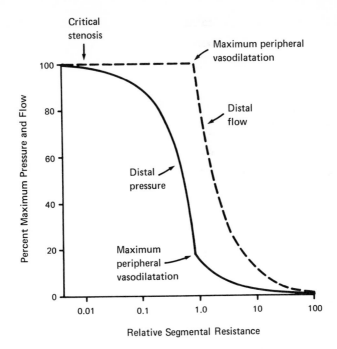

Fig. 6 Effect of increasing segmental resistance on pressure and flow distal to a stenotic artery and its collaterals.

segmental resistance low enough to maintain an adequate peripheral blood flow; maximum arteriolar dilatation is not attained; and a drop in distal pressure is the only physiologic indication of circulatory impairment. It is for these reasons that measurement of pressure distal to a stenosis has proved to be a much more reliable indicator of the presence of arterial disease than measurement of peripheral flow, especially under basal conditions.

Although peripheral blood flow (Q_T) may remain constant despite increasing segmental resistance, flow through the stenosis itself (Q_s in Fig. 5), will decrease as the diameter of the arterial lumen diminishes. The relationship between the pressure gradient across and the flow through the stenosis will continue to resemble that depicted in Fig. 2. However, when collaterals are well developed, the magnitude of the pressure drop will be less and decrease in flow will be more than it would be in the absence of a parallel circuit. For example, even when an artery is

totally occluded and there is no flow; the pressure distal to the
stenosis will not be zero, but will be decreased commensurate with
the resistance of the collaterals.

Effect of Stress

Under normal conditions, the peripheral arterioles have the
capacity to dilate sufficiently to meet the increased flow requirements imposed by stress such as exercise, infection, or a
period of ischemia. In the resting lower limbs, for example, the
segmental resistance (R_{cs}) is quite low and the peripheral resistance (R_p) is relatively high. With exercise, the peripheral
resistance falls as a result of arteriolar dilatation, while the
segmental resistance remains fairly constant. As a result, the
total resistance ($R_{cs} + R_p$) is markedly reduced, and there is a
great increase in flow to the exercising muscles (Formula 5 and
Fig. 7). Because the segmental resistance is low, there is
ordinarily little drop in the mean arterial pressure in the distal
parts of the leg (Formula 6 and Fig. 8).

The situation is distinctly different in the presence of
arterial disease that elevates the segmental resistance (10).
Even at rest the peripheral arterioles are partially dilated to
maintain resting blood flow at normal values. With exercise,
further arteriolar dilation occurs; but despite the fact that
dilation may be maximal, the total resistance remains high.
Therefore, blood flow, though increased, is less than that observed in the normal extremity (Fig. 7). If the magnitude of the
flow increase is insufficient to sustain the metabolism of the
exercising muscle, claudication develops. Because there is almost
always some increase in flow through the diseased segment and its
collaterals, the peripheral pressure falls (Fig. 8).

The decrease in peripheral pressure that follows exercise is
one of the most sensitive indicators of the presence of arterial
disease. For example, in some limbs the distal pressure may be
normal at rest; yet after exercise, the pressure will fall,

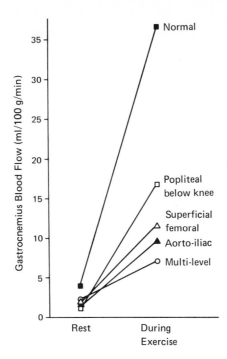

Fig. 7   Muscle blood flow at rest and after exercise in normal
subjects and in patients with occlusive arterial disease at the
indicated sites.   (From Ref. 23.)

confirming the presence of an arterial obstruction that is subcritical at low flow rates, but critical under conditions of
increased flow.

In normal extremities, little "flow debt" is incurred during
exercise and that which develops is rapidly repaid. Within a few
minutes the postexercise hyperemia rapidly subsides to preexercise
flow levels (Fig. 9). Because of the inadequate flow generated during exercise in limbs with arterial obstruction, a large "flow debt"
develops, and because the postexercise arterial inflow is restricted
by the high proximal resistance, this large debt may require many
minutes to repay (Fig. 10). As a result, in limbs with arterial
obstruction, the peak postexercise flow level is less than that
seen in normal limbs; but the hyperemia lasts much longer (10).

Persistence of the increased flow in the postexercise period
causes a prolonged decrease in the pressure distal to the diseased

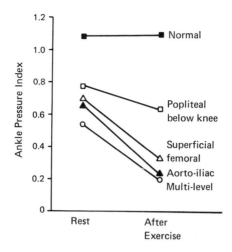

Fig. 8 Ankle pressure indices (the ratio of ankle systolic blood pressure to brachial systolic blood pressure) at rest and after exercise in normal subjects and in patients with arterial occlusions. (From Ref. 23.)

arterial segment. Peripheral pressure rises as the hyperemia gradually subsides, reaching preexercise levels only after blood flow has returned to resting values (Fig. 10). These pressure-flow patterns are valuable indicators of the functional severity of the obstructive process (10).

Similar changes in pressure and flow occur after a period of ischemia. The resulting reactive hyperemia reaches higher peak levels in normal limbs than it does in diseased limbs, but the hyperemia is more persistent in abnormal limbs than it is in normal limbs.

Steal Phenomena

The physiologic impact of multilevel arterial lesions is often greater than that which would be predicted based on the arithmetical sum of the segmental resistances. Tissues deriving their blood supply from more proximally located arterial segments may divert blood away from those that are located further distally, especially during conditions of stress, thus causing an apparent increase in the resistance of the inflow vessels (11). A situation

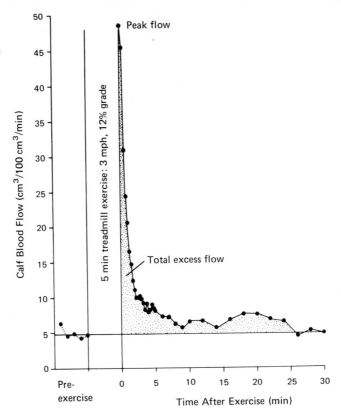

Fig. 9   Blood flow before and after exercise in a normal human
calf.   (From Ref. 25.)

commonly encountered by the vascular surgeon is combined obstructive disease of the iliac and superficial femoral arteries.   The
hydraulic model illustrated in Fig. 11 helps explain the effects
of this combination on peripheral pressure and flow.   At rest,
normal blood flow to the calf and thigh muscles is maintained by
nearly complete vasodilatation in the calf (R_c).

This results in an increased flow through the stenotic iliac
artery (R_I), which causes a drop in pressure in the common femoral
artery (P_2).   Because the resistance in the superficial femoral
artery (R_{SF}) has not changed and because the pressure head (P_2)
perfusing the calf falls, blood flow to the calf decreases.   Thus,
the effect of exercise is to increase flow to the thigh, to

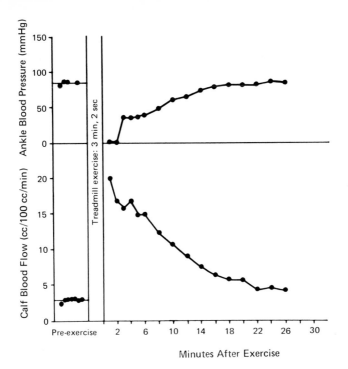

Fig. 10   Calf blood flow and ankle pressure before and after exercise in a patient with stenosis of the superficial femoral artery.   (From Ref. 10.)

decrease flow to the calf, and to decrease peripheral blood pressure (P_3).   In other words, the proximal vascular bed <u>steals</u> blood from the distal bed.   Since the pressure gradient ($P_1 - P_3$) is increased and the calf flow is decreased, the resistance of the limb appears to rise with exercise.

Following exercise, calf blood flow and peripheral pressure will increase only after the flow to the thigh has begun to decrease (Fig. 12).   Thus, the onset of hyperemia in the calf muscle will be delayed and the period of hyperemia will be prolonged when there are multiple levels of obstruction.

Because there are many possible combinations of multiple stenoses, each with side branches to separate vascular beds, the response to exercise can vary from a mild reduction in peripheral flow to total extinction.   Similarly, the delay in recovery of

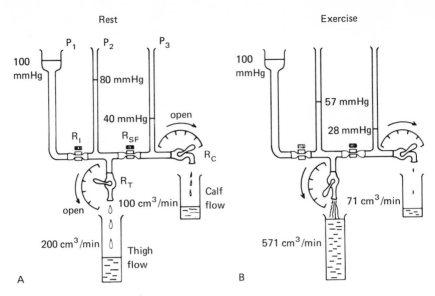

Fig. 11 Hydraulic model illustrating vascular steal. See text
for explanation. (From Ref. 23.)

peripheral pressure and flow in the postexercise period may
be brief or it may be quite prolonged. There may be some postexercise hyperemia in the most distal vascular bed or there may
be none, flow merely returning gradually to the preexercise
level.

Moreover, steals are sometimes evident even when there is
only one level of arterial disease. For example, flow to the
foot may decrease during exercise in the presence of isolated
femoral arterial obstruction and flow to the calf may be impaired
when there is obstruction of the iliac artery (10,11). In these
situations, the multiple proximal vascular beds, with their
enormous capacity to absorb blood flow coupled with the normal
resistance of a long segment of peripheral artery, create conditions that are analogous to those existing with multiple level
occlusions.

Steals will also occur in response to reactive hyperemia
produced by a period of ischemia or may result from arteriovenous
fistulae located at some proximal site.

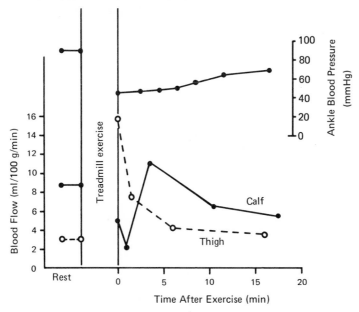

Fig. 12   Ankle pressure, calf and thigh blood flow before and after exercise in a patient with combined iliac and superficial femoral arterial obstructions.   (From Ref. 26.)

FUNCTIONAL SIGNIFICANCE: HEMODYNAMIC EFFECTS

While it may be feasible to characterize the resistance of a particular arterial lesion under rigidly defined conditions of pressure, flow, pulse rate, peripheral impedance, etc., it is seldom possible to predict its functional significance with any degree of certainty. However, as a rule, one can safely say that an isolated lesion that does not reduce the arterial diameter by more than 50% is quite unlikely to affect peripheral pressure and flow. On the other hand, it is impossible to say whether a severe stenosis or even occlusion will have any detrimental effect on the peripheral circulation.

Collaterals provide the only physiologic means of completely obviating the effects of an arterial lesion. In many areas of the body, the preexisting collaterals are so well established that complete occlusion of an artery has no perceptible effect. For example, occlusion of the radial artery ordinarily produces no

change in hand blood flow provided the ulnar artery is intact.
Similarly, gradual occlusion of one or two of the major branches
of the popliteal artery (anterior tibial, posterior tibial, pero-
neal) will have little effect. The digital artery on one side of
a finger can be occluded without causing difficulty if the other
is patent. Even the internal carotid artery may be severely narrowed or occluded without causing a decrease in pressure or flow
in the ipsilateral cerebral hemisphere if the opposite carotid is
patent, the circle of Willis is complete, and/or the vast collateral network furnished by the branches of the external carotid is
well established. Nevertheless, in other areas of the body--
especially those supplied by an unpaired artery--collaterals, even
when well developed, prove incapable of sustaining normal circulatory dynamics. Examples include severe stenoses of the aorta,
iliac, femoral, popliteal, and brachial arteries. Finally, occlusions that develop in terminal arteries, beyond the last communication of any potential collateral artery, will usually produce marked
impairment of the circulation to the tissues that they supply.

Except in the areas where there are paired arteries of roughly
comparable size, the rapidity with which the artery becomes
occluded is of importance in determining the extent of collateral
development. For this reason emboli, which cause sudden occlusion, almost invariably cause more functional impairment than a
gradually developing arteriosclerotic lesion at the same site. A
thrombus, forming at the site of a preexisting arterial stenosis,
ordinarily has less effect on the peripheral circulation than an
embolus would to the same area of a previously normal artery,
because collateral development has already been stimulated by the
longstanding arterial disease.

Stenoses or occlusions located at branch points in an artery
(such as the common femoral artery where it divides into the
profunda femoris and superficial femoral arteries) are usually
much more significant than lesions of similar severity that are
located in the mid-portion of the artery (e.g., superficial
femoral at the adductor canal). Occlusions in these locations not

only block the main artery but also block major inflow channels from potential collaterals. In effect, this creates a multilevel occlusion. Since emboli almost invariably lodge at branch points, they tend to obliterate potential collaterals that might have served to ameliorate their effect.

As discussed previously, vasodilatation of the peripheral vascular bed is often capable of maintaining normal flow to the tissues despite the increased proximal resistance imposed by a stenotic or occluded artery and its high-resistance collaterals. This ability to autoregulate functions until the perfusion pressure drops below 20-30 mmHg in skeletal muscle or below 50-60 mmHg in the brain. Further reduction in perfusion pressure will cause comparable reduction in flow, and ischemia will result. On the other hand, when the tissues are ischemic and autoregulation is abolished, an increase in systemic pressure will improve flow. But even when flow is adequate under resting conditions, it may not be capable of increasing enough to satisfy the demands imposed by exercise or other stress, such as trauma or infection. Steal phenomena also interfere with peripheral circulation, especially when there is disease at multiple levels.

In summary, the functional effects of arterial disease are determined by the degree of stenosis, the number of affected sites, the location of the obstructive process, steal phenomena, collateral development, the ability of the peripheral arterioles to dilate, the demands imposed by stress, the acuteness or chronicity of the occlusion, and the systemic blood pressure.

FUNCTIONAL SIGNIFICANCE: INDIRECT EFFECTS

Lesions that cause no perceptible change in mean pressure or flow may, nevertheless, have important clinical implications. Platelet thrombi or clots developing on the surface of the plaque, in areas of stasis proximal or distal to the plaque, or in "ulcerations" within the plaque, may be carried downstream where they may obliterate a terminal artery. If these emboli land in a sensitive

area such as the brain or retina, infarction may result causing
a stroke or blindness. In the legs, such emboli commonly lodge
in the distal pedal vessels or digital arteries, causing the
"blue toe syndrome." When the ultimate resting place is in a
silent area of the brain or in the skeletal muscle of the legs,
there may be no evident functional impairment.

INDIRECT METHODS FOR EVALUATING THE FUNCTIONAL SIGNIFICANCE
OF ARTERIAL LESIONS

The hemodynamic effects of an arterial lesion (or lesions) are
most easily and accurately evaluated by measurement of arterial
pressure (10). Although direct pressure measurements can be made
by cannulating the artery, it is often possible to obtain reasonably reliable results, noninvasively, with a pneumatic cuff and a
flow sensor (Doppler or plethysmograph). Pressures can be measured at multiple levels of the arm or legs, including the fingers
and toes. Any decrease in pressure with the extremity at rest
signifies the presence of a hemodynamically significant arterial
lesion at some point proximal to the site of measurement. Although
the magnitude of the pressure decrease correlates only moderately
well with the anatomical extent of the disease (Fig. 13), it
correlates quite well with the functional significance of the
obstructive process (Fig. 14). For example, the likelihood of a
foot lesion healing is markedly reduced when the ankle pressure is
less than 55 mmHg or the toe pressure is less than 30 mmHg (12,13).
When the pressure is less than 30 mmHg, blood flow is also likely
to be reduced. The drop in peripheral pressure that follows
exercise (or reactive hyperemia) provides a sensitive method for
detecting lesions that produce no perceptible decrease in resting
pressure, either because the stenosis is not quite critical at
rest or because collaterals are sufficiently developed to maintain
a normal resting pressure but are not adequate to carry the
increased flow generated by exercise (or reactive hyperemia)
without a concomitant pressure drop. Also, the magnitude of the

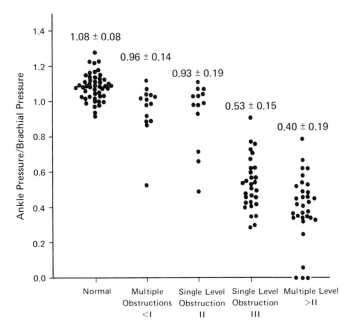

Fig. 13 Relationship of ankle pressure index to extent of occlusive arterial disease. Degree of obstruction is indicated by I, stenosis by less than 50%; II, stenosis by greater than 50% diameter; and III, total occlusion. Note wide range of values and extensive overlap.

postexercise or postischemic pressure drop and the time required for the pressure to return to prestress levels correlates with the degree of physiologic impairment.

Under resting conditions, measurement of mean flow is of less value than pressure measurement (10). As pointed out above, flow decreases only when the peripheral pressure falls to very low levels. Moreover, the range of normal resting flow values is quite large, depending upon the ambient temperature, the metabolic activity of the tissue being served, and the volume of the tissue bed. However, under certain circumstances, resting flow measurements may prove valuable in predicting the likelihood that skin lesions or amputations may heal (14).

Because the increase in flow that follows exercise or a period of ischemia is less in tissues fed by an obstructed artery than it

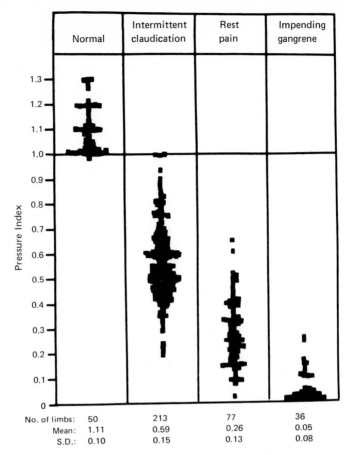

Fig. 14 Relationship of ankle pressure index to functional impairment. (From Ref. 27.)

it is in tissues with normal inflow, flow measurements made under conditions that induce peripheral vasodilation can be used to detect an arterial lesion and assess its functional severity. Delay in the return of flow, delay in the peak hyperemic response, and persistance of hyperemia are all factors that can be used to estimate the degree of physiologic impairment; but all of these measurements are rather imprecise, since there is no way of assuring a standard stress. Moreover, flow measurements are rather cumbersome, requiring the application of an electromagnetic probe to the

vessel, quantifying the Doppler frequency shift, using venous
occlusion plethysmography, or employing isotope techniques.
Thermographic methods are merely a crude way of estimating flow.
Thus, pressure measurements are usually equally meaningful and
much less difficult to perform than flow measurements, and,
consequently, are to be preferred in most clinical situations.

Pressure pulses can be recorded directly with a transducer
or indirectly by the use of plethysmography. Flow pulses can
be recorded with a noncannulating electromagnetic flow probe
or with a Doppler velocity detector. This distortion of the
pulsatile information produced by a proximally or distally located
obstructive process can be observed directly, can be roughly
quantified by the use of various pulsatility indices, or can be
more precisely defined by means of an analysis of the moduli
and phase relationships of the harmonic components of the pulse
(15,16). Configurational changes in the pulse occur with lesser
degrees of stenosis than are required to produce changes in mean
flow, and seem to provide a sensitivity roughly comparable to
that of pressure measurements. Transfer function analysis of
the Doppler shift waveform from the femoral artery has proved
to be an accurate method for assessing the severity of iliac
lesions even in the presence of superficial femoral arterial
obstruction (22).

Tests that attempt a more precise definition of defects in
the nutritional circulation or in the metabolic activity of the
capillary bed--including isotope clearance studies, measurement
of skin blood pressure, and transcutaneous oxygen determinations--
may have important clinical applications, but their utility has
not been firmly established (14,17-19).

DIRECT METHODS FOR EVALUATING LESION CONFIGURATION

Measurement of pressure or flow in the involved artery just distal
to a stenosis has little chance of accurately describing the
degree of narrowing and much less the configuration of the lesion.

There will be no perceptible change in these parameters until the
stenosis reaches critical dimensions, and with further narrowing
the changes are so precipitous that minor decreases in the diameter of the arterial lumen have major repercussions in terms of
hemodynamic parameters. Moreover, alterations in peripheral
resistance shift the curves that describe the relationship between pressure-flow parameters and the degree of arterial stenosis. As indicated by the curves in Fig. 2, a given pressure
gradient may be compatible with a rather wide range of arterial
radii.

Velocity measurements should be linearly correlated with
reduction of luminal diameter until critical stenosis is reached
(Fig. 4); beyond this point the ratio of the mean velocity of flow
within the stenosis to that farther downstream (or upstream)
should continue to correlate with the dimensions of the stenosis
in an unbranched system (5,6).

Flow disturbances alter the velocity profile and create multiple flow vectors that can be detected when the Doppler frequency
spectrum is analyzed (7,8). Minor degrees of stenosis can often
be detected by this method and the degree of stenosis can be estimated with some accuracy. Vibrations of the arterial wall created
by flow disturbances can also be analyzed to provide an estimation
of the degree of stenosis (9). However, precise characterization
of the configuration of an arterial lesion is not possible by any
physiologic means. Imaging techniques are required. Although
recent results with both Doppler and echo imaging have been
promising; at present, the most reliable technique continues
to be contrast arteriography (7,20,21).

CONCLUSIONS

The quantitative evaluation of atherosclerosis cannot be accomplished reliably with tests that evaluate hemodynamic parameters
at sites remote from the lesion. Unless the lesions are extensive, those that reduce the arterial cross section by less than

75% are seldom detected. Any observed improvement in function is more likely to be due to collateral development, thrombus dissolution, or metabolic changes than to regression of the atherosclerotic lesion. On the other hand, deterioration in function is often associated with advancing disease; but here again, the observed changes could be due to thrombus formation or collateral obliteration.

Tests that directly interrogate the region of the atheromatous plaque are more likely to yield quantitative information. Within limits that remain to be defined, tests that analyze the frequency spectrum of bruits or Doppler shifts, compare flow velocities, or provide noninvasive images of the plaque are capable of characterizing lesions in terms of their morphology, extent, location, and physical composition. Even at the present nascent state of technological development, gross changes in degree of stenosis can be recognized with a modicum of accuracy.

In contrast, functional significance is best evaluated by means of tests that quantitate perfusion of the tissues supplied by the arteries involved with atherosclerosis. Currently available invasive and noninvasive tests provide a fairly good estimation of the perfusion deficit. When properly employed in the appropriate clinical context, they have proved to be particularly valuable for assessing functional impairment, for planning therapy, for evaluating the results of therapy, and for following patients with atherosclerosis. Because any individual artery with an atherosclerotic plaque is but one part of a complex hydraulic circuit, direct tests shed little light on functional significance. As emphasized earlier in this chapter, low-grade lesions that have little or no effect on pressure or flow may be highly significant. At the other end of the scale, a large lesion that increases the pressure gradient and restricts or disturbs flow may be completely asymptomatic.

Therefore the choice of tests must depend on the questions being asked by the clinician or clinical investigator.

RECOMMENDATIONS

Functional tests would prove more informative if the measurements of physiologic changes in the distal arteries could be supplemented by more precise characterization of the nutritional deficit experienced by the target organ and by more precise definition of the boundaries of the nutritionally deprived tissues. Isotope flow studies and transcutaneous PO_2 measurements are tentative steps in this direction. From the therapeutic standpoint, identification of which lesion or lesions are most responsible for the observed physiologic deficit is of immense practical importance. Most of the noninvasive tests have proved to be woefully inadequate in this regard, but the more elegant computer-assisted methods for analyzing pulsatile data have shown some promise.

For evaluating the lesion itself, the initial results of the various imaging and spectral analysis methods have proved encouraging. Further development of these modalities is recommended. However, we still need better methods for identifying the boundary phenomena that determine which atherosclerotic plaques are apt to serve as sources for emboli.

SUMMARY

Stenoses within the arterial system have no appreciable effect on mean pressure and flow unless the cross-sectional area of the artery is reduced by approximately 75%. Beyond this point, further narrowing produces a marked drop in flow and an equally marked increase in the pressure gradient. However, stenoses in the arterial system are part of a complex hemodynamic circuit that includes collateral arteries and the peripheral vascular bed. Collateral development reduces the effective inflow resistance, and dilatation of the peripheral arterioles reduces the outflow resistance. Unless the stenosis is very severe and the collaterals are poorly developed, blood flow at rest is maintained within normal limits; but the peripheral pressure is reduced.

Although flow may be adequate under basal conditions, it may prove inadequate when the system is stressed by exercise, infection, or trauma.

Tests that measure hemodynamic parameters distal to the arterial lesion accurately reflect the extent of the functional disability, but cannot be relied upon to detect the presence of a plaque, estimate the degree of stenosis, or recognize progression or regression of atherosclerosis. On the other hand, tests that detect hemodynamic alterations in the immediate vicinity of the plaque may yield quantitative information regarding degree of stenosis and configurational changes, but cannot determine the functional significance of the lesion.

BIBLIOGRAPHY

Bernstein EF (ed) (1982) Noninvasive diagnostic techniques in vascular disease, 2nd Edn. CV Mosby Co, St Louis
Shepherd JT (1963) Physiology of the circulation in human limbs in health and disease. WB Saunders, Philadelphia
Strandness DE Jr (1969) Peripheral arterial disease, a physiologic approach. Little Brown, Boston
Strandness DE Jr, Sumner DS (1975) Hemodynamics for surgeons. Grune & Stratton, New York
Sumner DS (1977) The hemodynamics and pathophysiology of arterial disease. In: Rutherford RB (ed) Vascular Surgery, WB Saunders, Philadelphia, pp 25-46

REFERENCES

1. Berguer R, Hwang NHC (1974) Critical arterial stenosis. A theoretical and experimental solution. Ann Surg 180:39-50
2. May AG, DeWeese JA, Rob CG (1963) Hemodynamic effects of arterial stenosis. Surgery 53:513-524
3. Kindt GW, Youmans JR (1969) The effect of stricture length on critical arterial stenosis. Surg Gynecol Obstet 128:729-734
4. Flanigan DP, Tullis JP, Streeter VL, Whithouse WM Jr, Fry WJ, Stanley JC (1977) Multiple subcritical stenoses: effect on post-stenotic pressure and flow. Ann Surg 186:663-668
5. Spencer MP, Reid JM (1979) Quantitation of carotid stenosis with continuous-wave (C-W) Doppler ultrasound. Stroke 10: 326-330
6. Blackshear WM, Phillips DJ, Chikos PM, Harley JD, Thiele BL, Strandness DE Jr (1980) Carotid artery velocity patterns in normal and stenotic vessels. Stroke 11:67-71

7. Fell G, Phillips DJ, Chikos PM, Harley JD, Thiele BL, Strandness DE Jr (1981) Ultrasonic duplex scanning for disease of the carotid artery. Circulation 64:1191-1195

8. Giddens DP, Mabon RF, Cassanova RA (1976) Measurement of disordered flows distal to subtotal vascular stenosis in the thoracic aortas of dogs. Circ Res 39:112-119

9. Miller A, Lees RS, Kistler JP, Abbott WM (1980) Spectral analysis of arterial bruits (phonoangiography): experimental validation. Circulation 61:515-520

10. Sumner DS, Strandness DE Jr (1969) The relationship between calf blood flow and ankle pressure in patients with intermittent claudication. Surgery 65:763-771

11. Angelides NS, Nicolaides AN (1979) Simultaneous isotope clearance from the muscles of the calf and thigh. In: Puel P, Boccalon H, Enjalbert A (eds) Hemodynamics of the limbs - 1. GEPESC, Toulouse, pp 547-562

12. Raines JK, Darling RG, Buth J, Brewster DC, Austen WG (1976) Vascular laboratory criteria for the management of peripheral vascular disease of the lower extremities. Surgery 79:21-29

13. Tønnesen KH, Noer I, Paaske W, Sager Ph (1980) Classification of peripheral occlusive arterial disease based on symptoms, signs, and distal blood pressure measurements. Acta Chir Scand 146:101-104

14. Moore WS, Henry RE, Malone JM, Daly MJ, Patton D, Childers SJ (1981) Prospective use of xenon Xc 133 clearance for amputation level selection. Arch Surg 116:86-88

15. Evans DH, Barrie WW, Asher MJ, Bentley S, Bell PRF (1980) The relationship between ultrasonic pulsatility index and proximal arterial stenosis in a canine model. Circ Res 46:470-475

16. Johnston KW, Maruzzo BC, Cobbold RSC (1978) Doppler methods for quantitative measurement and localization of peripheral arterial occlusive disease by analysis of the blood velocity waveform. Ultrasound Med Biol 4:209-223

17. Olsen TS, Larsen B, Skriver EB, Enevoldsen E, Lassen NA (1981) Focal cerebral ischemia measured by the intra-arterial ^{133}xenon method. Stroke 12:736-744

18. Franzeck UK, Talke P, Bernstein EF, Goldbranson FL, Fronek A (1982) Transcutaneous PO_2 measurements in health and peripheral arterial occlusive disease. Surgery 91:156-163

19. Holstein P, Sager P, Lassen NA (1979) Wound healing in below knee amputations in relation to skin perfusion pressure. Acta Orthop Scand 50:49-58

20. Comerota AJ, Cranley JJ, Cook SE (1981) Real-time B-mode carotid imaging in diagnosis of cerebrovascular disease. Surgery 89:718-729

21. Sumner DS, Russell JB, Ramsey DE, Hajjar WM, Miles RD (1979) Noninvasive diagnosis of extracranial carotid arterial disease. A prospective evaluation of pulse-Doppler imaging and oculoplethysmography. Arch Surg 114:1222-1229

22. Baird RN, Bird DR, Clifford PC, Lusby RJ, Skidmore R, Woodcock JP (1980) Upstream stenosis: its diagnosis by Doppler signals from the femoral artery. Arch Surg 115:1316-1322

23. Sumner DS (1977) The hemodynamics and pathophysiology of arterial disease. In: Rutherford RB (ed) Vascular surgery. WB Saunders, Philadelphia
24. Russell JB, Miles RD, Ramsey DE, Sumner DS (1979) Effect of arterial stenosis on Doppler frequency spectrum. Proc. 32nd ACEMB 45 (Abstr 6.1)
25. Strandness DE Jr, Sumner DS (1975) Hemodynamics for surgeons. Grune & Stratton, New York
26. Sumner DS, Ramsey DE (1979) The relationship of segmental pressure measurements and calf blood flow to arteriographic findings. In: Puel P, Boccalon H, Enjalbert A (eds) Hemodynamics of the limbs - 1. GEPESC, Toulouse, pp 463-471
27. Yao ST (1970) Hemodynamic studies in peripheral arterial disease. Br J Surg 57:761-766

DISCUSSION: DON P. GIDDENS

Rather than discussing specific points of Dr. Sumner's excellent presentation, I would like to spend the next few minutes in what might be thought of as a continuation of his report. If we focus attention, for the moment, on an axisymmetric model of a localized lesion, additional insight may be gleaned regarding the effect of stenoses upon fluid dynamic behavior.

One experiment that is useful in defining departures from normal hemodynamics is that of measuring the velocity distal to a constriction while the degree of area reduction is increased. Fig. A.1 illustrates typical results found in the dog aorta when employing invasive instrumentation to measure velocity as a function of time. As the degree of constriction increases velocity disturbances can be noted, and the level of disturbance appears to increase as the stenosis area decreases. Several observations may be made. First, the disturbance character and level depends upon the site of measurement; and strong variations in both radial and axial position may be expected. Second, the results at a given measurement site are a function of the Reynolds number and frequency parameter of the flow and of the degree and contour of the constriction. Third, there is not a particularly simple way of classifying the nature of disturbances. For example, the underlying waveform may be altered with increasing stenosis as shown in Fig. A.2 (the underlying waveform is determined by ensemble averaging a number of beats using the EKG as a time reference). Additionally, the disturbances may be random and therefore expressed as a "turbulence" level as illustrated in Fig. A.3.

From the fluid dynamics viewpoint, then, several problems arise:
1. How may flow disturbances be characterized, particularly with regard to quantification?
2. How are these disturbances related to the lesion and to the severity of disease?
3. What are the most informative methods for treating flow and/or velocity data?
4. How can flow/velocity data be obtained noninvasively with sufficient accuracy to enable a practical application of answers to the three problems posed above?

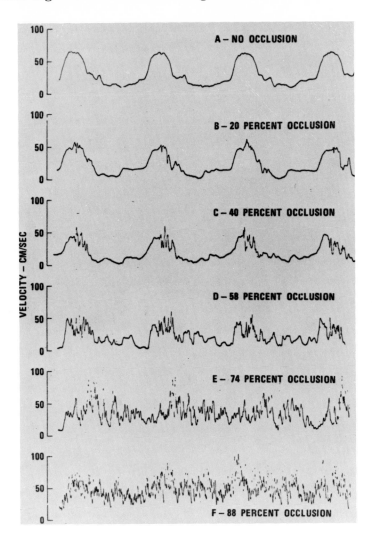

Fig. A.1   Typical results found in the dog aorta when employing invasive instrumentation to measure velocity as a function of time.

I would like to illustrate these problems with the aid of experimental data gained in laboratory models, where careful control of flow conditions and very precise measurements of velocity are possible.   Fig. A.4 illustrates measurements of velocity waveforms taken by laser Doppler anemometer at several locations

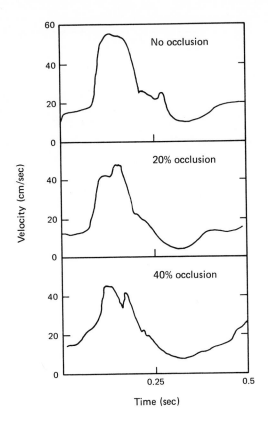

Fig. A.2 Changes in underlying hemodynamic waveform with
increasing stenosis.

distal to a smoothly contoured 50% stenosis model. Analysis of
these data using ensemble averaging, autocorrelation, and power
spectra techniques reveals that, for Reynolds numbers and frequency parameters typical of the dog aorta, three types of disturbance
patterns exist: coherent structures, shear layer instabilities,
and turbulence. Furthermore, all of these phenomena occur before
a constriction is sufficiently advanced to cause a significant
pressure gradient or flow reduction.

We may therefore list several "functional" disturbances in
velocity patterns in an order of appearance as the degree of stenosis increases: coherent structures, shear layer instabilities,

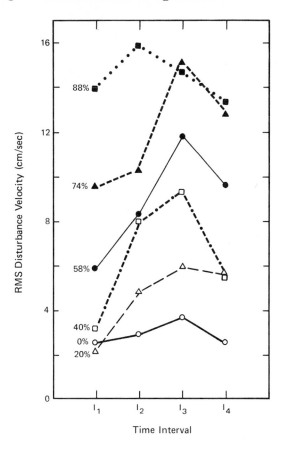

Fig. A.3   Variation of rms disturbance velocity as a function of time interval.

turbulence, waveform change, pressure drop, and flow reduction. If we are interested in detecting the mild lesion, then it is perhaps the presence of coherent disturbance structures we should be seeking.

In the real-life situation the picture presented above is complicated by several factors--one of the most dominant being the fact that atherosclerotic lesions tend to occur within complex vessel configurations such as bifurcations. Consequently, "undisturbed" flow patterns may not be well known, with the result that flow disturbances due to early lesions are difficult to identify.

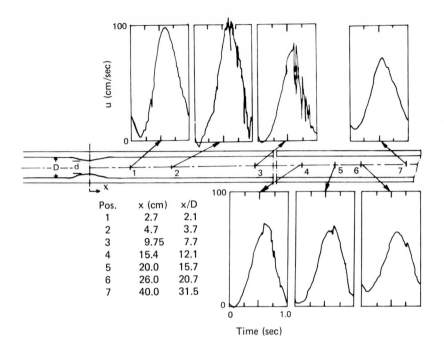

Fig. A.4 Measurements of velocity waveforms taken by laser Doppler anemometer at several locations distal to a smoothly contoured 50% stenosis model.

Fig. A.5 gives such an example using hydrogen bubble flow visualization in a model of the human carotid bifurcation. The Reynolds number and flow division for this photograph are within the range of normal human physiology, and the very strong secondary flow patterns are clearly evident. A composite schematic representation of velocity profiles measured by laser Doppler anemometer in this model is presented in Fig. A.6, and it is seen that the bifurcation contains regions of high velocity and low velocity in close proximity, as well as circumferential flow patterns.

In case there is any doubt that these detailed flow patterns may have "functional" significance, Fig. A.7 presents morphologic data taken from a human carotid bifurcation in a joint research project with Zarins and Glagov from the University of Chicago, we have shown that there exists a strong correlation between the

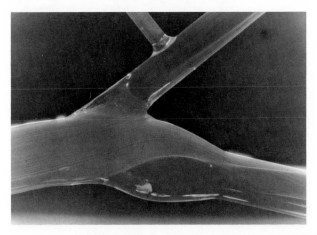

Fig. A.5 Hydrogen bubble flow visualization in a model of the human carotid bifurcation.

localization of lesions within the bifurcation and the sites of low flow velocity and wall shear stress.

To summarize I would like to suggest that the factors defining the "functional significance" of lesions might well be extended to include, not only reductions in flow, but also the various types of flow disturbances discussed here. To understand these phenomena

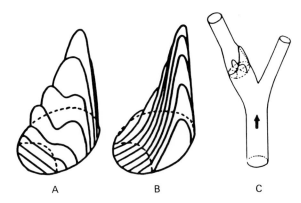

A   B   C

Fig. A.6 Composite schematic representation of velocity profiles measured by laser Doppler anemometer in a model of the human carotid bifurcation.

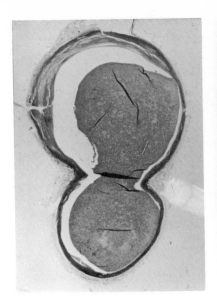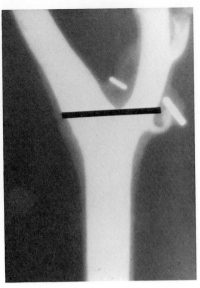

Fig. A.7 Atherosclerotic human carotid bifurcation. A strong
correlation exists between the localization of lesions within
the bifurcation and the sites of low flow velocity and wall
shear stress.

and their significance further, research must comprise detailed

fluid dynamic study of "normal" flow patterns, in addition to study

of departures from normalcy once lesions develop. Certainly,

improvement in noninvasive velocity measurement techniques to

allow more accurate data to be acquired in vivo is a corequisite

for advancement.

12

Correlation of Antemortem Angiography with Pathology

C. MILLER FISHER

In this workshop the long-range focus is on the use of arteriography in the study of the biology of atherosclerosis--its origin, evolution, and response to therapeutic measures. Information on the subject is meager, and to approach the problem we are obliged to turn to the vast experience of clinical radiology and the use of angiography in the diagnosis and treatment of vascular disease.

Arteriography is the most reliable and in many instances the only available method for the delineation of atherosclerosis in the living patient. It reveals arterial disease almost solely by alterations in the profile and contours of a column of dye; variations in the density of the column are of relatively little help to the radiologist. Clinically we know arteriography is good, but just how good is it?

THE CORONARY SYSTEM

In the past 19 years there have been eight studies in which coronary atherosclerosis visualized on conventional angiograms made in life has been compared with the postmortem findings. Hale and Jefferson (1) studied four cases within 6 months of angiography and concluded that arteriographic interpretation may underestimate the extent of the disease. Kemp et al. (2) reported the

Supported by a grant from the Freed Foundation, Washington, D.C.

findings in 29 patients who died from 1 day to 22 months after angiography. The angiographic estimations of the degree of stenosis were based on conversion of the diameters of the residual lumen judged in two projections into the area of cross section for comparison with the pathological estimate. There was agreement in 22 of 27 studies of the right coronary artery. The only significant error was a 30% underestimation. In four cases there was a minor underestimation of the disease. There was agreement in 25 of 26 studies of the left main coronary artery.

Vlodaver et al. (3) studied 10 patients, dividing each coronary tree into 19 gross segments. In addition, 55 histologic sections were prepared. The lumen was graded as <50% narrowing or >50% narrowing. Of 135 segments compared, there was agreement in 64%, underestimation in 32.5%, and overestimation in 3.5%. The segments particularly prone to underestimation were the intermediate segment of the right coronary artery, the left main coronary artery, and the proximal half of the left circumflex artery. The errors were attributed to failure to project X rays from an adequate number of directions, the presence of diffuse atheroma, and the occurrence of crescentic residual lumens.

Grondin et al.(4) studied 23 cases dying within 30 days of the angiographic examination, thereby avoiding the criticism of other studies in which a much longer period had elapsed. In 11 instances involving 9 patients there was a significant underestimation, 3 involving the right coronary artery and 8 involving the left coronary artery. Shrinkage due to postmortem fixation technique was deemed of no significance. Of a total of 145 angiographically significant lesions in the 23 cases, there was a discrepancy in only 11 (7.5%). However, in four cases underestimation of the severity of the lesion resulted in surgical decisions that contributed to failure. Schwartz et al. (5) studied the findings in 25 patients, 23 of whom had died within 4 months of angiography. Of 226 coronary segments studied, there was agreement in 79%, underestimation in 15%, and overestimation in 6%. The underestimations of 75% or more involved only 6% of cases. Major errors were attributed to crescent-shaped lumens, stenosis of 75% or more in the artery proximal to the segment being evaluated--i.e., significant obstruction of flow, the presence of prosthetic valves, and a uniform deposit of atheroma over long segments. Accuracy was less in the more distal parts of the tree. Hutchins et al. (6) reported on 28 patients, 23 of whom had died within 1 month of angiography. Of 315 arterial segments studied, in 294 (93%) the difference was 50% or less; in 21 segments (7%) the difference was greater than 50%. Underestimations occurred in 15 (5%) and overestimations in 6 (2%). Errors were attributed to overlapping of vessels and vasospasm at the catheter tip.

Arnett et al. (7) reported the findings in 61 coronary arteries from 10 patients who died within 57 days of cardiac operation. The arteries were cut into a total of 476 5-mm segments from each of which two histologic sections were prepared. The percentage reduction in diameter of the lumen in the angiogram was compared with the percentage reduction in the cross-sectional area on pathologic examination. Each coronary tree was divided into nine major subdivisions. In 61 major divisions analyzed there were no overestimations. No underestimations were made when the degree of histologic narrowing was 50% or less. Underestimations by one or more experienced angiographers were frequent in the group with 51-75% narrowing (7 of 8 divisions) and in the group with greater than 75% narrowing (17 of 42 divisions). Underestimations were more frequent in the left main and proximal left circumflex coronary arteries. Of the 10 patients studied, all had narrowings missed by at least one angiographer. In 4 of 10, more than one severe narrowing was missed. The error rate for severe narrowing was 40% (17 of 42). The presence of diffuse atherosclerosis seemed to account for most of the angiographically missed narrowings.

Isner et al. (8) studied the left main coronary artery (LMCA) alone in 28 patients. In 13 of the 28 patients the degree of narrowing of the LMCA was underestimated by two of three

experienced angiographers, and in 10 patients it was overestimated, making a total of 71% with errors. Of 12 LMCAs narrowed
76-100% histologically, 6 were underestimated at angiography. Of
12 LMCAs narrowed 51-75% histologically all 12 were either under-
or overestimated. Of four LMCAs narrowed 26-50% histologically,
two were overestimated by two of three angiographers. The errors
were attributed to diffuse narrowing, crescentic lumen, the short
length and varying course of the LMCA, and an inadequate number
of projections. The discrepancies in the overestimates were not
as wide as in the underestimates.

In summary, angiographic underestimation of the degree of
coronary narrowing was more common than overestimation. The
several explanations of errors included: diffuse atherosclerosis,
an inadequate number of projections, crescentic lumen, overlapping
of arteries, observer variation, severe and more proximal stenosis,
prosthetic valves, vasospasm, prolonged period between angiography
and death, peripheral location of the plaque, and shrinkage
artifact during fixation of tissue.

In angiography is the plaque visualized as plain atherosclerosis or is it complicated by hemorrhage into plaque, ulceration,
or mural thrombus? None of these was described by Arnett et al.
(7) who referred only to irregularity of the surfaces of the
plaques. Ridolfi and Hutchins (9) using serial sections of
coronary plaques found intimal ulceration; plaque erosion, disruption, and rupture; or mural thrombus in 90% of plaques associated with myocardial infarction days to weeks old (81 or 90
lesions). These plaque changes were focal and measured roughly
0.3 mm. Clearly, the plaque revealed by angiography may not be
uncomplicated "pure" atheroma.

Is coronary angiography accurate enough to be used to monitor
the progression or regression of atherosclerosis? The answer is
yes, but only if the changes are in the range of 25% of the
original lumen, a goal somewhat beyond current expectations. Is

angiography sensitive enough to be used to detect premature or early deposition of atheroma which may signal a special proclivity? In the series of Arnett et al. (7), estimations were more accurate with luminal narrowings of 50% or less. It is conceivable therefore that angiography would be useful for this purpose. Are certain coronary arteries or segments thereof sites of predilection for atherosclerosis and therefore likely to provide especially favorable conditions for monitoring? Montenegro and Eggen (10) in a pathology study found the pattern of distribution of lesions strikingly similar in 2964 sets of coronary arteries. Is a particular coronary artery segment visualized by angiography with a special or regular reliability and therefore more dependable for monitoring? In the study of Hutchins et al. (6), all the larger proximal arterial segments were equally subject to errors in interpretation.

Interobserver variability is not a seriously limiting factor, and consistency of interpretation by each observer can be determined. It is acknowledged that reproducibility on successive angiograms is desirable, but generally it is not mentioned.

Last but not least, conventional coronary angiography is not entirely safe, a point of particular importance because of its proposed use in the detection of early, asymptomatic disease. Digital subtraction angiography, which has been introduced recently, does not have as good resolution as conventional angiography.

Although it is precisely in heart disease more than in any other organ that we are particularly dependent on indirect means of investigating the arteries, conventional angiography is not ideal for detecting early lesions that might serve as the basis for the introduction of preventive measures or therapeutic options before the lesions become advanced. It probably is not sufficiently sensitive for monitoring moderate degrees of the progression and regression of lesions.

THE CAROTID SYSTEM

The origin of the internal carotid artery (ICA) is a site of
special predilection for atheroma formation. Mehnert and Chiari
11) found atherosclerosis as severe in the ICA as in the aorta.
It is localized to the proximal 2.5 cm of the cervical segment
of the artery, and only very small plaques are ever found more
distally in the pre-petrous part of the artery. When the plaque
narrows the lumen of the ICA to 3.5 mm or less from its original
diameter of 7-9 mm, a systolic bruit is created, which is audible
with a stethoscope and can be evaluated by phonoangiography (12).
In the carotid system, therefore, unlike the coronary system,
correlation studies involve a single plaque in a large artery at
a predictable site.

From the time of Moniz it was clear that angiographic por-
trayal of the state of the carotid system was sufficiently accurate for practical purposes. With the introduction of surgery of
the ICA, examination of the endarterectomy specimen at the time
of operation showed good correlation between the residual lumen
demonstrated angiographically and the anatomical findings. There
seemed to be no need for a special investigation of the matter,
with the result that there have been only two systematic studies
comparing the accuracy of angiographic interpretation with the
findings on gross examination of the endarterectomy specimen.
Gryspeerdt (13) in 22 carotid specimens found that the appearances
in antemortem angiograms were exactly similar to those in postmortem angiograms and the histologic sections, accurately reflecting the pathological changes in the vessel wall and the
degree of luminal constriction. The second study is that of
Kistler et al. (14). At the Massachusetts General Hospital it
has been the custom to report carotid narrowing in terms of the
diameter of the residual lumen (in mm) rather than the percentage
reduction of the original lumen, and this method of reporting was
used in the latter study. Thirty-nine specimens were available.
Angiograms were taken in two planes, corrected for magnification,

and the diameter of the residual lumen was measured to the nearest 0.1 mm with a calibrated X7 magnifier. When the stenosis could be identified in two angiographic planes, the effective residual-lumen diameter was calculated as the square root of the product of the two orthogonal diameters. The endarterectomy specimens were obtained at the time of surgery and serial coronal sections were made in the fresh state. The residual lumen was measured in the coronal plane with a ruler graduated in mm. Subsequently, the specimens were placed in formalin and studied after fixation. Fixation did not appreciably change the residual-lumen diameter. In 35 of 39 cases the radiographic estimate of the residual-lumen diameter agreed to within 0.5 mm with the diameter measured in the endarterectomy specimen. The angiogram interpretation overestimated the residual lumen by 0.8 mm in one patient (2 vs 1.2 mm) and underestimated it by 0.8 mm in another patient (2 vs 2.8 mm). In two cases the angiogram was unsatisfactory.

All endarterectomy specimens had stenosis of the distal common carotid artery and proximal ICA. The residual-lumen diameter ranged from a pinpoint to greater than 2 mm, an indication of the great thickness of the plaque. Six of the 39 specimens contained an intraluminal thrombus at the time of endarterectomy. In each of these six the clot was not at the narrowest point of the lumen, but either proximal (one specimen) or immediately distal (five specimens), i.e., it did not contribute to the narrowing of the residual lumen. Fourteen specimens showed evidence of hemorrhage into the arteriosclerotic plaque. In none of these 14 did the hemorrhage produce further narrowing of the lumen at the point of maximal stenosis. Ten of the specimens had an elliptical lumen. In all specimens the majority of the atheromas were located at the posterior aspect of the bifurcation. The stenosis in all cases was located within 1 cm of the bifurcation of the common carotid artery. The length of the stenosis varied from 0.5 to 10 mm. In most specimens, however, the length of the most stenotic segment was quite short (0.5-1 mm). One specimen had an ulcer in the prestenotic portion of the lumen. Pathologically, the residual-

lumen diameter was less than 1.5 mm in 34 of 37 cases. The mean
difference between the angiographic and the pathological lumen was
calculated for all specimens that were not too small to measure
accurately, and was 0.26 mm. The accuracy of carotid angiography
when the lumen is severely narrowed is amply demonstrated.

There have been several pathological studies of carotid
endarterectomy specimens in which attention has been directed to
the occurrence of ulceration and hemorrhage into the carotid
plaque rather than the degree of stenosis, providing findings that
bear on the accuracy with which the atherosclerotic process itself
is being monitored. Julian et al. (15) in 17 cases of proved
ulceration on gross examination concluded that angiography failed
to show any consistent pattern. Blaisdell et al. (16) classified
surgical bifurcation plaque specimens according to the degree of
occlusion and the presence of macroscopic ulceration. Four
lesions narrowed the lumen by 10-29%, 2 of which were ulcerated
and 2 were not; 17 lesions narrowed the lumen by 30-59%, 13 of
which were ulcerated (76%) and 4 were not; 10 lesions narrowed
the lumen by 60-89%, of which 8 were ulcerated and 2 were not; and
19 lesions narrowed the lumen by 90-99% of which 15 were ulcerated
(79%) and 4 were not. Of the 50 lesions, 22 had large ulcerations
(4 mm in diameter or larger), 16 had smaller superficial ulcerations and 12 were not ulcerated. The radiologic diagnosis was
correct in 43 instances for an accuracy of 86%. When the lumen
was narrowed by more than 30%, four out of five lesions were
ulcerated. Houser et al. (17) observed that in 322 carotid
systems evaluated for surgical endarterectomy, a close correlation
was found between the predicted degree of stenosis and the surgical finding. Ulcerations identified on angiograms invariably were
confirmed in the specimens. Minor degrees of ulceration, although
present in most patients with marked stenosis, were not visualized
on the angiograms.

Olemann et al. (18), studying 40 carotid endarterectomy
specimens microscopically, found that the main occluding mass was
an atheromatous plaque in 75%, hemorrhage into the plaque in 15%,

and a fibrin mass in 10%. Sixty percent of the 33 specimens from patients with cerebrovascular symptoms showed hemorrhage into the main plaque. In only one-third of these did it add appreciably to the mass of the occluding tissue, but in some cases it furnished the nidus for the deposition of a mural thrombus that finally occluded the lumen. A fibrin mural thrombus was present on the surface of the plaque in 10 of 12 patients with severe stenosis and a history of cerebrovascular transient ischemic attacks.

Hertzer et al. (19), using scanning electron microscopy, studied the luminal surface of seven carotid endarterectomy specimens and demonstrated surface abnormalities that were not visible in preoperative angiograms or by direct inspection after surgery. Five specimens contained distinct atheromatous ulcers that measured between 80 and 550 μm in diameter. Two specimens contained adherent intraluminal thrombi measuring 400 to 600 μm in diameter. The other two specimens both showed severe carotid stenosis, but had normal endothelium. Aspirin but not heparin had been used preoperatively. Correlation studies using transmission EM and light microscopy were not made. In all likelihood such minor abnormalities would not be relevant in angiographic monitoring of carotid plaques.

Edwards et al. (20), analyzing the findings in 50 surgical carotid specimens, found grossly visible ulceration in 20. Twelve of these were diagnosed angiographically and eight were not, giving an accuracy of only 60%. The degree of stenosis was not a factor. Of the 30 carotid specimens that were grossly free of ulceration, 17 (57%) had been incorrectly interpreted as showing ulceration. Ten of the 17 had intramural hemorrhage and subintimal hematoma into an atherosclerotic plaque. Edwards et al. (21) further described the subintimal hematomas into atherosclerotic plaques in 12 of the 50 carotid endarterectomy specimens. Eight had no associated ulceration, while four had shallow ulceration. Ten hematomas were associated with carotid stenosis of greater than 70%, two with carotid stenosis of less than 70%. Seven of the hematomas appeared angiographically as sharply demarcated, rounded filling defects with smooth contours and could be eccentrically or concentrically placed. The presence of hemosiderin indicated that the hemorrhages predated surgery and were not the result of surgery. In all cases surgery was performed between 24 and 48 h after angiography. In 4 specimens the hemorrhage had produced a false picture of ulceration on the angiogram. The authors attributed the hemorrhage to rupture of a small artery or venule within the plaque, rather than to dissection into the artery from the base of an ulcer.

It seems that the presence of subintimal hemorrhage would have to be considered in the interpretation of changes in size when monitoring the progression or regression of carotid plaques.

An angiography-pathology correlation of moderate degrees of carotid stenosis has not been reported. Because carotid atherosclerosis is a herald of disease elsewhere, it could conceivably be used as an early warning signal that preventive measures were indicated. However, conventional angiography of the carotid system is not an entirely safe procedure, and a series of several invasive studies would not be justified. Digital subtraction angiography produces images that fall short of those obtained by conventional angiograms, but it is possible that it could reliably detect moderate stenosis and serve for monitoring purposes.

What about the rest of the cerebral arterial system? First of all, the cerebral arteries are not sites of high predilection for atherosclerosis. Furthermore, I was unable to find reports of an angiography-pathology correlation for the common carotid, vertebral, basilar, intracranial internal carotid, middle cerebral, anterior cerebral, posterior cerebral, and ophthalmic arteries, or their outlying branches. At sites other than the carotid sinus non-atherosclerotic disease processes complicate the picture--dissection, fibromuscular dysplasia, embolism, arteritis, "primary" thrombosis, and processes of indeterminate nature--although atherosclerosis is still by far the most frequent. The carotid siphons in particular are subject to calcification which regularly is demonstrated in plain X rays of the skull. The calcification lies partly within the inner media and partly in shallow atherosclerotic plaques that seem not to evolve into severely stenotic plaques (22). It is remarkable that atheroma within the carotid sinus progresses regularly, often becoming occlusive while, 5 inches distally, atheroma that also appears very early usually remains small and poses no threat. The carotid siphon has the distinctive feature of lying within a venous channel, the cavernous sinus. Because of its sinuous shape the siphon is a difficult place in which to determine the degree of arterial narrowing. Also, in several cases the main occluding tissue has been multilayered thrombus rather than atheroma. Similarly thrombotic occluding masses have been found in the basilar artery. To be sure, monitoring the cerebral arteries for atherosclerosis poses many uncertainties. Atheroma in the outlying convexity branches of the cerebral arteries reflects the presence of severe hypertension plus an atheromatous diathesis, and even though monitoring were accurate, it would be at the end-stage of the disease. Fluorscein angiography can be used to depict the retinal arteries, but atherosclerosis has not been recognized in arteries of this size.

ARTERIES OF THE LOWER EXTREMITIES

Despite our vast knowledge of disease of the aorta and iliac, femoral, popliteal, and tibial arteries, not a single account of a between-antemortem angiography and methodical pathology correlation was found. Certainly angiography has proved sufficiently accurate for clinical purposes. Lindbom (23) included in his extensive investigation one case in which there had been an arteriogram three weeks before death. The appearance was the same as in the postmortem angiogram, but it was not clear if there had also been a postmortem pathology study. He concluded that an intimal thickening of 0.5 mm in the femoral artery could be detected angiographically when seen in profile. It is a common impression among surgeons that the size of the atheromatous plaque is much greater than the apparent degree of stenosis shown by angiography (24).

The arteries of the lower extremities are sites of predilection for atherosclerosis, and in Lindbom's series (23) the lower extremity was more often the site of arterial thrombosis than the coronary system. Early atherosclerotic formation occurred more often in the thigh than in the leg. There were two particular sites of predilection, the superficial femoral artery in Hunter's canal (the middle third of the thigh) and the proximal part of the popliteal artery. Either or both of these sites could be monitored for early discovery of premature atherosclerosis or the detection of progression and regression of the atherosclerotic process. Digital subtraction angiography might well prove adequate for this purpose.

Again, in the case of femoral and popliteal plaques, intimal hemorrhages were widespread and large, a reminder that not all arteriographic filling defects mean pure lipid. Lindbom (23) was of the opinion that these hemorrhages were the factor that caused intimal thickenings to grow and encroach upon the lumen. Histologic preparations suggested that the hemorrhage was intramural and did not signify transintimal penetration from the lumen.

Pathology studies of atherosclerosis formed in saphenous vein grafts used in aorto-coronary bypass surgery have not been coupled with antemortem angiography (25).

As already mentioned, no investigations of a correlation between antemortem arteriography and pathology have been performed with the aorta as subject. Such an investigation would help determine with what proficiency plaques of slight to moderate thickness might be delineated. Unfortunately, digital subtraction angiography of the aorta and iliac arteries has had limited success because of movement artifact.

There are no reports of correlative studies of the renal, mesenteric, and coeliac arteries. However, neither are they sites of special predilection for atherosclerosis. The arteries of the upper extremities, except for the subclavian artery, usually show only very shallow plaques despite severe atherosclerosis elsewhere.

CONCLUSION

Conventional arteriography is highly efficient in the clinical delineation of atherosclerotic disease, particularly when the process is advanced. Assuming that thick fibrous plaques will be more resistant to reversal than plaques at an earlier stage, focus must be on the detection of less advanced disease. From a clinical point of view it would be desirable to discover an individual proclivity to disease at the earliest time. Our goal, therefore, is to find sentinel or tell-tale plaques that can be monitored with safe, relatively noninvasive techniques in patients with a family history of atherosclerosis. If conventional angiography or digital subtraction angiography is to be used, the two most likely sites appear to be the femoral artery in Hunter's canal and the origin of the internal carotid artery. It is possible, however, that plaques of predilection may be less susceptible to reversal and hence less sensitive for monitoring purposes than plaques at other sites. But where these secondary sites are located remains unknown.

SUMMARY

Studies comparing antemortem angiographic appearances with pathologic findings are not numerous. There have been eight such studies of the coronary arteries and two of the internal carotid artery. There have been no studies of the aorta, iliac, femoral, renal, vertebral, basilar, cerebral, and brachial arteries. In the coronary system underestimation of the degree of arterial narrowing is more common than overestimation, even with generous allowances for discrepancies. In the carotid system angiography provides an accurate picture when the stenosis is severe. In the internal carotid artery, hemorrhages into plaque, ulceration, and mural thrombus complicate the interpretation of changes in a plaque in terms of pure atheroma.

Conventional angiography could be used for monitoring early plaque formation and the progression and regression of plaques, but its invasive and less than perfectly safe character precludes routine serial examinations. Digital angiography may well be adequate for monitoring carotid and femoral atherosclerosis.

REFERENCES

1. Hale G, Jefferson K (1963) Technique and interpretation of selective coronary arteriography in man. Br Heart J 25:644-654
2. Kemp HG, Evans H, Elliott WC, Gorlin R (1967) Diagnostic accuracy of selective coronary cinearteriography. Circulation 36:526-533
3. Vlodaver Z, Frech R, Van Tassel RA, Edwards JE (1973) Correlation of the antemortem coronary arteriogram and the postmortem specimen. Circulation 47:162-169
4. Grondin CM, Dyrda I, Pasternac A, Campeau L, Bourassa MG, Lesperance J (1974) Discrepancies between cineangiographic and postmortem findings in patients with coronary artery disease and recent myocardial revascularization. Circulation 49:703-708
5. Schwartz JN, Kong Y, Hackel DB, Bartel AG (1975) Comparison of angiographic and postmortem findings in patients with coronary artery disease. Am J Cardiol 36:174-178
6. Hutchins GM, Bulkley BH, Ridolfi RL, Griffith LSC, Lohr FT, Piasio MA (1977) Correlation of coronary arteriograms and left ventriculograms with postmortem studies. Circulation 56:32-37
7. Arnett EN, Isner JM, Redwood DR, Kent KM, Baker WP, Ackerstein H, Roberts WC (1979) Coronary artery narrowing in coronary heart disease: Comparison of cineangiographic and necropsy findings. Ann Int Med 91:350-356
8. Isner JM, Kishel J, Kent KM, Ronan JA, Ross AM, Roberts WC (1981) Accuracy of angiographic determination of left main coronary arterial narrowing. Circulation 63:1056-1064
9. Ridolfi RL, Hutchins GM (1977) The relationship between coronary artery lesions and myocardial infarcts. Ulceration of atherosclerotic plaques precipitating coronary thrombosis. Am Heart J 93:468-486
10. Montenegro MR, Eggen DA (1968) Topography of atherosclerosis in the coronary arteries. Lab Invest 18:586-593
11. Chiari H (1905) Ueber das Verhalten des Teilungswinkels der Carotis communis bei der Endarteriitis chronica deformans. Verh Dtsch Pathol Ges 9:326-330

12. Duncan GW, Gruber JO, Dewey CF, Myers GS, Lees RS (1975) Evaluation of carotid stenosis by phonoangiography. N Engl J Med 293:1124-1128
13. Gryspeerdt GL (1968) Comparison of angiographic and pathological appearances in atherosclerosis of the carotid artery. Br J Radiol 41:805 (abstract)
14. Kistler JP, Lees RS, Miller A, Crowell RM, Roberson G (1981) Correlation of spectral phonoangiography and carotid angiography with gross pathology in carotid stenosis. N Engl J Med 305:417-419
15. Julian OC, Dye WS, Javid H, Hunter JA (1963) Ulcerative lesions of the carotid artery bifurcation. Arch Surg 86:803-809
16. Blaisdell FW, Glickman M, Trunkey DD (1974) Ulcerated atheroma of the carotid artery. Arch Surg 108:491-496
17. Houser OW, Sundt TMN, Holman CB, Sandok BA, Burton RC (1974) Atherosclerotic disease of the carotid artery. Correlation of angiographic, clinical and surgical findings. J Neurosurg 41:321-331
18. Olemann RG, Crowell RM, Roberson GH, Fisher CM (1975) Surgical treatment of extracranial carotid occlusive disease. Clin Neurosurg 22:214-263
19. Hertzer NR, Beven EG, Benjamin SP (1977) Ultramicroscopic ulcerations and thrombi of the carotid bifurcation. Arch Surg 112:1394-1402
20. Edwards JH, Kricheff II, Riles T, Imparato A (1979) Angiographically undetected ulceration of the carotid bifurcation as a cause of embolic stroke. Radiology 132:369-373
21. Edwards JH, Kricheff II, Gorstein F, Riles T, Imparato A (1979) Atherosclerotic subintimal hematoma of the carotid artery. Radiology 133:123-129
22. Fisher CM, Gore I, Okake N, White PD (1965) Calcification of the carotid siphon. Circulation 32:538-548
23. Lindbom A (1950) Arteriosclerosis and arterial thrombosis in the lower limb. A roentgenological study. Acta Radiol [Suppl] (Stockh) 80:1-80
24. Haimovici H (1968) Patterns of arteriosclerotic lesions of the lower extremity. Ann NY Acad Sci 149:997-1021
25. Lie JT, Lawrie GM, Morris GC (1977) Aortacoronary bypass saphenous vein graft atherosclerosis. Am J Cardiol 40:906-914

DISCUSSION: JAMES DEWEESE

Dr. Fisher is to be complimented on his extensive review of
reported correlations of antemortem angiography with pathology.
The atherosclerotic lesions most frequently evaluated have been
in the coronary vessels, in the internal carotid artery at the
carotid bifurcation, and in the femoral-popliteal arteries as
they pass through Hunter's canal (1). These lesions may produce
narrowing of the blood vessel with the potential for decreasing
blood flow or may ulcerate, providing a nidus for peripheral
embolization.

Dr. Miller has reviewed eight reports that indicate there is
good correlation between the angiographic identification of a
narrowing of a coronary artery and the pathologic findings. It
is rare for an angiographer to miss a significant lesion. On the
other hand, the degree of stenosis is underestimated by the
angiographer in 11-33% of cases and overestimated in 3-6%. It
has not been possible to routinely demonstrate ulcerations of
coronary arteries by current angiographic techniques.

We have been primarily interested in studying lesions of the
carotid artery. The lesions are usually sharply localized to the
distal common carotid and proximal external and internal carotid
arteries. The entire lesion can be removed intact at carotid
endarterectomy. The vessel can be intubated, fixed, and then
longitudinal sectioning of the vessel allows direct visual
correlation with the angiogram and with histologic appearance.
Alternatively, multiple cross sections can be made for histologic
correlation.

In 1970 we reported the results of angiographic and pathologic changes in 34 carotid endarterectomy specimens (2). The
cross-sectional area percent stenosis produced by the lesion was
estimated on the angiograms and endarterectomy specimens. The
correlation was within 10% in 82% of the specimens. Twelve
percent of the angiograms overestimated the degree of the stenosis and 6% underestimated it. A possible explanation for the

lack of correlation is that on occasions the residual lumen is elliptical or crescent-shaped rather than circular. An accurate angiographic demonstration of the luminal size would require radiographs in multiple projections. We were not as successful as Blaisdell and Edwards in demonstrating ulcerations. This may have been related to the fact that our angiograms at that time were four vessel arch aortograms and not carotid arteriograms. On the other hand, Edward's 59% false positive rate and 38% false negative rate for angiographic demonstration of ulcerations would indicate that even current radiographic techniques may not be accurate in the diagnosis of ulcerations.

The most frequent site of atherosclerotic narrowing of the femoral-popliteal arteries is in Hunter's canal. Although these lesions may appear sharply localized on angiograms at the time of operation it is usually necessary to endarterectomize a 10-15 cm segment of vessel to find a more normal site to end the endarterectomy.

It is possible to make multiple cross-sectional cuts of these specimens and compare the luminal size to that seen on angiograms. We have done this on four occasions and found there was a very close correlation between the angiographic measurements and the pathologic measurements. As Dr. Fisher has indicated, this may be a fruitful area for future studies.

I would like to mention one other lesion that may lend itself to angiographic and pathologic correlation. This is the localized lesion of the proximal renal artery, frequently responsible for reno-vascular hypertension.

In conclusion I would like to review the reported reasons for poor correlation of angiography and pathology which are not related to technique. These include (1) inadequate opacification, usually secondary to proximal critical stenosis, (2) the presence of crescent shaped lesions, (3) a uniform, diffuse intimal thickening, (4) uncontrollable distractors, such as prosthetic valves or overlapping vessels, and (5) (?) shrinking during fixation.   I put this question mark here because I think it requires further discussion.   Most observers have not felt that this contributes to lack of correlation.

REFERENCES

1. DeWeese JA, Van de Berg L, May AG, Rob CG (1964)   Stenoses of arteries of the lower extremity.   Arch Surg 89:806-816
2. DeWeese JA, May AG, Lipchik EG, Rob CG (1970)   Anatomic and hemodynamic correlations in carotid artery stenosis.   Stroke 1:149-157

13

Correlation of Postmortem Angiography with Pathologic Anatomy
Quantitation of Atherosclerotic Lesions

CHRISTOPHER K. ZARINS, MICHAEL A. ZATINA,
AND SEYMOUR GLAGOV

Angiography is a useful and specific clinical means for identifying and assessing atherosclerotic lesions. However, since it provides images only of the arterial lumen, quantitative assessment of the extent and complexity of atherosclerotic disease can only be surmised indirectly. Accurate evaluation of lumen contour by angiography in vivo is complicated by vessel motion, angulation, branching, and overlapping as well as by variations in x-ray technique, magnification, projection, and dye concentration. Inconsistencies in imaging are compounded by observer variability in interpretation of angiographic images (1), making quantitative angiographic assessment of disease difficult. In an effort to gauge the accuracy of angiography, a number of investigators have compared the degree of lumen stenosis as seen on angiography in vivo to the degree of stenosis as seen at postmortem examination, and have come to the conclusion that angiography in vivo underestimates stenoses (2-6). This discrepancy is thought to occur because plaques cause arterial lumens to be "eccentric and slit-like" (2,6) rather than rounded, so that many angiographic projections may show deceptively wide lumens. In most validation studies, excised arteries were fixed by simple immersion without

Supported in part by HL 15062-08 (IVe), NSF CME 7921551, and T32 HL 7237

restoration of in vivo vessel configuration. Errors introduced by
fixation of collapsed vessels may be considerable (8) and the assumption that examination of such vessels provides a suitable standard by which to validate angiography has not been substantiated.

The purpose of this report is to delineate the problems
encountered in attempting to establish a consistent methodology
for making comparisons between angiographic images and atherosclerotic disease. We will consider two aspects of the problem.
First, what are the technical problems encountered in preparing
anatomic specimens for validation studies of angiographic findings
and second, to what extent can atherosclerosis be quantitated by
angiographic or by histologic examination. We will compare data
obtained from postmortem angiograms with data obtained from microscopic sections of arteries fixed while distended at physiologic
pressures. We will set forth the precautions required for validating in vivo measurements from postmortem specimens. In particular, we will demonstrate the pitfalls encountered in specimen
preparation and in the quantitative assessment of extent, severity,
progression, and regression of atherosclerotic disease by angiography. We will show how measurements on light microscopic cross
sections of arteries fixed while distended may be related to
extent, severity, and complication of atherosclerotic disease.

VALIDATION OF ANGIOGRAPHIC FINDINGS FROM THE STUDY
OF ANATOMIC SPECIMENS: METHODS OF PREPARATION

Restoring Lumen and Lesion Configuration

Arterial lumens visualized by angiography in vivo are distended
by a mean intraluminal pressure of at least 80 mmHg, while most
postmortem examinations are usually performed on undistended,
collapsed arteries. Examination of atherosclerotic arteries fixed
while distended reveals that lumen cross sections are almost
always round (7,8) (Fig. 1) and only rarely have the irregular,
triangular or slit-like lumen contours so often seen in immersion-
fixed vessels (2,6).

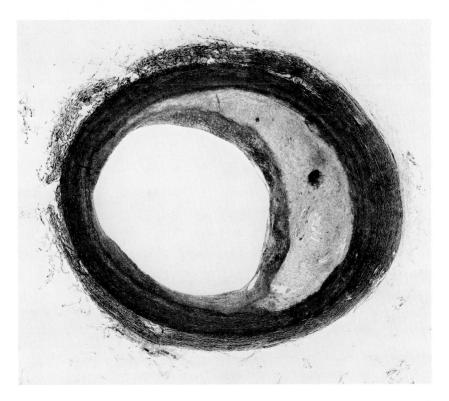

Fig. 1 Cross section of perfusion-fixed human carotid artery with
a large intimal plaque occupying more than 50% of the area bounded
by the internal elastic lamina. Verhoeff van Gieson stain. Note
the eccentric nature of the plaque and the round lumen. The
subendothelial "fibrous cap" appears as a well-organized, layered
structure comparable in thickness to and continuous with the
adjacent media. The external contour of the artery is oval and
the lesion appears to be sequestered to one side.

Wolinsky and Glagov (7) redistended rabbit aortas at various
intraluminal pressures from 0 to 200 mmHg and found that aortic
radius increased and wall thickness decreased markedly until
diastolic blood pressure levels were achieved. They noted a
two-fold increase in aortic radius from 0 mmHg to 100 mmHg, which
represents a four-fold increase in lumen cross-sectional area.
At higher pressures there was little further change; diastolic
pressure levels were sufficient to distend vessels completely.
While vessel dimension changes between zero and diastolic pressure

may be somewhat less when the artery wall is thickened by rigid
intimal lesions, significant change in dimensions can, nevertheless, be expected when intraluminal distending pressure is below
diastolic levels. It is, therefore, prudent to maintain at least
diastolic pressures during fixation. Differences in distending
pressures above diastolic levels will introduce little error while
variations below diastolic levels are likely to result in poor
reproduction of in vivo configurations.

Perfusion Fixation

Redistention of arteries to normal dimensions may be accomplished
in situ or after excision of the vessel. The artery should be
cannulated at each end or at two points in the arterial tree: one
proximal and one distal to the segment under study. One cannula
is used for introduction of contrast medium or fixative and the
other is used to control the rate of fluid runoff and to monitor
the pressure in the vessel to be studied. We routinely use an
intraluminal pressure of 100 mmHg to distend vessels during
postmortem angiography and during fixation. Intraluminal pressure
should be measured directly when possible, for pressure within the
artery lumen may be considerably lower than the pressure in the
system proximal to the inflow cannula due to resistance in the
cannula, runoff into the capillary bed, and leaks from unligated
branches. Perfusion fixation of an entire arterial tree can be
accomplished in situ, but because of rapid fluid runoff (9) such
a procedure usually requires relatively high flow rates to maintain
adequate distending pressure. In general, the more branches that
are ligated and the smaller the segment of arterial tree being
perfused, the more successful the redistension. Redistension
with adequate pressure will restore both circumferential and
longitudinal arterial dimensions.

In studies where careful postmortem perfusion fixation of
coronary arteries was carried out, there was good correlation
between angiography and pathology and the coronary artery lumens

were noted to be round (8,10). Schwartz (11) studied coronary
arteries that were fixed under pressure and noted that angiography
occasionally underestimated the percent stenosis and that in four
instances the lumen was "slit-like." Such errors are probably
due to failure to monitor intraluminal pressure during the course
of vessel fixation and probably could be eliminated by maintaining
intraluminal arterial pressure during perfusion.

Arteries obtained at autopsy have usually been cooled to
temperatures ranging from 4°C (morgue refrigerator) to room
temperature before redistention and fixation procedures are
carried out. It is reasonable to assume that lesion components
such as lipids are likely to vary in consistency and physical
state depending on temperature. Such differences may affect
distensibility. Although there are as yet no studies which
document or quantitate such an effect, we have taken the precau-
tion to perfuse with contrast medium or fixative maintained at
37°C. Depending on the thickness of the arterial wall under
study, fixation under pressure is carried out for 30-120 min.
Fixation is enhanced by simultaneous immersion in fixative once
stable distending pressures have been established. For ultrastructural studies, buffering of the perfusate may be important
for minimizing cytologic artifacts.

Shrinkage Due to Tissue Processing

Fixation in formalin and paraffin processing for histologic
examination results in tissue shrinkage of 30-40% (12). Thus,
measurements obtained from fixed and processed postmortem tissues
will be smaller than the same dimensions measured in vivo.
Shrinkage does not affect all dimensions equally. In 10 human
superficial femoral arteries we found that the wall thickness
decreased 36% due to shrinkage, but that lumen diameter decreased
only 20% (Table 1).

Shrinkage rates may vary from artery to artery and in relation
to the extent of disease or composition of lesions. For example,

288 C. K. Zarins, M. A. Zatina, and S. Glagov

Table 1. Dimension Changes in the Human Superficial Femoral Artery Due to Fixation and Tissue Processing

	External Diameter (mm)	Lumen Diameter (mm)	Wall Thickness (mm)
Prefixation angiography	8.6 ± 0.5	5.9 ± 1.1	1.4 ± 0.5
Histologic sections[a]	6.6 ± 0.9	4.7 ± 1.2	0.9 ± 0.4
Percent difference	-23%	-20%	-36%

[a] $p < .005$, compared to prefixation dimension.
Note: Values are mean ± SD; n = 10.

in a study of coarcted monkey thoracic aortas (13,14), we compared lumen diameters measured on angiograms made in vivo with lumen diameters measured at identical sites on angiograms of the perfusion- fixed postmortem specimens as well as on the corresponding histologic sections. There was a 31% decrease in lumen diameter on the microscopic sections compared to the in vivo dimensions (Table 2). The major portion of the shrinkage occurred with fixation, for there was a 22% difference in lumen diameter between in vivo and postmortem angiograms and only an 11% further decrease on light microscopic sections.

Thoracic aortic coarctations were produced in these animals by wrapping the aorta with a dacron band (13). The decrease in lumen diameter caused by coarctation in these nine monkeys was estimated to be 50% on the in vivo angiogram. Perfusion fixation and tissue processing resulted in different degrees of shrinkage in the proximal aorta and the coarctation channel. The calculated percent stenosis based on lumen diameter of tissue sections was only 36% (p = 0.001).

Table 2. Cynomolgus Monkey Aorta Lumen Diameter (mm)

	In Vivo Angiography	Postmortem Angiography	Histologic Section
Proximal aorta	6.8 ± 0.5	5.3 ± 0.5	4.7 ± 0.4
Coarct channel	3.4 ± 1.6	3.1 ± 1.0	3.0 ± 0.4
Percent stenosis	50%	42%	36%

Note: Values are mean ± SD; n = 9.

This was due to the greater shrinkage rate of the proximal aorta
(31%) compared to the coarctation site (12%). Thus, dimensions
are markedly altered by fixation and processing may also vary
depending on the composition of vessels and lesions.

Quantitation of Histologic Sections

Direct measurement of dimensions on light microscopic sections
can be performed using an ocular micrometer fitted with a point
counting grid, but recent introduction of computer-assisted planimetric techniques (15-17) have improved efficiency, accuracy,
and reproducibility. The technique consists of tracing the lumen,
internal elastic lamina, and outer limit of the media, and is
programmed for immediate computation of lumen, lesion, and media
areas as well as diameters, lesion thickness, and media thickness.
Contour tracing also permits evaluation of sections that may have
become somewhat distorted during embedding, sectioning, or mounting.
For example, the internal elastic lamina can be traced on a technically distorted section and the length used to recreate a circle
for subsequent calculation of the lumen cross-sectional area (16).
A number of measurements have been used to quantitate atherosclerosis on histologic sections. These include percent lumen area
reduction by intimal lesion based on the area encompassed by the
internal elastic lamina (2,5), ratio of the area of intima to the
area of media area (18), and absolute intimal lesion area (19).

Postmortem Angiography

As with angiography in vivo, evaluation of atherosclerosis from
postmortem angiograms depends mainly on the assessment of lumen
diameters and contours. Postmortem angiography, however, permits
a more detailed appraisal of the limits of angiography for the
quantitation of atherosclerosis. Not only are contrast and
resolution optimal, but projection and magnification can be controlled. In addition, if periarterial tissues are dissected away,

estimates of artery wall thickness can be made and special soft-
tissue radiologic techniques might be developed to obtain information related to the composition of artery walls and lesions.
The angiogram may then be used to select precise levels of
sampling for the preparation of histologic sections.

Since postmortem angiography under controlled pressure can be
performed either before or after perfusion fixation, significant
discrepancies may occur when dimensions on such angiograms are
compared to direct measurements on histologic preparations. For
example, we redistended 10 human superficial femoral arteries
at 37°C with an intraluminal pressure of 100 mmHg, filled the
lumen with angiographic contrast material and obtained multiple
projection x rays (20). Perfusion fixation, at an intraluminal
pressure of 100 mmHg, was carried out after the angiogram. Lumen
diameter on angiography was 5.9 mm ± 1.1 mm (SD) but was 20% less
on histologic examination (4.7 mm ± 1.2 mm, p < .001) due to
tissue shrinkage.

On the other hand, we fixed 13 human common carotid arteries
at an intraluminal pressure of 100 mmHg and subsequently filled
the lumen with a liquid micropaque-gelatin mixture at 37°C and
100 mmHg and then allowed it to solidify at 25°C (21). The lumen
diameter on post-fixation angiography was 6.0 mm ± 1.1 mm (SD)
and on histologic sections was only 7% less (5.6 mm ± 1.0 mm)
indicating that most tissue shrinkage had occurred before the
angiographic x-ray films were taken.

Thus, in human as well as monkey vessels, fixation had a
greater effect on dimensions than processing to produce histologic
sections and angiograms made before fixation were closer to in
vivo dimensions than those made after fixation. These findings
emphasize the importance of defining the precise conditions of
postmortem study and the need to apply suitable correction factors
for shrinkage before making quantitative comparisons. This is
particularly important because inaccuracies in measuring linear
dimensions will be greatly magnified when area calculations are

made. More than one correction factor may need to be calculated for
each experimental condition. For example, angiographic data must
be corrected for magnification due to divergence of the x-ray beam
and positioning of the artery relative to the x-ray beam and the
film cassette. This is most conveniently done by placing a radio-
paque scale adjacent to and in the plane of the artery under study.

QUANTITATION OF ATHEROSCLEROSIS: COMPARISON OF POSTMORTEM
ANGIOGRAPHIC IMAGES WITH HISTOLOGIC SECTIONS

Meaningful quantitative comparison between angiographic images
of atherosclerotic plaques and actual atherosclerotic lesions
are possible when the technical problems of specimen preparation
and imaging are understood and controlled and measurements and
definitions are standardized.   Measurements from postmortem
angiograms can then be compared to measurements from precisely
located histologic sections; the usefulness of each technique
for assessing the severity, extent, composition, or complication
of atherosclerotic lesions can be judged.

    The severity of a lesion refers to its effect in obstructing
the arterial lumen and is usually expressed as the degree of lumen
stenosis. Both the length of a lesion and its effect on the
residual lumen cross-sectional area are important in determining
its influence on blood flow. The extent of atherosclerosis refers
to the quantity of atherosclerotic disease present regardless of
its effect on blood flow, and is important for assessing the
progression or regression of the disease.   The composition of
lesions may vary and may be an important factor in detecting or
predicting complications such as ulceration or thrombosis.
Changes in composition may also be important in evaluating
progression and regression of atherosclerosis.

    In order to better illustrate the methods and problems of
quantitation and correlation, let us consider an example of a
straight, uniform, and unbranched human artery segment, the common
carotid artery. (See Figs. 2 and 3 and Tables 3 and 4.) Our
sample vessel is the left common carotid artery of a 66-year-old

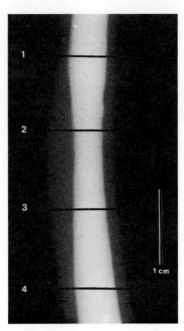

Fig. 2 Postmortem angiogram of a 4-cm segment of perfusion-fixed
common carotid artery. A smooth, tapered plaque is visible
producing a mild stenosis with 45% reduction in lumen cross-
sectional area.   Artery cross sections were taken as indicated.
Section 1 is proximal, section 4 is distal.

male who died of metastatic colon cancer with no clinical evidence

of vascular disease.   The artery was perfusion-fixed with formalin

at 37° and at an intraluminal pressure of 100 mmHg.   It was then

filled with a barium-gelatin mixture and multiple projection x-ray

pictures were obtained.   The angiogram revealed a smooth-surfaced,

tapering plaque that had produced a mild reduction in lumen

diameter.   Tissue sections were taken at 0.5 cm intervals with

each location marked on the angiogram.   Representative sections

proximal to, through and distal to the narrowest lumen are shown

in Fig. 3.   Measurements of lumen diameter and wall thickness were

made on the angiogram using an ocular micrometer and corrected for

x-ray magnification.   Tissue sections were analyzed by contour

tracing and computer assisted planimetry (15).   The results are

shown in Table 3.

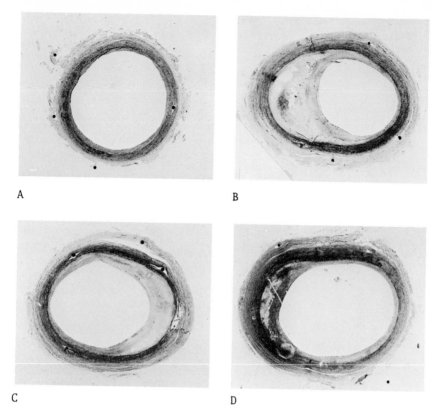

A   B

C   D

Fig. 3 Cross sections of perfusion-fixed common carotid artery.
Gomoritrichrome aldehyde fuchsin stain. A: Minimal intimal
plaque is seen. B: Marked increase in intimal plaque, which now
occupies 53% of the area encompassed by the IEL. Note the increase
in artery wall diameter and sequestration of the plaque to one
side. The lumen contour remains round and the area encompassed
by the IEL is enlarged to limit the effect of plaque size on the
lumen. C: Moderate amount of intimal plaque, but relatively
little effect on lumen cross-sectional area, compared to section
1, due to dilatation of the artery wall. D: Intimal plaque area
is similar to that seen in section 3 but because of greater arterial dilatation, the lumen cross-sectional area is larger than
that seen in section 1, which has the least involvement.

Lumen Diameter and Wall Thickness

There was good correlation between lumen diameter measurement in

postmortem angiograms and in histologic sections with a less than

5% disparity in results (Table 3). However, there was a large

Table 3. Postmortem Angiography and Histology of a Human Carotid Artery (See Figs. 2 and 3)

Section	Lumen Diameter on Angio (mm)	Diameter (mm)			Cross-sectional Area (mm^2)				Medial Thickness (mm)	Intima Area/ Media Area
		Lumen	IEL	External	Lumen	Lesion	IEL	Media		
1	4.9	4.7	5.0	5.8	17.0	1.6	19.6	7.6	0.46	0.2
2	3.9	3.9	5.5	6.4	10.5	12.1	23.8	8.5	0.47	1.4
3	4.5	4.4	5.5	6.4	14.4	8.5	23.8	8.3	0.45	1.0
4	5.2	5.0	5.9	7.0	19.2	7.3	27.3	10.5	0.53	0.7

Table 4. Severity of Atherosclerosis in Human Carotid Artery:
Percent Stenosis

Section	Lumen Area Relative to "Normal" Lumen		Intima Area as Part of IEL Area (Histology)
	Angiogram	Histology	
1	11%	11%	8%
2	45%	47%	53%
3	25%	25%	37%
4	--	--	28%

discrepancy in the measurement of wall thickness between postmortem angiography and histology. This was due to eccentricity
of the plaque and limited x-ray projections and to the variable
amount of adventitia surrounding the artery. Adventitia is
indistinguishable from media and plaque on standard x-ray images;
thus wall thickness measurements, while useful in evaluating
histologic sections, were not reliable measures on postmortem
angiography. In the future, the use of improved, multiplane
x-ray techniques on specimens in which adventitia is completely
removed may provide more reliable measurements of wall thickness.

Percent Stenosis Estimated From Changes in Lumen Diameter

Calculation of percent stenosis from angiographic images is
usually accomplished by comparing the smallest lumen diameter
to the nearest adjacent, presumably "normal" segment of the same
vessel. The widest diameter in our segment of common carotid
artery was 5.2 mm at section 4. Using this as the reference,
there was a 27% diameter reduction at the narrowest point (section
2), representing a 45% reduction in lumen cross-sectional area
(Table 4). There was a close correlation between postmortem
angiography and histology using this method. Tissue sections
revealed a 22% diameter reduction and 45% lumen cross-sectional
area reduction. Thus, comparable data on changes in lumen area
are provided by both techniques.

Percent Stenosis Estimated From Tissue Sections

Quantitation of the severity of atherosclerosis from artery cross
sections is usually based on the assumption that the internal
elastic lamina (IEL) represents the original lumen diameter and
that the area of intimal lesion found within the area encompassed
by the IEL represents the true degree of lumen obstruction (2,5).
This assumption seems reasonable enough, but it may lead to substantial errors in estimation of lesion severity. It is well
known that arteries dilate with age and may also dilate in response to the development of the plaque itself (12,22). The most
uninvolved portion of the carotid artery was at section 1, where
intimal lesion area was only 1.6 mm^2. One centimeter was more
distal in the artery at section 2, there was a substantial increase in lesion area to 12.1 mm^2, which represented a 53%
stenosis as calculated from the reduction in the IEL circumscribed
cross-sectional area (Table 4). However, there was an increase in
the diameter of the artery at this level, producing a 21% increase
in IEL cross-sectional area resulting in a decrease in the calculated percent stenosis (Fig. 3). The true original artery wall
diameter is probably closer to that seen in section 1 than in
section 2. If artery dilatation had not taken place, then the
percent stenosis at section 2 would have been 62% rather than the
53% observed. Dilatation at section 3 was such that little lumen
narrowing occurred despite 8.5 mm^2 lesion area and dilatation at
section 4 was such that lumen cross-sectional area exceeded that
observed at section 1 by 13% despite a more than four-fold increase in lesion area. Thus, arterial dilatation can result in
underestimation of the severity of arterial lesions if one uses
lumen diameter measurements. This source of error must be
considered in serial evaluations using angiography to assess
progression or regression of atherosclerosis.

A second source of error in using this technique to compare
tissue section measurements to angiographic findings occurs if
pressure-perfusion fixation is not carried out. The collapsed

artery wall will cause the intimal plaque to bulge into the empty
lumen space producing an irregular, often "slit-like" lumen
contour. Intimal cross-sectional area may be unaffected, but
the area encompassed by the IEL will be decreased and the net
effect would be to overestimate the percent stenosis. In order
to appreciate the magnitude of error possible from failure to fix
arteries under pressure, let us assume a 25% decrease in lumen
diameter due to collapse of the artery after death. This is a
conservative estimate since Wolinsky and Glagov measured a 50%
decrease in lumen diameter of collapsed rabbit aortas (7). A
25% decrease in lumen diameter would cause a 25% cross-sectional
area stenosis in vivo to appear as a 45% stenosis in the postmortem specimen (an error of 80%). Similarly, a 50% area stenosis
in vivo would erroneously be measured as a 90% stenosis on a
nonperfusion-fixed postmortem specimen (70% overestimation). This
may account for the discrepancies found by most investigators in
comparing in vivo angiography to postmortem measurements of
vessels (2-5).

Extent of Atherosclerosis

It is apparent that quantitative assessment of the extent or amount
of atherosclerosis cannot be judged from visualization of the
arterial lumen alone, but requires direct measurement of the
lesion itself. Intimal lesion area is the best reflection of the
quantity of atherosclerosis present, but does not necessarily
provide information on lumen encroachment. Thus the same amount
of lesion may have little effect on the lumen of a large artery,
but have a substantial effect on the lumen of a small artery.

   In an effort to correct for variation in artery size, intimal
lesion area has been related to the area of media using the ratio
intima area:media area, assuming that the area of media is a
reasonable index of vessel size (18). This is subject to error
because it assumes that the media is unaffected by the disease.
Medial area may increase or decrease with increasing plaque and

in our carotid artery we noted that the medial area actually
increased in the most dilated portion of artery (section 4).
Thus, while this measure may be useful, it is subject to several
sources of error.

Estimates of overall extent of atherosclerosis using intimal
lesion area on artery cross sections is subject to substantial
sampling error due to the focal nature of atherosclerotic disease.
As can be seen in our example, there was an eight-fold difference
in intimal lesion area between section 1 and section 2, located
only 1 cm apart. Thus, it is important to compare tissue sections
to postmortem angiograms so that sampling errors may be minimized
and information obtained from tissue sections can be generalized
for the artery as a whole. By integrating the lesion area over
the length of the artery, assessment of the extent of atherosclerotic lesion for a given vessel is possible. Thus, for our 4-cm
segment of carotid artery, the average area of lesion was 7.4 mm^2.
Multiplication of lesion area by the length (40 mm) produces a
lesion volume of 296 mm^3. This represents 74 mm^3/cm of carotid
artery. Such measures would be useful for quantitating the total
volume of atherosclerotic lesion in a test segment and would be
an important measure for determining the true rates of progression
and regression of atherosclerosis, particularly in experimental
models.

Precision of Sampling: Arterial Branch Points

Quantitation of atherosclerotic lesions at arterial branch sites
is much more complex than for straight portions of arteries.
Plaques commonly occur at arterial branch points and are very
important in the overall consideration of disease state. Lesions
at branches may be difficult to evaluate by angiography due to
overlapping of vessels (8). Similarly, errors in quantitation of
lesions from histologic sections may occur even in well distended
vessels due to the plane of section at branch points. For example,
Fig. 4 indicates the plane of section of the common carotid artery

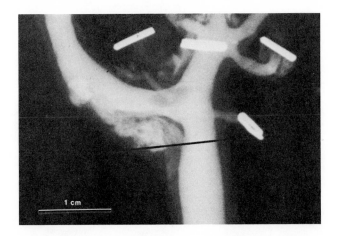

Fig. 4 Postmortem angiogram of perfusion-fixed human carotid
bifurcation. Note extensive, calcified plaque at origin of
internal carotid artery with minimal encroachment on the lumen.
Plane of section is indicated by the black line (see Fig. 5).

just proximal to the bifurcation into internal and external
carotid. The artery cross section reveals a very large intimal
plaque (Fig. 5). This plaque does not arise from the common
carotid as it appears on the tissue section, but from the internal
carotid artery, as can be seen on the angiogram. Plaques have
specific localization patterns at branch points and the tissue
sections must be precisely selected using the angiographic image
as a guide for full understanding. Plaques at branch points pose
difficult problems in quantitation, but cannot be ignored in
evaluating the total extent of atherosclerosis since the disease
is so common in these locations.

Lesion Complication

Lesion complications, such as ulceration and thrombosis, can be
seen on postmortem angiograms as well as on histologic sections.
Both methods offer advantages and disadvantages. For example,
plaque ulcerations and irregularities can be seen on postmortem
angiography, especially when multiple projections are taken.
Single-plane angiograms may frequently miss ulcerations.

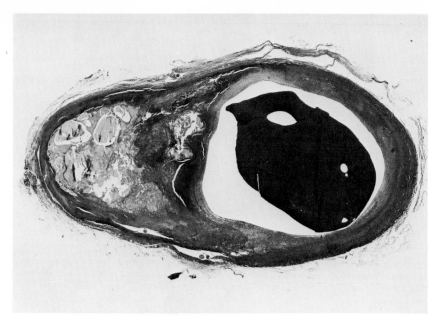

Fig. 5 Cross section of carotid artery seen in Fig. 4. Note
extensive intimal plaque, which is related to the internal carotid
artery but appears with the common carotid artery due to plane of
sectioning.

Similarly, even interval cross sections may miss lesions, since
complications are frequently quite focal. Quantitation of histologic sections and careful correlation with intimal lumen contour
on postmortem angiograms should lead to more precise recognition
and characterization of lumen contour irregularities on angiograms
made in vivo. This would enhance the application of computerized
techniques for estimating long-term sequential changes in the
arterial wall (23). Further developments in computerized x-ray
technology and B-mode ultrasound imaging should permit such
assessment of soft tissue densities and more precise evaluation
of plaque composition in the living subject.

CONCLUSIONS

1. Arterial lumens are normally circular even in the presence of
   advanced lesions. The impression that lumens are frequently

triangular, crescent-shaped, or slit-like probably arises from postmortem examination of undistended, collapsed vessels. Quantitation of such material leads to overestimation of the degree of stenosis. Discrepancies in lumen diameter between angiograms made in vivo and pathologic examination of undistended vessels is due mainly to overestimation by the pathologist rather than underestimation by the angiographer. Fixation under conditions of controlled pressure distension should be carried out with pressure maintained above diastolic levels.

2. In addition to reductions in lumen diameter attributable to vessel collapse, fixation results in tissue shrinkage. This occurs whether vessels have been fixed while collapsed or distended. External diameter, internal diameter, and wall or lesion thickness do not shrink to the same degree. Preparation of tissue sections for light microscopy examination results in further shrinkage. These effects must be taken into account when quantitative validation comparisons are made with angiograms taken in vivo.

3. The angle of section and the presence of arterial branches may confound the configuration and location of plaques and interfere with accurate correlation of anatomic specimens with angiograms. Planes of section must correspond to precisely identified locations on angiograms.

4. The severity of stenosis is estimated on angiograms by establishing a ratio between the narrowed channel and an adjacent lumen of presumed normal dimensions. On the other hand, the severity of stenosis is estimated on tissue sections by comparing the cross-sectional area of the lesion with the area encompassed by the internal elastic lamina, i.e., the presumed original lumen before disease developed. This difference in definition, along with possible dilatation of the IEL-defined area as plaques develop can account for a discrepancy in results between the two methods.

5. Angiographic estimates of percent stenosis are not an accurate index of the extent of atherosclerosis and may not be a reliable measure for use in studies of progression and regression of atherosclerosis.

6. Estimates of the extent of disease are best made using the actual area of intimal lesion on arterial cross sections. Multiple cross sections can then be integrated so that the mass of intimal lesion can be established for a given segment of artery. Such a measure of intimal lesion mass would be the most reliable means for following progression and regression of atherosclerotic disease and hopefully will become available for in vivo determinations with the perfection of ultrasound imaging methods. Changes in lumen diameter and contour on angiography may prove to be insufficient.

7. Lesion complication can be studied best by a combination of postmortem angiography and histologic cross sections, since postmortem angiography in several projections can be used to

define lumen irregularities and ulcerations and tissue cross sections can be used to validate and quantitate the corresponding changes in lesion composition.
8. Postmortem angiography combined with histologic study are complementary in expanding our understanding of the limits and possibilities of angiography in vivo.

REFERENCES

1. Slot HB, Strijbosch L, Greep JM (1981) Interobserver variability in single-plane aortography. Surgery 90:497-503
2. Isner JM, Kishel J, Kent KM, Ronan JA Jr, Ross MA, Roberts WC (1981) Accuracy of angiographic determination of left main coronary arterial narrowing. Circulation 63:1056-1064
3. Vlodaver Z, Frech R, Van Tassel RA, Edwards JE (1972) Correlation of the antemortem coronary arteriogram and the postmortem specimen. Circulation 47:162-169
4. Grondin CM, Dyrda I, Pasternac A, Campeau L, Bourassa MG, Lesperance J (1974) Discrepancies between cineangiographic and postmortem findings in patients with coronary artery disease and recent myocardial revascularization. Circulation 49:703-708
5. Arnett EN, Isner JM, Redwood DR, Kent KM, Baker WP, Ackerstein H, Roberts WC (1979) Coronary artery narrowing in coronary heart disease: comparison of cineangiographic and necropsy findings. Ann Intern Med 91:350-356
6. Vlodaver Z, Edwards JE (1971) Pathology of coronary atherosclerosis. Prog Cardiovasc Dis 14:256-274
7. Wolinsky H, Glagov S (1964) Structural basis for the static mechanical properties of the aortic media. Circ Res 14:400-413
8. Hutchins GM, Bulkley BH, Ridolfi RL, Griffith LSC, Lohr FT, Piasio MA (1979) Correlation of coronary arteriograms and left ventriculograms with postmortem studies. Circulation 56:32-37
9. McNamara JJ, Norenberg RG, Goebert HW III, Soeter JR (1976) Distribution and severity of atherosclerosis in the coronary arteries. J Thorac Cardiovasc Surg 71:637-640
10. Bulkley BH, Hutchins GM (1977) Accelerated "atherosclerosis": A morphologic study of 97 saphenous vein coronary artery bypass grafts. Circulation 55:163-169
11. Schwartz JN, Kong Y, Hackel DB, Bartel AG (1975) Comparison of angiographic and postmortem findings in patients with coronary artery disease. Am J Cardiol 36:174-178
12. Bahr GF, Bloom G, Friberg U (1957) Volume changes of tissues in physiological fluids during fixation in osmium tetroxide or formaldehyde and during subsequent treatment. Exp Cell Res 12:342-343
13. Zarins CK, Bomberger RA, Taylor KE, Glagov S (1980) Artery stenosis inhibits regression of diet-induced atherosclerosis. Surgery 88:86-90

14. Zarins CK, Bomberger RA, Glagov S (1981) Local effects of stenoses: Increased flow velocity inhibits atherogenesis. Circulation 64(Suppl II):221-227

15. Glagov S, Grande J, Vesselinovitch D, Zarins CK (1981) Quantitation of cells and fibers in histologic sections of arterial walls: Advantages of contour tracing on a digitizing plate. In: McDonald TF, Chandler AB (eds) Connective tissues in arterial and pulmonary disease. Springer-Verlag, New York, pp 57-93

16. Clarkson TB, Bond MG, Marzetta CA, Bullock BC (1980) Approaches to the study of atherosclerosis regression in rhesus monkeys: Interpretation of morphometric measurements of coronary arteries. In: Gotto AM Jr, Smith LC, Allen B (eds) Atherosclerosis V. Springer-Verlag, New York, pp 739-748

17. Wissler RW, Vesselinovitch D, Schaffner TJ, Glagov S (1980) Quantitating rhesus monkey atherosclerosis progression and regression with time. In: Gotto AM Jr, Smith LC, Allen B (eds) Atherosclerosis V. Springer-Verlag, New York, pp 757-761

18. Bomberger RA, Zarins CK, Glagov S (1981) Subcritical arterial stenosis enhances distal atherosclerosis. Resident Research Award. J Surg Res 30:205-212

19. Bond MG, Adams MR, Bullock BC (1981) Complicating factors in evaluating coronary artery atherosclerosis. Artery 9:21-29

20. Lyon RT, Zarins CK, Lu CT, Yang CF, Glagov S (1981) Arterial wall disruption by balloon dilatation: Quantitative comparison of normal, stenotic and occluded vessels. Surg Forum 32:326-328

21. Zarins CK, Giddens DP, Balasubramanian K, Sottiurai V, Mabon RF, Glagov S (1981) Carotid plaques localize in regions of low flow velocity and shear stress. Circulation 64 (Suppl IV):44

22. Young W, Gofman JW, Tandy R, Malamud N, Walter ESG (1960) The quantitation of atherosclerosis. I. Relationship to artery size. Am J Cardiol 6:288-293

23. Crawford DW, Brooks SH, Barndt R Jr, Blankenhorn DH (1977) Measurement of atherosclerotic luminal irregularity and obstruction by radiographic densitometry. Invest Radiol 12:307-313

DISCUSSION: M. GENE BOND

The studies reported by Dr. Zarins have focused on several important factors that must be considered when attempting to validate different techniques used to evaluate atherosclerosis.

The most traditional and widely used characteristic to document atherosclerosis severity has been "percent lumen stenosis," derived from either longitudinal arteriographic images or from cross-sectional histological specimens. The majority of studies that have compared data from these methods have described discrepancies, most typically characterized as a tendency for arteriography to underestimate lesion severity or for pathology evaluation to overestimate the degree of atherosclerosis. Dr. Zarins has pointed out very clearly the major reasons for these discrepancies which include the different methods used to define "percent lumen stenosis," and the effects of tissue shrinkage artifact and pressure fixation versus immersion fixation on arterial size characteristics.

The observation that plaques do not "protrude" into the lumen, at least when evaluated on cross sections of moderately atherosclerotic common carotid arteries fixed under lumen pressures found in vivo, is consistent with similar studies of human aorta and iliac arteries (1,2), human coronary arteries (3,4), and animal arteries (5). These findings support the notion that atherosclerotic plaques may extend outwardly toward the adventitia with the result that the arterial lumen maintains a circular or eliptical shape, at least during the early stages of atherosclerosis progression.

In addition to the demonstrated effects of pressure fixation and tissue processing on arterial size and contour, Dr. Zarin's studies have presented a second important and thought-provoking observation. Briefly stated, Tables 3 and 4 suggest that atherosclerosis may influence arterial size focally, and may do so in such a way that lumen size becomes less accurate as a predictor

of the amount of atherosclerosis per se (lesion area). Stated
in another way, because of arterial enlargement there may not be
a 1:1 inverse relationship between increasing plaque size and
decreasing lumen caliber.

The relationship between atherosclerosis and artery size has
been investigated in immersion-fixed coronary arteries from human
beings and in pressure fixed arteries of animals. In the human
studies, a significant relationship was noted between atherosclerosis (defined as the ratio of intimal area to the area within
the external elastic lamina), and the radius of coronary and
cerebral arteries , i.e., the larger arteries had more atherosclerosis (6). In the animal studies, high correlations were
observed between intimal area and the area enclosed within the
internal elastic lamina in pressure-fixed coronary arteries from
atherosclerotic rhesus monkeys that were part of a large atherosclerosis regression experiment (7). Also in a comparative study
of atherosclerosis among three species of nonhuman primates in
which test and control animals were matched for gender, age, body
weight, and heart weight, significant arterial enlargement
occurred in the coronary arteries of some test animals that were
hypercholesterolemic for 3 years (8). In that study even though
severe and complicated lesions were induced, the effect of
arterial enlargement resulted in some atherosclerotic test animals
having considerably larger coronary artery lumens than were
present in controls.

A study of coronary artery atherosclerosis in the Masai people
of East Africa has shown that men in this society have a very low
clinical incidence of coronary heart disease (9) even though the
amount of atherosclerosis in older males is as great as that found
in an age-matched cohort of California men (10). In that study,
the apparent reason for the protection against the development of
ischemic heart disease was that the coronary arteries became
larger with age, and presumably in part, because of exercise.

For whatever reason(s), increasing artery size and the effect of that change on lumen contour or caliber are potential complicating factors in serial evaluations of atherosclerosis progression and regression, especially in studies that rely only on evaluation of lumen characteristics (11).

REFERENCES

1. Thoma R (1886)   Ueber die Abhangigkeit der Bindegewebsneubildung in der Arterienintima von den Mechanischen Bedingungen des Blutumlaufes. Virchows Arch [Path Anat] 104:209-241
2. Crawford T, Levene CI (1953)   Medial thinning in atheroma. J Pathol Bacteriol 66:19-23
3. Harrison CV, Wood P (1949)   Hypertensive and ischaemic heart disease: a comparative clinical and pathological study. Br Heart J 11:205-229
4. Stewart JD, Birchwood E, Wells HG (1935)   The effect of atherosclerotic plaques on the diameter of the lumen of coronary arteries.   JAMA 104:730-733
5. Bunce DFM (1964)   Effect of intimal thickening on vascular capacity in vivo.   JAOA 63:869-870
6. Young W, Gofman JW, Tandy R (1960)   The quantitation of atherosclerosis.   1.   Relationship to artery size.   Am J Cardiol 6:288-293
7. Clarkson TB, Bond MG, Bullock BC, Marzetta CA (1981)   A study of atherosclerosis regression in Macaca mulatta.   IV.   Changes in coronary arteries from animals with atherosclerosis induced for 19 months and then regressed for 24 or 48 months at plasma cholesterol concentrations of 300 or 200 mg/dl.   Exp Mol Pathol 34:345-368
8. Bond MG, Adams MR, Kaduck JM, Bullock BC (1981)   Effects of atherosclerosis on coronary artery size.   Fed Proc 40:773 (abstract)
9. Mann GV, Shaffer RD, Anderson RS, Sandstead HH (1964)   Cardiovascular disease in the Masai.   J Atheroscler Res 4:289-312
10. Mann GV, Spoerry A, Gray M, Jarashow D (1972)   Atherosclerosis in the Masai.   Am J Epidemiol 95:26-37
11. Bond MG, Adams MR, Bullock BC (1981)   Complicating factors in evaluating coronary artery atherosclerosis.   Artery 9:21-29

14

Correlation of Doppler Ultrasound with Arteriography in the Quantitative Evaluation of Atherosclerosis

CHRISTOPHER P. L. WOOD

To the interested observer it may seem a paradox that a technique based on the detection of small moving targets should have been compared for validation almost exclusively to a method that outlines large, fixed structures. Yet in comparing the various Doppler ultrasound methods of detecting blood flow through normal and arteriosclerotic arteries with conventional contrast arteriography, this is precisely what has been attempted.

How well has Doppler ultrasound performed in these tests, how well has this correlation of a technique detecting red blood cell motion with a method outlining the impingement of atherosclerotic plaques upon the vessel lumen worked in practice, and, perhaps of more importance, if this correlation method is lacking in precision, how can future studies using Doppler ultrasound to quantify atherosclerosis be planned and validated? This review will try to answer the first two questions and to provide some recommendations as a basis for answering the last question.

VALIDATION STUDIES IN ANIMALS

It may seem astonishing, but it would appear that no prospective studies have been done to validate any form of Doppler method in the detection and quantification of atherosclerotic lesions induced in animals. Yet when the difficulties in human studies

are considered it is perhaps not surprising. The small size of
most available laboratory animals and the consequent small size
of their arteries and atherosclerotic lesions makes hard demands
on the resolution of Doppler ultrasound systems as well as on
conventional arteriography. It is perhaps because of the apparent
safety of the technique and the limits of the ultrasound systems
that the method has been used from the start in human beings.
This has allowed many studies to be performed in which the severity of a lesion has been defined by one of the forms of Doppler
ultrasound and then compared to the findings of conventional
contrast arteriography. These validation studies using arteriography have been extremely useful but suffer from the limitation
that the process is essentially a once-only diagnostic test,
because of the risks and morbidity inherent in using repeated
contrast arteriography, without follow-up testing over a period
of time to observe change.

DETECTION OF DOPPLER ULTRASOUND STUDIES AND ADVANCED
ATHEROSCLEROSIS IN HUMANS

The question of definition of advanced atherosclerosis is addressed
in Chap. 2. Nevertheless it is worth emphasizing that the very
nature of most Doppler techniques for detecting the effects of
atherosclerosis limits the method to measuring the overall severity of a single or several lesions rather than the overall extent
of the disease in one or both limbs or in the head or neck. This
has obvious drawbacks in that there may be a large mass of atheroma
spread throughout the main vessels of a limb but causing little if
any local, severe stenosis. This form of disease, although
advanced, may not be detected by many of the ultrasound techniques.
However, a lesser mass of atherosclerosis with one or two severe
local lesions will almost certainly be detected by Doppler ultrasound.

The intimate relationship between structure and function in
the artery is the basis of several Doppler-derived methods for

detecting advanced atherosclerosis. Thus, the complete or partial
intrusion of plaque into the lumen at a specific site (or sites)
may cause a drop in the blood pressure distal to the site. In the
situation of a complete occlusion, the vessel patency beyond may
be assured by its refilling from collateral vessels of supply,
bypassing the occlusion. Doppler ultrasound has been used to
detect these conditions in several ways: (1) measurement of
distal systolic blood pressure, (2) compression of collateral
vessels and observation of the subsequent flow pattern and direction in the artery under investigation, and (3) analysis of the
blood flow waveform pattern to observe any alteration caused by
the effects of local atherosclerosis. The design limits of
Doppler instruments in the presence of attenuation and reflection
by tissues like muscle, bone, and gas-containing organs like lung
and bowel have restricted most Doppler arterial studies to the
head and neck and to the limbs. Some work has been done on the
aorta.

Lower Limbs

The simplest, most widely used and clinically trusted application
of Doppler ultrasound is in the determination of systemic arterial
blood pressure. In the basic test the resting systolic blood
pressure is measured at the ankle and compared to the pressure
recorded from the upper arm. In the normal individual the pressure at the ankle is equal to or greater than the pressure at the
arm and the ratio of these two pressures is therefore one or more.
When the aortoiliac or femoropopliteal segment is occluded this
ratio is between 0.5 and 1, but with more than one level of
occlusion the ratio is usually less than 0.5.

Carter was among the first to report the assessment of atherosclerotic patients with ankle pressures measured by Doppler
ultrasound (1-3). In these studies he insisted on standardized
basal conditions for measurement and also reported on the reproducibility of his measurements. Many investigators reporting

their work since then have not been so forthcoming in the description of their technique. Carter commented on what is a recurring problem in many subsequent series--the difficulty in assessing accurately the severity of an atherosclerotic stenosis from a single x-ray projection--and suspected that this was the reason for the apparent lack of difference in mean ankle pressure between limbs with mild and severe stenosis.

In an important study reported in 1972 (2), it was demonstrated that abnormal responses of ankle pressure to exercise were present in many of the limbs in which pressures measured at rest were within normal limits. This pressure drop with exercise allowed the detection of stenoses with as little as 25% reduction in lumen diameter. Although showing an important principle, the numbers in this report were small (arteriographic confirmation in only 12 limbs), the exercise workload to induce the pressure drop was not completely standardized, the relative pressure drop with a 25% as opposed to a 50% stenosis was not described, and neither was the level of the patient's disease process (either proximal, distal, or both).

Similar results were obtained in a large series by Yao, Hobbs, and Irvine (4) who compared ankle systolic Doppler pressure measurements with single plane arteriography in 183 limbs of patients with angiographic evidence of atheroma in the distal aorta and leg arteries. They included a control group of 25 healthy young adults without evidence of cardiovascular disease who did not undergo arteriography. Of interest was that in 25 limbs they compared systolic pressure measurements made by ultrasound with those made by strain-gauge plethysmography and found an excellent correlation between the two.

The results of Carter (2) and of Yao, Hobbs, and Irvine (4) showed overlap in ankle systolic pressure ratios between various grades of disease and in various levels of the extremities (proximal and distal). This overlap was due both to the difference between patients in the extent of their collateral pathways around partial or complete stenosis and to the difficulty in accurately assessing the tightness of a stenosis from a single-plane arteriographic view.

To improve the sensitivity of detecting atherosclerosis and to measure more precisely its effect on blood flow, stress testing by inducing hyperemia in the limbs, either through standard exercise regimens or through cuff-induced reactive hyperemia, has become commonplace.

In a detailed investigation into the effects of cuff-induced reactive hyperemia on the limbs of atherosclerotic patients, Johnson (5) highlighted both the virtues of the method and its deficiencies in the accurate assessment of atherosclerosis. He showed that ankle pressure measurement alone, with or without reactive hyperemia, was unable to distinguish between iliac or femoral, or combined iliofemoral stenotic or occlusive disease, or indeed to ascertain which of two or more stenoses was exerting the most significant adverse effect on blood flow. It was unfortunate that Johnson did not include in his study patients with mild atheromatous changes and stenoses between 0 and 40% to confirm the earlier findings of Carter and Yao et al. in the success of this technique in detecting "early" atherosclerosis.

This not unexpected failure of ankle pressure ratio to localize the disease has prompted the use of measurements of pressure at several levels in the lower limb to provide more information on the site and extent of the atherosclerotic lesions. Several groups have reported encouraging results. In a series of 66 limbs undergoing arteriography Allan and Terry (6) had an 83% success rate in predicting the correct anatomical level of the disease. From a slightly larger series of 60 patients and 30 controls Cutajar and colleagues (7) drew guidelines for estimating the level and severity of disease. Heintz et al. (8) in a smaller study had a 78% success rate in localizing disease to the aorto-

iliac or femoropopliteal or both regions, and were completely
successful in establishing the level in limbs with isolated
aortoiliac or femoropopliteal disease.

Colt (9) reported an interesting variation in the measurement
of segmental pressures to localize arterial disease in the leg.
He avoided the use of a high thigh cuff by applying pressure (with
a simple portable apparatus) directly over the femoral artery in
the groin, and compressed the vessel against the underlying pubic
ramus. Popliteal artery pressure was measured by using a large,
low thigh cuff placed just above the knee. He used the segmental
pressures to plot a family of pressure curves, each curve having
a specific shape depending on the location of the disease in the
limb. The correlation with arteriography in the iliac region was
excellent with 94% agreement; was good in the superficial femoral
region with 79% agreement; and only fair at 63% in the tibial
region. The decline in accuracy more distal in the extremity was
thought to be due to collateral flow affecting local pressures.
He noted the problems that resulted from obesity and calcification
of the arterial wall that produced an incompressible vessel. This
occurred in the iliofemoral vessels of patients with atherosclerosis and in the tibial arteries of diabetic patients. These
factors may potentially reduce correlations with arteriography.

An important contribution towards validating Doppler ultrasound
in quantifying peripheral arterial disease was a study reported by
Rutherford and colleagues in 1979 (10). They compared segmental
systolic limb pressures and segmental pulse volume plethysmography
recordings to arteriography and used a computer to subject the
large mass of data to discriminant analysis to provide objective
criteria for the identification of significant arterial stenotic
lesions (defined as stenosis of greater than 50% by diameter).
Doppler limb pressures and pulse volume recordings were approximately equal in their ability to define accurately the site and
significance of arterial disease in the limb in 86% of cases.
Combining the two techniques raised the overall diagnostic

accuracy from 86% for each, to 97% for both. This improvement was probably a reflection of the complementary nature of the two techniques, one of which measures arterial pressure, the second reflecting arterial flow. The authors noted that if the patient population studied had included more normal patients or patients with isolated lesions rather than many patients with severe multilevel occlusive disease, the accuracy of the combined tests would have been higher. The use of multiplanar arteriography and the introduction of a further category for classifying arteries with stenosis of less than 50% by diameter would have given greater insight into the ability of Doppler segmental pressures to identify and characterize all grades of arterial lesions.

Although the inaccuracy of arteriography, particularly in defining the severity of stenotic disease in the aortoiliac segment, has been known for some time, it is only now that the use of Doppler-derived segmental limb pressures is beginning to be validated against another and probably better "gold standard" than arteriography. Flanigan et al. (11) have correlated the accuracy of Doppler-derived, high-thigh, wide-cuff occlusion pressure against the baseline of direct intraarterial pressure measurement in the assessment of aortoiliac disease. Acknowledging the more accurate localization of disease to the aortoiliac segment with a narrow-cuff technique, they wished to validate the supposedly more accurate measurement of pressure using the wide cuff on the thigh. The intraarterial pressures were measured at the time of arteriography. Despite the use of several pelvic and groin views there was a wide variance in the correlation between direct common femoral arterial pressure and the degree of aortoiliac stenosis measured on the arteriogram. They indicated that this variance could be explained by the failure of the arteriogram to demonstrate the true degree of stenosis, the presence of excellent collaterals, and vessel incompressibility. Comparison of the high-thigh Doppler measurement with the direct pressure measurement showed the Doppler technique to be 79% sensitive, 56%

specific, and 63% accurate in the evaluation of hemodynamically significant aortoiliac disease. Unfortunately they omitted their definition of what constituted a hemodynamic change across a stenosis, but one assumes a pressure drop of 10 mmHg. This is an important study in that it indicates the rather poor performance of Doppler-derived, wide-cuff, high-thigh pressure as an indicator of hemodynamically significant aortoiliac artery occlusive disease. However, it by no means negates the ability of Doppler-derived limb pressures to accurately define atherosclerotic disease, because they were testing one technique only (single segmental limb pressure) and at rest, without the benefit of the increased sensitivity provided by hyperemia. The results of their further investigations, which will hopefully include validation of the narrow multiple cuff technique, are awaited with interest.

So far this review has dealt with the simplest application of Doppler ultrasound in the form of local pressure measurement. This technique has been shown to be inexpensive, easy to perform, and has been surprisingly successful in detecting and quantifying moderate to severe atherosclerosis. However, it has long been realized that the velocity waveform contains valuable physiological information within it. Thus the encroachment of plaque upon the vessel lumen, if severe enough, may alter the shape and characteristics of the waveform. Much attention has been devoted to both the qualitative and quantitative assessment of flow waveforms detected by the Doppler ultrasound. This work has been done simultaneously with pressure studies in many centers and has increased our ability in diagnosing and localizing atherosclerosis. Use of the simple zero-crossing continuous wave Doppler ultrasound instruments are an easy and practical way of obtaining velocity waveform data. The techniques of using a calibrated, directionally sensitive Doppler instrument have been well standardized by Fronek and his colleagues (12) who have analyzed the waveform for peak forward flow, peak, mean velocity ratio, and deceleration of the instantaneous velocity curve. They have monitored a post-cuff-occlusion reactive hyperemia by measuring the mean femoral artery flow velocity during this procedure. Thus they have combined velocity information gained from examination of the limb at rest and after hyperemia. In their studies using multisegment pressures and femoral artery velocity waveform information, only 3.4% of limbs with proximal aortoiliac arterial disease were misclassified as normal. It would be interesting if this group would extend the scope of their investigation to include patients with angiographic lesions of less than 50% diameter reduction and plot in graphic form the angiographic appearance (preferably derived from multiplanar angiographic views) against the values obtained from segmental limb indices and quantitative velocity measurements. A cautionary note in attempting to quantify and standardize velocity waveform information obtained from the arteries of the limb using simple continuous wave Doppler instruments has been sounded by Fish (13).

A similar but even simpler approach has been taken by Nicolaides and Angelides (14) in which they derived various empirical indices from common femoral and posterior tibial waveforms. These were obtained by a simple continuous wave Doppler ultrasound instrument standardized prior to each recording by a built-in 1000-Hz calibration pulse. The indices, which include waveform height, acceleration time, initial deceleration time, presence or absence of turbulence at the insonation site after exercise, and value of a waveform "index," were subjected to multivariate analysis. In comparison with uniplanar arteriography, this method could determine with a high probability the condition of the aortoiliac segment in 86% of limbs and could define the status of the superficial femoral artery even in the presence of aortoiliac disease.

Important new concepts relating to velocity waveform dampening by local atherosclerosis were conceived and underwent early validation study by the group from Guy's Hospital (15,16). To avoid the built-in inaccuracies of the zero-crossing technique in

measuring Doppler frequency they used real-time spectral analysis
to produce sonograms that were essentially independent of beam-
to-vessel angle thus permitting identification of the waveform
even with poor signal-to-noise ratio. They derived a parameter
called the "pulsatility index," which was defined as the peak-to-
peak sonogram waveform excursion, allowing for reverse flow,
divided by the algebraic mean height over one cardiac cycle. An
arterial segment could be defined further by a "damping factor,"
which was defined as the pulsatility index at the inlet to the
segment divided by the pulsatility index at the outlet from the
segment. They used transit time, which was the foot-to-foot delay
between sonograms, obtained by two separate Doppler probes placed
at either end of a vessel segment for the same heart beat, as a
measure of the pulse wave transmission velocity. After early
investigations they realized that the sensitivity of these parameters could be improved if the damping factor and transit time
were corrected for the age and blood pressure of the subject. The
corrections were supplied by collecting data from a large number
of normal subjects of different age groups. Segmental Doppler-
derived limb pressures were an essential part of the examination
protocol, not only for their help in giving pressure indices but
also for the derivation of the mean perfusion pressure in a
segment that was used to help normalize the transit time for that
segment. The normalized transit time and damping factor were
collated with arteriography in 386 arterial pathways to provide
diagnostic thresholds for categorizing vessel segments as normal,
stenosed, occluded, or unusually widened or narrowed. The plotting of damping factor against transit time gave agreement with
the x-rays in more than 90% of the ultrasound values obtained.
They assessed proximal, distal, and combined disease and classified collateral circulation into four different grades ranging
from short, wide-diameter vessels to long, narrow-diameter collateral vessels. These important concepts were validated in series
by Fitzgerald and Carr (17), in which biplanar arteriography was

used as the standard, and by Harris et al. (18), using single-plane arteriography.

Pulsatility index has been investigated extensively by Johnston and colleagues (19). In comparing pulsatility index from the common femoral, popliteal, dorsalis pedis, and posterior tibial arteries with arteriograms (biplanar with oblique views) in 155 limbs, the pulsatility index accurately assessed the severity of arterial disease and localized it to the correct segment even in the presence of coexisting disease in proximal or distal segments. Minor degrees of stenosis, not defined but probably less than 50%, were not consistently detected. Accurate grading of arterial disease into stenosis of less than 50%, greater than 50%, and complete occlusion was regularly achieved, although patients with major arterial stenoses were separated poorly from those with complete occlusion. Of interest is that studies using pulsatility index have been done in patients at rest and have not required the use of reactive hyperemia or exercise testing to improve their sensitivity.

Presumably stimulated by the same reasons as Flanigan et al. (11), Demorais and Johnston (20) have collated pulsatility index in assessment of aortofemoral atherosclerosis with direct measurement of the pressure gradient across this segment at the time of angiography. Forty-five patients were studied, including six normal subjects. An inverse relationship was found between common femoral artery pulsatility index and the aortofemoral systolic pressure gradient. Thus when the inverse of the femoral pulsatility index was plotted against the pressure gradient a linear relationship was found. The correlation coefficient was r=0.82. Of interest in this study was that 20% of the single-plane arteriograms were incorrectly interpreted when collated with the intraarterial pressure measurements of gradient. This form of validation study using direct measurement of pressure gradients across atherosclerotic arteries is needed not only to assess the Doppler tests, but also to point out the inadequacies of the

angiographic atherosclerosis assessment as performed in most
clinical settings. It is unfortunate in this study that no
details were given about the presence or absence of significant
distal atherosclerosis in the 39 patients with aortoiliac disease.
If patients were selected because they had proximal disease only,
an opportunity was lost to vindicate pulsatility index in its
ability to assess the quantity and site of disease in the lower
limb using this excellent validation method. This is unfortunate
in view of the findings of Evans et al. (21), who used dogs with
stenoses of different severity implanted into the iliac artery and
found under controlled experimental conditions that although reduction of pulsatility index in the vessel distal to the stenosis
correlated broadly with the severity of that stenosis, the scatter
of results was wide and only a very tight stenosis of greater than
86% area reduction produced a pulsatility index low enough to be
diagnostic of a significant proximal lesion. This discrepancy
between these two studies illustrates the difficulty of applying
models developed in vivo to the study of pathology in patients.

A search for further simple methods of interpreting Doppler
velocity waveform information has produced several variations of
the techniques already described. Investigators have reported
good results using velocity waveform measurements in assessing
peripheral atherosclerosis. Waters et al. (22) defined a term
called "proximal damping quotient"; Craxford and Chamberlain (23)
used a velocity ratio as did Thomas and Cotton (24), and all
tested the validity of these concepts against arteriography. Each
of these methods has yet to be tested by other groups.

The recent advent of easy-to-use real-time spectrum frequency
analyzers and the relatively inexpensive microcomputers has
prompted a further search for more complex ways of defining
Doppler-derived velocity waveforms from arteries. Several of
these methods are essentially complex forms of pattern recognition.
Two promising new methods of waveform analysis are transfer
function analysis (TFA) (25) and principle component analysis

(PCA) (26). Critical assessment of these two new techniques is still at a very early stage, with both groups reporting results in small preliminary series of patients undergoing conventional arteriography. Of interest is the apparent capacity of the transfer function, derived by a three-pole Laplace transform method, to be sensitive to changes in the elastic modulus of proximal vessels and to changes in distal impedance. Future evaluation and validation of this index are vital to assess whether a waveform obtained from a single point in an artery can indeed describe with good sensitivity and specificity the influence of atherosclerosis in that artery both proximal and distal to the point of interrogation. Early work (27) has found that in comparison with single plane arteriography, PCA is 100% sensitive and 94% specific in identifying diameter stenosis of less than 50% at the origin of the internal carotid artery (27). A study by Evans et al. (28) using an animal model suggests partial validation of the PCA concept. Using a technique similar to a previous investigation of pulsatility index (21) they compared the ability of PCA, TFA, and pulsatility index to differentiate between various grades of stenosis implanted in iliac arteries of dogs. They found that the transfer function damping factor and pulsatility index distinguished only stenoses of greater than 85% area reduction. PCA proved more sensitive and was able to distinguish stenoses of 65% and 70% area reduction from stenoses of less than 51% area reduction. Despite the difficulties of providing an adequate model test-bed in vivo to simulate atherosclerosis in human beings, these studies are important as a method of investigating the validity of the Doppler-derived analysis for evaluating atherosclerosis.

Carotid Arteries

Variations of Doppler techniques in detecting and quantifying atherosclerosis in the legs have been used to assess disease in carotid arteries. Doppler ultrasound has been used to detect the directional flow in collateral vessels supplying the intracranial internal carotid artery after the original direction of flow had been reversed by changes in pressure secondary to hemodynamically significant disease in the proximal internal carotid artery. Further tests have included detection of changes in pulse wave velocity and in the maximum frequency envelope of the Doppler waveform secondary to atherosclerosis. The first of these methods is known as the Doppler supraorbital test, which is positive in the presence of a pressure drop across stenosis of 50% or greater in the internal carotid artery. Many investigators have compared this test with arteriography including Wise et al. (29), Barnes et al. (30) and Moore et al. (31). In the most successful attempt (30) the test is 98.7% accurate in identifying the presence or absence of stenosis of greater than 50% in the internal carotid artery, but by no means are all reports as encouraging. Indeed in a later report from Barnes et al. (32) the test was only 52% sensitive in detecting stenosis of greater than 50%, although it was 97% sensitive in detecting complete occlusion of the internal carotid artery.

An interesting use of pulse wave transit time was reported by Horrocks et al. (33). Transit time in the carotid artery was measured by using two continuous-wave Doppler instruments simultaneously, with one overlying the proximal common carotid artery at the root of the neck and the second overlying the supraorbital artery above the eye. The transit time between the two probes was subsequently normalized for the patient's age and blood pressure by dividing it by the transit time between the common carotid artery and the brachial artery. The transit time in 31 carotid arteries was correlated with biplanar carotid arteriograms obtained by direct puncture of the carotid artery. Although the numbers of patients studied was small, this was a well-designed study with good assessment of the arteriograms by three independent observers. The values of percent stenosis obtained by each observer for each vessel segment were averaged to produce a mean

figure for the correlation. When there was significant disagreement in the interpretation of the x-ray, particularly if it was of
poor quality, the case was excluded from the study. The Doppler-
derived information was measured by three independent observers to
produce a series of mean values. The use of Doppler-derived
transit time was able to separate patients with minimal disease
(less than 20% diameter stenosis), moderate disease (21-50%
diameter stenosis) and severe disease (greater than 51% diameter
stenosis). There was a highly significant separation among these
three groups using this technique. They do not report on the
sensitivity or specificity of the method but noted that a transit
time ratio of greater than 2.75 was 85% correct in predicting a
greater than 50% diameter stenosis. It is unfortunate that no
other investigators have repeated this study to see whether the
original findings are valid. Nevertheless, considerable support
for their method was produced by an experimental attempt to test
the validity of the concept of increasing ocular pulse wave delays
with increasing degrees of carotid artery atherosclerosis. Walden
et al. (34) examined the phenomenon in 12 dogs into whose carotid
arteries they inserted machined plastic stenoses of different
lumen diameters. They used the technique of oculoplethysmography
and carotid phonoangiography to detect delay and disturbance in
carotid artery flow due to the artificial stenoses. They found
a delay in pulse wave velocity with increasing area reduction and
discussed the possible biophysical explanations for this. This
was an important study illustrating the use of complementary
methods to provide evidence for the validity of the concept of
pulse wave delay in atherosclerosis.

A relatively simple analysis of the systolic peak of the
velocity waveform in the common carotid and supraorbital artery,
derived from Doppler spectral analysis, has been tested by Baskett
et al. (35). They devised a ratio of the primary peak (A) to the
secondary peak (B) in systole and found that when the A:B ratio
was less than 1.05 there was an 88% probability of disease at the

carotid bifurcation. If the A:B ratio was greater than this value there was an 80% probability of a normal carotid bifurcation. The basis of this critical value of the A:B ratio was determined in a correlation study in which 101 uniplanar carotid arteriograms were compared with ultrasound findings. Direct carotid puncture or arch arteriography was performed and in most cases within 24 h of the Doppler study. Although the sensitivity of the technique was poor in detecting both low-grade stenosis and stenosis of less than 60%, the specificity for detecting a normal junction was good at 91%. The validity of the A:B ratio of the sonogram has been established in another study by Aukland and Hurlow (36). They improved the sensitivity of the test by including an A:B ratio for the internal carotid artery at the bifurcation as well as at the common carotid and supraorbital arteries. These ratios were correlated with the angiographic interpretation in 63 carotid arteries. No details of the angiogram technique were given. There was a high specificity and sensitivity for discriminating between normal carotid bifurcations and stenosis of greater than 50%. Stenoses greater than 20% were detected with a sensitivity of 83%. They emphasized that insonation of the internal carotid artery was essential to distinguish between high-grade stenosis and complete occlusion.

The more sophisticated recognition of abnormalities in the velocity waveform envelope by the principle component analysis (PCA) technique has already been mentioned (26). It is of interest that Martin and coworkers are expanding the technique to analyze and detect principle components not only in the waveform envelope but also in the spectrally analyzed data contained within the envelope. This opens up considerable possibilities for improving the already good sensitivity and discrimination of the test.

Another form of analysis of the Doppler velocity waveform envelope has been proposed and tested in a series of studies by Rutherford and Kreutzer (37). Measurement of various dimensions of the waveform produces ratios that allow the presence or absence of atherosclerosis at the carotid bifurcation to be detected and quantified. In their latest series of 77 patients with arteriographic comparison, discriminant analysis of the ratios was able to detect a stenotic lesion of greater than 25% (diameter) in 76% of the carotid arteries. The specificity was 92%.

The principle of Doppler detection of increased blood velocity as it flows through arterial stenoses has been demonstrated graphically in one continuous wave Doppler imaging instrument, in which colors of the constructed flow map are proportional to the speed of the moving blood. Curry and White (38) have collated over 100 carotid angiograms against the Doppler system. They have noted a 94% specificity in detecting normal carotid artery bifurcations and an excellent sensitivity of 94% in detecting carotid stenoses of over 50% of the arterial diameter. Their ability to detect 85% of stenoses between 25% and 49% (39) has not been reproduced in other careful but considerably smaller studies (40,41).

The continuous wave Doppler imaging instrument introduced originally by Spencer et al. (42) has found extensive use in the clinical assessment of carotid artery disease, yet only a few validation studies utilizing arteriography have been reported. The instrument produces an ultrasound arteriogram equivalent, for instance of the carotid bifurcation, which is then used as a "reference map" from which Doppler signals are derived. The operator's interpretation of these signals provides the basis for classifying the underlying atherosclerosis. Bloch et al. (43) and Zwiebel and Crummy (44) collated the system with biplanar arteriography and found a sensitivity of 83% and specificity of 96% for a stenosis of greater than 50% diameter (the former group) and a 92% sensitivity in detecting lumen area reduction greater than 90% (the latter group). A more precise use of the continuous wave Doppler ultrasound has been attempted by Lewis et al. (45) using an instrument similar in concept to that of Spencer et al. (42). In a small preliminary series they compared 20 carotid arteriograms with a carefully produced continuous wave angiogram.

The degree of plaque intrusion shown on both the x-ray and ultrasound image was expressed as the percent diameter reduction at the tightest point of the lesion when compared to the normal artery beyond the lesion. They classified a severe lesion as having a reduction in diameter of 50% or more. They were able to define all nine complete occlusions, detected all four severe lesions, and missed only one lesion, which was a 20% stenosis. Although an extremely preliminary attempt at validation, this technique is encouraging particularly in view of its relative simplicity.

DETECTION OF EARLY ATHEROSCLEROSIS IN HUMANS

So far this review has concentrated mainly on the ability of Doppler-derived measurements to detect atherosclerosis ranging from stenosis of 50% or more to complete occlusion of the artery. The validation studies reviewed form a basis for establishing the accuracy of Doppler ultrasound in the assessment of what is really quite severe atherosclerosis. Is there any evidence to suggest that Doppler ultrasound may be used to detect the smaller lesions of atherosclerosis? Several possible methods exist.

The first method of detecting early atherosclerosis suffers from the extreme difficulty of finding a technique with which to validate it. From the basis that very early atherosclerosis might change the compliance of an artery, Gosling (16) has derived an ingenious and essentially simple technique for noninvasive measurement of the compliance of a length of artery, rather than an individual point. This technique involves the measurement of pulse wave velocity between two points a known distance apart on the artery. King et al. (15) have studied nearly 800 subjects to establish the compliance of the aorta in normal individuals from children 3 years old to adults. These normal values of compliance have been used as a basis for comparison with other groups of patients suffering from atherosclerosis, connective tissue disorders, and diabetes mellitus.

The difficulties in establishing a validation test for measurements of compliance are self-evident. Scarpello et al. (46) and Cairns et al. (47) have investigated changes in compliance derived by pulse wave velocity in patients with diabetes mellitus. Interesting differences were seen among the various clinical groups. Although arteriograms or other forms of validation tests were not done, the investigators concluded that increases in pulse wave velocity in some of their patient groups resulted from an underlying, clinically undetectable diffuse atherosclerosis. One possible method of confirming that changes in compliance occur with the development of early atherosclerosis would be to compare measurements of compliance derived by this ultrasound technique with serial arteriograms of a specific arterial segment using a precise technique such as that proposed by Blankenhorn (48). A study of this kind could be done both in human beings and in suitable animal models. If the concept of measurement of compliance by Doppler ultrasound were validated it could prove to be an extremely useful clinical technique for following atherosclerosis progression and regression, and in establishing the effect of therapeutic intervention.

A second method that has the potential for detecting moderately early atherosclerosis stenosis of less than 50% in diameter is real-time spectrum analysis of Doppler signals to detect flow disturbance. In the simplest and most inexpensive application Barnes et al. (49) used a continuous wave transducer which was manually scanned over the carotid bifurcation and in which the Doppler signals were analyzed by a real-time spectrum analyzer. No imaging system was used. In a prospective validation study comparing biplanar contrast angiography with a qualitative grading of the spectral information the accuracy of the technique was good: 70% of stenoses with less than 50% and all of the stenoses greater than 50% were identified. The specificity in identifying normal carotid arteries was low at 53%. They had noticed a mild flow disturbance in false positive patients: it is possible that this was due to boundary layer separation, which may be present in normal carotid artery bifurcations.

With increasing clinical interest in Doppler spectral analysis in the last 5 years, investigators are beginning to validate both the theory and practice of the technique for quantifying disturbances of blood flow and thus atherosclerosis. Handa et al. (50) published the results of a small but important study in which they attempted to determine the relationship between spectral disturbances and the degree of stenosis. They performed model experiments in vitro with stenoses of known severity with both steady and pulsatile flow using a blood analog and then extended their experiments to dog studies in vivo and finally human studies. This early validation study was able to show the increasing disturbance in the spectral pattern with increasing degrees of stenosis both in vitro and in the dog and patient studies.

Forster and Knapp (51) performed a careful investigation both in vitro and with canine preparations in vivo to compare pulsed-Doppler-derived spectral data with hot-film anemometer data for the same degrees of stenosis. The maximum disturbance level (calculated from the spectral broadening for the Doppler) was compared for the two techniques. The results showed that the Doppler instrument gave evidence of more flow disturbance than did the hot-film method. Forster noted that this was due to the difference in the two techniques: The Doppler can detect periodic disturbances such as vortex shedding as well as random turbulent events, whereas hot-film data measure only random disturbance.

Validation of another technique derived from Doppler spectral analysis for quantifying stenosis (the relationship between detected peak Doppler frequency at a stenosis and the tightness of the stenosis) has been performed in both clinical studies and in experiments in vitro using continuous wave Doppler systems. Spencer and Reid (52) compared 95 carotid arteriograms, which were carefully assessed using a micrometer to measure the minimum diameter at the origin of the internal carotid artery, with Doppler frequencies measured in the region of the carotid bifurcation. They were able to plot the maximum frequency detected in the vicinity of the stenosis (usually at the stenosis exit) against the residual internal carotid artery diameter. The clinical relationship was close to the theoretical relationship until small residual lumens were encountered. At this point turbulence probably caused reduced velocities. They made the important point that most stenotic atherosclerotic lesions may be asymmetrical and that this was the probable reason for the finding that the Doppler frequency ratio (peak distal velocity at the stenosis exit divided by proximal velocity) gave a better prediction of the least diameter in the x-ray image. In measuring the arteriograms they found that the least measurable diameter in the x-ray image, using phantom wires, was 0.8 mm. They considered this limitation in the measurement and interpretation of arteriograms to be an important reason for the discrepancy between Doppler and x-ray correlation. A recent study in vitro by Brown et al. (53) has validated the concept of maximum frequency ratio at the stenosis, using a model with pulsatile flow and inserted stenoses of increasing tightness in the model tube section. Real-time spectral analysis was performed on recordings made with a continuous wave 5 MHz Doppler instrument. There was excellent agreement between the frequency ratio and the actual stenosis present. A preliminary clinical study using the measured angiographic stenosis in 18 carotid arteries found that the frequency ratio correlated within ±15%. Of course the assumption in this ratio is that the Doppler beam-to-vessel angle does not change significantly when moving from the region of the stenosis to the artery beyond. A change in angle will change the received Doppler frequency even though the actual blood velocity is unchanged. This was probably the explanation for the clinical results in this study which showed not quite such a good agreement as did the experiments in vitro. In the experiments in vitro the beam-to-vessel angle was kept constant, whereas this cannot be done in clinical studies.

The final part of this review summarizes the experience of
several groups who have used the most expensive and complex of
all Doppler instrumentation for arterial examination. These
pulsed Doppler instruments have been used to generate ultrasonic
angiograms similar to those of the continuous wave imaging systems,
but with the important difference that extra views are generated
including anteroposterior, lateral, and cross-sectional, and to
obtain spectral information from the flow stream with the interrogation point being selected by either Doppler image or a simultaneously generated dynamic ultrasonic B-mode image.

Barnes et al. (32,54), Sumner et al. (55), O'Donnell et al.
(56), Hobson et al. (57) and Blackshear and Strandness (58) have
reported detailed validation studies using contrast arteriography
compared with a six-channel pulsed Doppler instrument. Most of
these studies utilized biplanar carotid arteriography with independent assessment of both the arteriogram and the ultrasonic
image in a prospective manner. Sumner et al. (55) found that 81%
of the ultrasonic images agreed within ±20% of the angiographic
quantitation of stenosis. O'Donnell et al. (56) produced an
important assessment of the method and an interesting statistical
approach in which the dynamic relationship between sensitivity and
specificity of the technique was analyzed on receiver-operator
characteristic curves. With a significant stenosis defined as a
50% diameter reduction the test had only 50% sensitivity and 80%
specificity. This compares to the 92% sensitivity and 65% specificity found by Barnes et al. (54). This latter group's most
recent experience showed the specificity and sensitivity to have
improved to 100% each for this test, but these recent data are
derived from an extremely limited series of only 19 carotid
arteries where angiography was available for validation. Hobson's
group (57) showed a specificity of 81% and a sensitivity of 87% in
differentiating patients with normal and mildly stenosed carotid
arteries (less than 50%) from patients with greater than 50%
stenosis or occlusion and have published in detail their findings

of the capabilities and limitations of this technique (59).
Blackshear and Strandness (58) found the technique to be 88%
specific, and 75% sensitive for detecting any degree of stenosis
or occlusion. With subdivision of the categories of stenosis they
found the technique to be 59% sensitive in detecting stenoses of
between 10% and 49% and 91% sensitive in detecting stenoses of
greater than 50%.

An interesting innovation in the use of the six-channel pulsed
Doppler instrument has been described by Miles et al. (60). They
utilized a microcomputer attached to the instrument in order to
generate a simultaneous lateral, anteroposterior, and transverse
cross-sectional image. A program plots out the cross-sectional
vessel area as it is being scanned. Stenoses are seen as a change
in an area histogram plot. They have correlated this technique
with 94 biplanar carotid arteriograms. The test was 85% specific
and 100% sensitive for detecting greater than 40% reduction in the
lumen diameter. This is a promising new technique for quantifying
atherosclerosis and potentially can be used to follow the progress
of individual lesions over time.

Utilizing a sophisticated 30-channel pulsed Doppler instrument
Warlow and Fish (61) in an unblinded study of 50 patients have
compared the results of the ultrasound arteriogram with selective
biplanar carotid angiography. They found the test to be 94%
specific with an overall sensitivity of 76%. The instrument
identified 30% of patients with stenosis of less than 25% by diameter, 80% of patients with stenosis of 25-49%, 100% of patients
with stenosis of 50-74%, and 100% of patients with stenosis of
75-99%. All six occluded carotid arteries were correctly identified. In a prospective trial of this instrument Lusby et al.
(62) detected 90% of all stenoses of less than 50% diameter
reduction and all total occlusions of the internal carotid artery.
The overall sensitivity was 93% and specificity 100%.

The Duplex system has been investigated almost exclusively
by the group at the University of Washington School of Medicine,

Seattle (63).   It has been collated with angiography through the
various phases of development.   The technique involves interrogation of blood flow in the center of the vessel with the position
of the pulsed Doppler beam guided by the operator using the self-
contained real-time B-mode scanner.   The Doppler data were passed
through a real-time frequency spectrum analyzer, and analyzed
using several indices that were empirically derived from retrospective studies.   Their most recent data have shown a specificity
of 100%, and remarkably good sensitivity for detecting various
grades of atherosclerotic intrusion on the lumen of the internal
carotid artery.   Thus it detected 67% of stenoses of 0-10%, 78% of
stenoses of 10-49%, and 100% of stenoses of 50-99%.   This team of
investigators is still searching for improvement, despite these
excellent results, by further analysis of the information contained
within the spectral waveform.   Computer-based pattern recognition
methods are being used to assess a variety of spectral features,
and these are being subjected to discriminant analysis to improve
the objective interpretation.   Future developments in this effort
are awaited with interest.   Most of the work in detecting early
atherosclerosis with these complex instruments has been directed
to the carotid artery, but there is no reason why they could not
be used to study the natural history of atherosclerosis in the
lower limb arteries.

REASONS FOR FAILURE OF THE DOPPLER TEST TO CORRELATE WITH
THE ANGIOGRAM

Lack of correlation of Doppler techniques with baseline arteriograms is mostly secondary to procedural and technical problems.
Calcification in atheromatous plaques may have prevented successful imaging of the atheroma deep to the calcium in about 11% of
patients in one study of ultrasound angiography (59).   To allow
correlation of this hidden segment of vessel with the arteriogram
the presence of any flow disturbance within the invisible section
must be searched for using spectral analysis of blood flow immediately distal this section.

Most Doppler imaging instruments produce an image of the blood flow in only one direction. This might result in a false over-estimate of the severity of a stenosis by failing to image the vortex or separation zones immediately beyond the stenosis exit in which the blood is flowing in the reverse direction to the main stream. This might be the case especially in stenoses with short exits or reverse venturi shape. The return Doppler power to the imaging instrument may vary as the ultrasound beam passes through tissue of different attenuation and reflectivity and through stenotic plaques (Fig. 1). This can produce variation in the size of the Doppler image and could be an important source of failure to correlate lesion dimensions with those found on arteriograms. The ability to maintain a constant return power while producing the image would minimize this source of error. The presence of the high-pass filter in all Doppler instruments which is used to screen out arterial wall movements, results in the loss of infor-mation about slowly moving blood near the vessel wall. This is likely to be important in patients with minimal plaque formation which produces localized areas of flow disturbance or vortex formation. The high-pass filter may cause complete failure of the instrument to detect this disturbed flow and so reduce its sensi-tivity in low-grade atherosclerosis. This problem needs further investigation. Excessive movement of the artery, for example in hypertensive patients, will cause the Doppler image to be over-sized. Thus, comparison of dimensions of both normal and diseased arterial segments with the arteriogram will produce a poor corre-lation, although the measurement of percent stenosis may not be adversely affected.

Significant errors can be caused by failure to perform the Doppler scan correctly: for example, not scanning over the edges of the artery and thus producing a narrow image, by excessive patient movement during the scan, and by using excessive pressure of the probe overlying the artery, which may not only produce artifactual increases in velocity and spectral disturbance but also move the vessel. These errors can be eliminated by attention

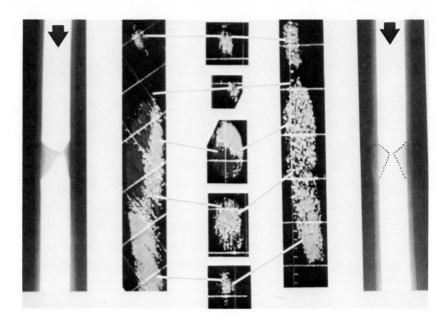

Fig. 1 Example of artifacts in the pulsed Doppler angiograms of blood flowing through a stenosis of 90% by diameter in an 8-mm latex tube. Three ultrasonic projections are shown: cross section (center), lateral (left), anteroposterior (right), with corresponding contrast arteriograms. Note: (1) narrow prestenotic blood stream image due to failure to detect the slowly moving blood near the wall secondary to high-pass filtering; (2) gap in ultrasonic image at the stenosis caused by attenuation of the material at the stenosis, simulating the effect of calcium in plaque; and (3) oversized image in poststenotic segment secondary to increase Doppler return power in region of blood flow turbulence and vortex formation. Arrows denote direction of blood flow.

to detail and by providing some form of immobilization of the patient's head during imaging. Investigators using Doppler ultrasound must be flexible enough to define unusual variations of pathology or anatomy by changing their scanning or interrogation technique as required. This will avoid failure to depict pathology often slightly removed from the immediate scanning site and thus improve correlation with the angiogram.

    A serious potential source of poor correlation is an often excessive time interval between the Doppler ultrasound study and the arteriogram. The local pathology might change dramatically in this time interval and thus result in total failure of the two tests to correlate.

In most of the studies reviewed above, uniplanar angiography was the baseline standard. This is totally inadequate to assess atherosclerotic lesions accurately and is an important source of the failure of the Doppler test to correlate. Further it is extremely difficult to produce an arteriographic view in exactly the same plane as the Doppler angiogram image for precise correlation. There is a lack of standardization of arteriographic procedure among various centers. For example, films may be taken in systole or diastole, which may produce between a 10% and 17% error in the measurement of arterial dimensions, particularly in the more normal arteries. The use of electrocardiographic triggering may help to avoid this source of error.

The most important source of error and thus lack of correlation is inter- and intraobserver variation in the interpretation of both the Doppler tests and the arteriograms. This has been noted to be particularly marked in the description of moderate stenoses (in the 50%-diameter-reduction range) (64). Most of the studies cited in this review have failed to address the problem of observer variation, and it certainly could be one explanation for lack of correlation where present.

Studies on the detection of atherosclerosis in the leg vessels are often difficult to interpret due to the lack of a standardized stress for inducing hyperemia. Furthermore, arteriography may produce inadequate filling of distal vessels beyond severe proximal disease in the legs, preventing accurate grading of the severity and extent of atherosclerosis present. These technically inadequate arteriograms should be withdrawn from any correlation study.

RECOMMENDATIONS FOR IMPROVING FUTURE DOPPLER VALIDATION STUDIES

It is perhaps because the management of patients is not a pure science that some of the diagnostic techniques upon which we base our management decisions have not been as rigorously tested for

accuracy as would be imperative in a purely scientific world.
Nevertheless it is surprising that investigators using the various
techniques reviewed above have not insisted on stricter conditions
for the validation of these methods. It is important to know
whether the relative failure of some techniques or the inconsistencies in others are due to the techniques themselves or to a
less than fair comparison with other methods. There is no ideal
baseline standard with which to compare Doppler studies of atherosclerosis, nor is there an ideal method of carrying out such a
comparison. Recent studies of chest x-rays of various pulmonary
conditions and of coronary angiograms for the estimation of coronary atherosclerosis have pointed out the difficulties involved in
interpreting data and provide some guidelines with which a more
scientific correlation of Doppler evaluation with arteriography
could be performed.

   Careful experimental design is imperative to reduce error due
to both the technical factors involved in performing the tests and
the human factors involved in their interpretation. Adequate
numbers of patients with all grades of atherosclerosis, from those
with completely normal arteries to those severely affected, must
be entered into the study from the beginning. The Doppler test
should be performed in the 24-hour period immediately before the
baseline arteriogram to avoid changes in the basic pathology that
might occur during any excessive interval between the two tests.
The Doppler study should be performed in a carefully controlled
and standardized way previously agreed upon by participants in the
study and preferably with the sonographer unaware of the clinical
status of the patient so that the test is performed blind. There
must be a standardized arteriographic technique for all patients
in the study, which should include guidelines for premedication
before the arteriogram and information on pressure and rate of
contrast injection. In the lower limbs the use of vasodilators at
the time of the arteriogram might improve the filling of the small
vessels of the calf and thus provide more accurate quantification

of atherosclerosis.   Only the highest-resolution angiographic
equipment should be used and technically poor studies should be
excluded from analysis.   Biplanar views of the target vessel
should be obtained routinely with added oblique projections as
required.   It would be ideal, although technically extremely
difficult, to obtain exactly the same views for the arteriogram
as were obtained by an ultrasound imaging system.   All measurements of arterial pathology on the arteriograms must be made
objectively using calipers or micrometers.

In at least 25% of patients the noninvasive Doppler test
should be repeated soon after the arteriogram to test the repro-
duciblity of the Doppler information.   The data from this re-
testing of randomly selected patients should be included in the
final statistical analysis of the accuracy of the technique.   In
only a few of the papers reviewed above (37,42) is the reproducibility of the technique formally mentioned.   In an attempt to
test the reproducibility of ankle pressure measurements after
standardized exercise to assess lower-limb atherosclerosis Clyne
et al. (65) found a considerable variation between two tests when
carried out one week apart.

The interpretation of the results of both the Doppler test
and the baseline test is a difficult task.   Accuracy may best be
served by the use of a consensus reading panel of at least three
observers, one panel for the Doppler test and one for the arteriogram.   Repine et al. (64) have suggested that a formal pilot trial
should be carried out before the major trial to discover any
discrepancies and the reasons for such discrepancies between
observers in interpretation of data.   This pilot trial would allow
the observers to come to final agreement on proper grading systems
for arteriograms.   A diagram of the vessel segment would be helpful to provide complete and standardized reporting by the observers.   Sketching of the location and shape of atheromatous plaque
and calculation of the degree of stenosis could be done with the
use of such an aid.   The pilot trial would have the benefit of

completely familiarizing the observers with any proposed classification system. Both this and perhaps the use of standard arteriographic films of different grades of disease might reduce the bias
of individual readers. However, if bias is displayed and detected
in the statistical analysis it can be utilized to increase the
precision of this analysis.

During the main trial tests intra- and interobserver variation
of interpretation must be carried out. This should be done by
random rereading of studies without the observer's knowledge that
he is in fact rereading a study. This variation should be tested
both over short and longer periods of time, for example, 3 months.
The number of random repeat interpretations in this study would
depend on the total number of patients planned for inclusion. If
the study is small then perhaps every single test should be reread
at random. By determining intra- and interobserver variability,
misreading rate and individual bias, statistical analysis would be
better able to describe the precision of the test and its range of
error in quantifying atherosclerosis and thus provide criteria by
which change in the noninvasive test as a result of change in the
atherosclerosis could be better defined. Calculation of sensitivity and specificity and perhaps a family of receiver operator
characteristic curves (56) would provide the evidence with which
to judge the individual Doppler test.

FURTHER STUDIES OF DOPPLER QUANTIFICATION OF ATHEROSCLEROSIS
WITH ANGIOGRAPHIC CONFIRMATION

This review has shown that the approach of investigators utilizing
Doppler techniques in the study of atherosclerosis has been
wide-based. Several of the techniques have been found to be
particularly promising both at the lower extreme of detecting
early disease and at the upper extreme of quantifying advanced
disease. It is obvious from the difficulties involved not just
in performing the Doppler studies but also the arteriogram that
far greater emphasis in future studies must be placed on developing

pathological examination of removed atherosclerotic specimens as the final arbiter of these correlation studies. This point has already been expressed extremely well in the summary of a 1980 workshop on noninvasive techniques for the assessment of atherosclerosis sponsored by the National Heart, Lung, and Blood Institute. Information on reproducibility of Doppler-derived data must be obtained in future studies and correlated with repeat angiography if necessary. The use of the recently introduced digital intravenous angiography may be extremely relevant to this form of reproducibility study because of its relative noninvasiveness and its acceptability to patients.

Studies comparing the relative performance of continuous wave and pulsed Doppler imaging systems must be initiated. The potentially greater sensitivity and precision of pulsed Doppler systems for detecting all grades of atherosclerosis will have to be proved and balanced against the increased cost of these instruments. It is quite likely that such a comparative trial would show that continuous wave systems could quantify severe disease more accurately than pulsed systems, whereas the latter systems would be more sensitive to the lower grades of disease and thus perhaps be more useful in natural history studies of atherosclerosis. The potential of several of the Doppler techniques for quantifying early atherosclerosis must be proved in larger trials in the future. Changes of vessel compliance in atherosclerosis described by pulse wave velocity measuring techniques must be validated by high resolution angiography of the type described by Blankenhorn (48) and in animal studies in which both angiographic and pathological confirmation of early atherosclerotic changes could be obtained. So far spectral information from both pulsed Doppler and Duplex imaging systems has tended to be taken only from the center of the moving blood stream within the artery. Work needs to be done to see whether information sampled from the vessel wall and from the vicinity of very small 1-mm plaques or less may show limited local flow disturbance.

The promise shown by the new, computer-based, sophisticated pattern recognition systems for identifying changes in Doppler waveform must be tested by further large-scale studies. The ability of principle component analysis, transfer function analysis and other derived indices must be validated in studies involving large numbers of normal patients of all age groups, including patients with hypertension, to see whether the changes in normal patients with aging and hypertension can be differentiated from the changes due to the development of early atherosclerosis. The techniques of waveform analysis and precision Doppler imaging could be tested with profit in suitable animal models of atherosclerosis in which adequate correlation between both angiography and pathology could be obtained.

FUTURE RESEARCH INTO THE QUANTIFICATION OF ATHEROSCLEROSIS
BY DOPPLER TECHNIQUES

With increasing advances in technology and in the understanding of Doppler physics there are many new areas where fruitful work could be carried out. The following suggestions are an expression of personal interest and preference. Of prime importance is the standardization of Doppler examination techniques, whether using the simplest or the most complex of instruments. Agreement must be reached among various centers as to how the procedures should be carried out and interpreted. Only then can real advances in understanding atherosclerosis be made.

Far more use must be made of phantoms to define the limits of the Doppler techniques, whether in imaging or describing changes in velocity spectra. This work should explore the potential for describing extremely early disease as well as accurately quantifying more advanced disease. In any long series of investigations, such as in clinical trials, it is of vital importance that instruments should be calibrated regularly. This does not seem to happen to any of the current Doppler instruments of whatever complexity. The use of phantoms would allow testing on a

regular basis to make certain that design specifications were
being maintained.

The large amount of information hidden within the spectrally
analyzed blood flow waveform needs to be accurately described and
quantified by both pattern recognition techniques and discriminant
analysis. This would allow objective quantification of the information and be less prone to subjective interpretation errors. In
addition, the influence of such important factors as the blood-
flow Reynolds number on spectral output must be defined. New
applications of Doppler techniques should be devised to improve
detection of dangerous, complex, ulcerating plaques. Some preliminary work done in vitro using pulsed Doppler imaging has shown
promise (see Fig. 2) (66). The large amount of data obtained by
Doppler techniques from individual stenotic plaques, both by
imaging and analysis of the local flow disturbance, should be
investigated to produce criteria that might define the risk of an
individual plaque, for example in the carotid, causing symptoms
in the patient. One might describe this as defining a "plaque
risk profile."

The increasing precision of the latest Doppler instruments,
particularly pulsed Doppler imaging and Duplex systems, should
provide a stimulus to investigate the subtle hemodynamics present
in normal and diseased circulation in regions where atheromatous
plaques develop. This might provide valuable information on the
cause of atherosclerosis and particularly its predilection for
certain sites.

To improve further the objectivity of Doppler scanning methods,
research into automating these ought to be done. The use of a
water bath containing a transducer attached to a stereotactic
probe arm might allow accurate, reproducible scanning, standardization of technique, and considerable reduction in operator
error. Furthermore, power return levels could be maintained
constant to reduce image artifact. Further work should be done
on investigating the potential of more tightly focused continuous

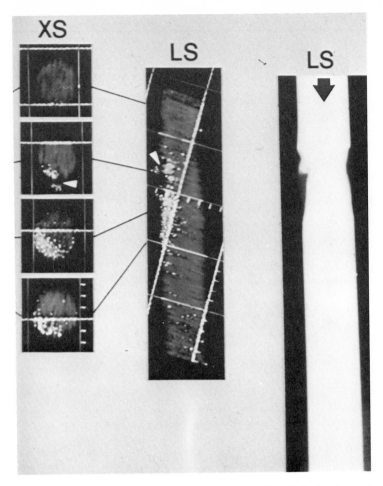

Fig. 2 Example of experimental detection of modeled ulcer in 30%
stenosis within 8-mm latex tube. The arteriogram on the right.
Color-coded 30-channel pulsed Doppler images [lateral (LS) and
cross section (XS) scans] in the center and on the left. Arrows
show the vortex imaged in the ulcer crater. Note the poststenotic
vortex depicted in both ultrasonic projections.

wave ultrasound beams and smaller pulsed-Doppler sample volumes to
detect local flow disturbances close to small plaques or areas of
intimal change in early atherosclerosis. These studies would need
to be validated by high-resolution angiography. The sensitivity
for detecting very low-grade lesions, for example in the carotid
arteries, may be improved by applying standardized stress tests to

see if spectral changes are incurred in the presence of minor plaque formation. This has worked well in a much cruder way for the detection of lesser grades of stenosis in the leg.

CONCLUSIONS

Rapid advances are being made in Doppler ultrasound, and the need to validate use of these techniques in the quantification of atherosclerosis remains a scientific imperative. Much progress in validation has been made already, but the studies could be improved considerably by better design and statistical analysis. Only then will we know how useful a tool Doppler ultrasound may become. These studies will require the utmost cooperation among clinicians, pathologists, radiologists, and ultrasound investigators.

REFERENCES

1. Carter SA (1969) Clinical measurement of systolic pressures in limbs with arterial occlusive disease. JAMA 207:1869-1874
2. Carter SA (1972) Response of ankle systolic pressure to leg exercise in mild or questionable arterial disease. N Engl J Med 287:578-582
3. Carter SA, Lezack JD (1971) Digital systolic pressures in the lower limb in arterial disease. Circulation 43:905-914
4. Yao ST, Hobbs JT, Irvine WT (1969) Ankle systolic pressure measurements in arterial disease affecting the lower extremities. Brit J Surg 56:676-679
5. Johnson WC (1975) Doppler ankle pressure and reactive hyperemia in the diagnosis of arterial insufficiency. J Surg Res 18:177-180
6. Allan JS, Terry HJ (1969) The evaluation of an ultrasonic flow detector for the assessment of peripheral vascular disease. Cardiovasc Res 3:503-509
7. Cutajar CL, Marston A, Newcombe JF (1973) Value of cuff occlusion pressures in assessment of peripheral vascular disease. Br Med J 2:392-395
8. Heintz SE, Bone GE, Slaymaker EE, Hayes AC, Barnes RW (1978) Value of arterial pressure measurements in the proximal and distal part of the thigh in arterial occlusive disease. Surg Gynecol Obstet 146:337-343
9. Colt JD (1978) New Doppler pressure indexes plotted as curves. Am J Surg 136:198-201
10. Rutherford RB, Lowenstein DH, Klein MF (1979) Combining segmental systolic pressures and plethysmography to diagnose arterial occlusive disease of the legs. Am J Surg 138:211-218

11. Flanigan DP, Gray B, Schuler JJ, Schwartz JA, Post KW (1981) Correlation of Doppler-derived high thigh pressure and intra-arterial pressure in the assessment of aorto-iliac occlusive disease. Br J Surg 68:423-425
12. Fronek A, Coel M, Bernstein EF (1978) The importance of combined multisegmental pressure and Doppler flow velocity studies in the diagnosis of peripheral arterial occlusive disease. Surgery 84:840-847
13. Fish PJ (1981) Recent advances in cardiovascular Doppler. In: Kurjak A (ed) Progress in medical ultrasound, vol 2. Excerpta Media, Amsterdam, pp 217-237
14. Nicolaides AN, Angelides NS (1981) Waveform index and resistance factor using directional Doppler ultrasound and a zero crossing detector. In: Nicolaides AN, Yao JST (eds) Investigation of vascular disorders. Churchill Livingstone, New York, pp 291-300
15. King DH, Coghlan B, Gosling RG, Pickup A, Newman DL, Woodcock JP (1972) Transcutaneous measurement of pulse wave velocity and mean blood pressure in man. In: Roberts C (ed) Blood flow measurement. Sector Publishing Limited, London, pp 40-43
16. Gosling RG (1976) IEE Medical Electronics Monograph 21, Extraction of Physiological Information From Spectrum-Analysed Doppler-Shifted Continuous-Wave Ultrasound Signals Obtained Noninvasively From the Arterial System. Peter Peregrinus Limited, Stevenage, pp 73-125
17. Fitzgerald DE, Carr J (1977) Peripheral arterial disease: assessment by arteriography and alternative noninvasive measurements. AJR 128:385-388
18. Harris PL, Taylor LA, Cave FD, Charlesworth D (1974) The relationship between Doppler ultrasound assessment and angiography in occlusive arterial disease of the lower limbs. Surg Gynecol Obstet 138:911-914
19. Johnston KW, Demorais D, Kassam M, Brown PM (1981) Cerebrovascular assessment using a Doppler carotid scanner and real-time frequency analysis. J Clin Ultrasound 9:443-449
20. Demorais D, Johnston KW (1981) Assessment of aorto-iliac disease by non-invasive quantitative Doppler waveform analysis. Br J Surg 68:789-792
21. Evans DH, Barrie WW, Asher MJ, Bentley S, Bell PRF (1980) The relationship between ultrasonic pulsatility index and proximal arterial stenosis in a canine model. Circ Res 46:470-475
22. Waters KJ, Chamberlain J, McNeill IF (1977) The significance of aorto-iliac atherosclerosis as assessed by Doppler ultrasound. Am J Surg 134:388-391
23. Craxford AD, Chamberlain J (1971) Pulse waveform transit ratios in the assessment of peripheral vascular disease. Br J Surg 64:449-452
24. Thomas MK, Cotton LT (1977) Assessment of arterial stenosis by pulse wave velocity measurements. Abstracts of 1977 meeting of the Vascular Surgical Society of Great Britain and Ireland. Edinburgh

25. Skidmore R, Woodcock JP, Wells PNT, Bird D, Baird RN (1980) Physiological interpretation of Doppler-shift waveforms--III. Ultrasound Med Biol 6:227-231
26. Martin TRP, Barber DC, Sherriff SB, Prichard DR (1980) Objective feature extraction applied to the diagnosis of carotid artery disease using a Doppler ultrasound technique. Clin Phys Physiol Meas 1:71-81
27. Sherriff SB, Barber DC, Martin TRP, Lakeman M, Dhillon P (1980) Mathematical feature extraction applied to the entire Doppler shifted frequency signal obtained from the common carotid artery. Abstracts of the International Conference on Blood Flow Theory and Practise, The Biological Engineering Society, London
28. Evans DH, MacPherson DS, Bentley S, Asher MJ, Bell PRF (1981) The effect of proximal stenosis on Doppler waveforms: a comparison of three methods of waveform analysis in an animal model. Clin Phys Physiol Meas 2:17-25
29. Wise G, Brockenbrough EC, Marty R, Griep R (1971) The detection of carotid artery obstruction: a correlation with arteriography. Stroke 2:105-113
30. Barnes RW, Russel HE, Bone GE, Slaymaker EE (1977) Doppler cerebrovascular examination: improved results with refinements in technique. Stroke 8:468-471
31. Moore WS, Bean B, Burton R, Goldstone J (1977) The use of ophthalmosonometry in the diagnosis of carotid artery stenosis. Surgery 82:107-115
32. Barnes RW, Rittgers SE, Thornhill B, Nix L, Marszalek P, Putney W (1981) Noninvasive cerebrovascular screening techniques; indirect versus direct carotid interrogation. In: Greenhalgh RM (ed) Smoking and arterial disease. Pitman Medical, Bath, pp 122-134
33. Horrocks M, Roberts VC, Cotton LT (1979) Assessment of carotid artery stenosis using pulse wave transit time. Br J Surg 66:265-268
34. Walden R, L'Italien G, Megerman J, Bouchier-Hayes D, Hanel K, Maloney R, Abbott W (1980) Complementary methods for evaluating carotid stenosis: a biophysical basis for ocular pulse wave delays. Surgery 88:162-167
35. Baskett JJ, Beasley MG, Murphy GJ, Hyams DE, Gosling RG (1977) Screening for carotid junction disease by spectral analysis of Doppler signals. Cardiovasc Res 11:147-155
36. Aukland A, Hurlow RA (1981) Detection of carotid bifurcation disease by spectral analysis of Doppler ultrasound. Abstracts of International Vascular Symposium, London
37. Rutherford RB, Kreutzer EW (1981) Doppler ultrasound techniques in the assessment of extracranial arterial occlusive disease. In: Nicolaides AN, Yao JST (eds) Investigation of vascular disorders. Churchill Livingstone, New York, pp 139-154
38. Curry GR, White DN (1978) Colour-coded ultrasonic differential velocity arterial scanner (Echoflow). Ultrasound Med Biol 4:27-35

39. White DN (1981)   Accuracy of colour-coded Doppler scans. Abstracts of Meeting of the International Cardiovascular Congress III, Arizona
40. O'Leary DH, Persson AV, Clouse ME (1981)   Noninvasive testing for carotid artery stenosis: 1. Prospective analysis of three methods.   AJR 137:1189-1194
41. Johnston KW, Maruzzo BC, Kassam M, Cobbold RSC (1981)   Quantitative analysis of Doppler blood flow velocity recordings using pulsatility index.   In: Nicolaides AN, Yao JST (eds) Investigation of vascular disorders.   Churchill Livingstone, New York, pp 274-290
42. Spencer MP, Reid JM, Davis DL, Paulson PS (1974)   Cervical carotid imaging with a continuous-wave Doppler flowmeter. Stroke 5:145-154
43. Bloch S, Baltaxe HA, Shoumaker RD (1979)   Reliability of Doppler scanning of the carotid bifurcation: angiographic correlation.   Radiology 132:687-691
44. Zwiebel WJ, Crummy AB (1981)   Sources of error in Doppler diagnosis of carotid occlusive disease.   AJR 137:1-12
45. Lewis RR, Beasley MG, Gosling RG (1980)   Detection of disease at the carotid bifurcation using ultrasound--including an imaging system.   J R Soc Med 73:172-179
46. Scarpello JHB, Martin TRP, Ward JD (1980)   Ultrasound measurements of pulse-wave velocity in the peripheral arteries of diabetic subjects.   Clin Sci 58:53-57
47. Cairns SA, Woodcock JP, Marshall AJ (1978)   Early arterial lesions in maturity onset diabetes mellitus detected by an ultrasonic technique.   Diabetologia 14:107-111
48. Blankenhorn DH (1978)   Progression and regression of femoral atherosclerosis in man.   Athero Rev 3:169-181
49. Barnes RW, Rittgers SE, Putney WW (1982)   Real-time Doppler spectrum analysis.   Predictive value in defining operable carotid artery disease.   Arch Surg 117:52-57
50. Handa H, Niimi H, Moritake K, Okumura A, Matsuda I, Hayashi K (1977)   Analysis of sound spectographic pattern for assessment of vascular occlusive disorders by continuous wave ultrasound Doppler flowmeter.   Arch Jpn Chir 46:214-225
51. Forster FK, Knapp CF (1980)   The assessment of pulsed Doppler with hot-film anemometry for measuring disturbed blood flow through stenoses in physiologic models and dogs.   Abstracts of 25th Annual Meeting of the American Institute of Ultrasound in Medicine
52. Spencer MP, Reid JM (1979)   Quantitation of carotid stenosis with continuous-wave (C-W) Doppler ultrasound.   Stroke 10: 326-330
53. Brown PM, Kassam M, Johnston KW (1981)   Real-time Doppler spectral analysis for the measurement of carotid stenosis. Abstracts of Meeting of the International Cardiovascular Congress III, Arizona
54. Barnes RW, Bone GE, Reinertson J, Slaymaker EE, Hokanson DE, Strandness DE (1976)   Noninvasive ultrasonic carotid angiography:

prospective validation by contrast arteriography. Surgery 80:328-335

55. Sumner DS, Russell JB, Ramsey DE, Hajjar WM, Miles RD (1979) Noninvasive diagnosis of extracranial carotid arterial disease. A prospective evaluation of pulsed-Doppler imaging and oculoplethysmography. Arch Surg 114:1222-1229

56. O'Donnell TF, Pauker SG, Callow AD, Kelly JJ, McBride KJ, Korwin S (1980) The relative value of carotid noninvasive testing as determined by receiver operator characteristic curves. Surgery 87:9-19

57. Hobson RW, Berry SM, Jamil Z, Mehta K, Hart L, Simpson H (1981) Oculoplethysmography and pulsed Doppler ultrasonic imaging in diagnosis of carotid arterial disease. Surg Gynecol Obstet 152:433-436

58. Blackshear WM, Strandness DE (1981) Angiographic imaging by ultrasound compared with indirect methods. In: Nicolaides AN, Yao JST (eds) Investigation of vascular disorders. Churchill Livingstone, New York, pp 165-200

59. Berry SM, O'Donnell JA, Hobson RW (1980) Capabilities and limitations of pulsed Doppler sonography in carotid imaging. J Clin Ultrasound 8:405-412

60. Miles RD, Russell JB, Sumner DS (1981) Simultaneous three-dimensional computerised imaging of the carotid bifurcation. Abstracts of Meeting of the International Vascular Symposium, London

61. Warlow CP, Fish PJ (1980) Pulsed Doppler imaging of the carotid artery. J Neurol Sci 45:135-141

62. Lusby RJ, Woodcock JP, Skidmore R, Jeans WD, Hope DT, Baird RN (1981) Carotid artery disease: a prospective evaluation of pulsed Doppler imaging. Ultrasound Med Biol 7:365-370

63. Thiele BL, Bodily KC, Blackshear WM, Phillips DT, Strandness DE (1981) Current status of ultrasonic imaging and spectral analysis in the detection of arterial stenosis. In: Greenhalgh RM (ed) Smoking and arterial disease. Pitman Medical, Bath, pp 142-152

64. Pepine CJ, Feldman RL, Nichols WW, Conti CR (1977) Coronary angiography: potentially serious sources of error in interpretation. Cardiovasc Med 2:747-756

65. Clyne CAC, Tripolitis A, Jamieson CW, Gustave R, Stuart F (1979) The reproducibility of the treadmill walking test for claudication. Surg Gynecol Obstet 149:727-728

66. Wood CPL, Smith BR (1981) A noninvasive method for detection of the complex ulcerated atheromatous plaque: experimental evaluation. Abstracts of Meeting of the International Vascular Symposium, London

DISCUSSION: MERRILL P. SPENCER

My comments pertain mainly to the carotid arteries. First, the problem of noninvasive detection of ulceration of the arterial intima is of paramount importance in stroke prevention, but at this time in history there is no method for detection of ulceration except direct inspection and histological sectioning. My definition of ulceration is that of a denuded intima. Arteriography can detect wall roughening and craters that may or may not be ulcerated, and no ultrasound technique has a signal which specifies ulceration. Doppler-shifted ultrasound itself offers little promise. It is my hope that B-scan imaging can, in the future, develop sufficient resolution to define with accuracy thrombus and fibrin and platelet strands adhering to the intimal lumen. Ultimately a new technique using radioisotope tagging or NMR may provide us with noninvasive detection of ulceration, intramural hemorrhage, and other substrata definition of the plaque. Meanwhile, continuous wave (CW) Doppler is the modality best suited to noninvasively detect and quantify carotid artery segmental stenosis. Stenosis, like cratering, is often associated with ulceration.

With respect to calcium deposits, which appear to present a problem to pulsed wave (PW) Doppler techniques in obscuring the Doppler ultrasound diagnostic signal, we have not found this to be a significant problem using CW Doppler. The CW Doppler with its high signal-to-noise ratio and interrogation of the entire arterial cross section vessel, without the problems of pulsed Doppler range gating, provides a clear signal of high velocity within a stenosis and the downstream turbulence. Our reason for enthusiasm for CW Doppler with imaging is that it does the best job of detecting all three features of a stenosis, including the primary high velocity within the stenosis, the secondary downstream turbulence, and tertiary effects of collateralization. Fig. A.1 illustrates the CW Doppler signal and image of a tight stenosis at the origin of the internal carotid, demonstrating both the primary and secondary

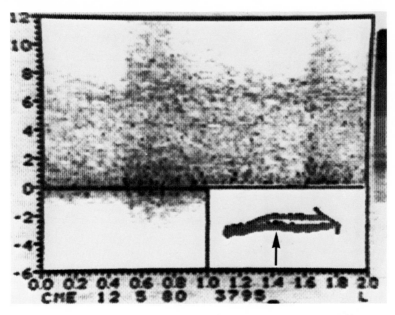

Fig. A.1 Continuous wave Doppler frequency spectral display of signals on the origin of the internal carotid artery representing high velocities of stenosis and low velocities of downstream turbulence.

features. The chances that the high frequencies and the downstream turbulence will both be obscured by calcium is remote.

Accuracy figures of our laboratory's most recent study (1981) of patients are illustrated in Fig. A.2. Two different grades of stenosis, 50% and 70%, were analyzed. The principal cause of the errors that we have made in Doppler correlations with angiography are those of degree when the interpreter overestimates the severity of stenosis. All eight false positives and one false negative were degree problems and not questions on presence or absence of stenosis. In two of the three remaining false negatives, a calcified plaque was diagnosed when in fact occlusion or extensive fibromuscular hyperplasia was present. No errors have been made in separating external carotid artery stenosis from internal stenosis since on-line spectral analysis has become available.

Fig. 3 provides accuracy figures for a special study to differentiate tight stenosis from total occlusion of the internal

348   C. P. L. Wood

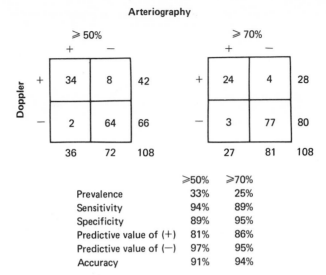

Fig. A.2 Decision matrix analysis at two levels of stenosis of
the internal carotid artery comparing continuous-wave Doppler
results with arteriography measurements.

carotid. Tight stenosis represents reduction in the lumen to less
than 1 mm in diameter, as indicated by either CW Doppler or
arteriography. We conclude from these studies that the CW Doppler
diagnosis of stenosis of the internal carotid artery increases in
accuracy with increasing severity of the lesions. We have always
recognized that Doppler does poorly in diagnosing minor degrees of
stenoses, but minor degrees of stenosis are not usually clinically
significant. Continuous-wave Doppler therefore provides a highly
accurate method of guiding the clinical decision concerning
patient management.

    Next, I would like to mention a new quantitative aspect of
continuous-wave Doppler detection of stenosis of the carotid
arteries. By means of the Bernoulli principle, and knowing the
angle between the Doppler beam and the arterial channel, the
pressure drop along the artery can be calculated in millimeters
of mercury. The equation for this is $\Delta p = 4v^2$, where v represents
blood velocity in m/s and Δp is in mmHg. Downstream turbulance
must be present for this relationship to hold.

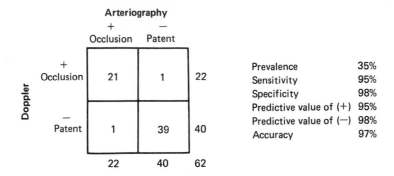

Fig. A.3 Decision matrix analysis illustrating the high predictive values and accuracy of continuous-wave Doppler in differentiating extremely tight stenosis of the internal carotid artery from total occlusion of that artery. (From West, Clark, and Spencer, Institute of Applied Physiology and Medicine, Seattle, Washington.)

Finally, I should like to comment on the excellent work being performed in the laboratories of Europe, including those of von Reutern of Freiburg, Pourcelot of Tours, France, and Müller of Basel, Switzerland. There are many others that are following the leadership of these workers. They have excellent results using hand-held techniques without Doppler imaging of the carotids. Their accuracy reaches to the 96-98 sensitivity/specificity range, but this degree of accuracy is achieved where there is a high disease prevalence, where the physician (often a neurologist) performs many of the examinations, and where the decisions concerning angiography are also made by the examining physician. This method of practice of medicine on the continent of Europe is not widely utilized in the United States, where we rely on paramedical personnel to collect the data for physician interpretation.

15

Correlation of B-Mode Ultrasound of the Carotid Artery with Arteriography and Pathology

Anthony J. Comerota

Carotid imaging techniques have become an increasingly popular part of the noninvasive cerebrovascular evaluation. Doppler ultrasound imaging diagrammatically recreates the vessel lumen when flow through that segment exceeds a threshold value, and anatomic information is inferred on the basis of this "physiologic image." Real-time B-mode ultrasound carotid imaging is a direct anatomic evaluation of the carotid artery. The vessel wall and plaque are visualized as the definitive structure. These structures are visualized by sound wave reflection from the interfaces of tissues with different acoustic impedence.

In 1969 Olinger published the first report on the visualization of the carotid arteries by B-mode ultrasound technique (1). Since that time a number of reports were published, with some of the most notable listed in Table 1 (1-8).

If one attempts to compare one series with another, or if one tries to draw a common conclusion, several problems with the previous literature surface:

I express appreciation to Dr. William Hayden and Dr. Thomas Fogarty for their assistance in gathering data at Sequoia Hospital, Redwood City, California, and to Dr. John Cranley, Good Samaritan Hospital, Cincinnati, Ohio, for his continuous encouragement and direction. I also recognize the great effort expended by the vascular technicians at Sequoia Hospital, Redwood City, California, Good Samaritan Hospital, Cincinnati, Ohio, and Temple University Hospital, Philadelphia, Pennsylvania.

352   A. J. Comerota

Table 1. Previous reports on visualization of the carotid
arteries by B-mode ultrasound technique.

Author	Year	No. Vessels	Transducer (MHz)
Olinger	1969	120	2
Blue	1972	30	2
Green	1978	15	10
Mercier	1978	21	2
Cooperberg	1979	52	5-7.5
Hobson	1980	84	6-11
Humber	1980	81	10
Fell	1981	270	5

1. Small numbers of patients in reported series
2. Lack of standard technique
3. Lack of consistent interpretation criteria
4. Transducers of varying frequency
5. Lack of uniform resolution
6. Lack of uniform image quality

   Realizing the previously encountered difficulties, an analysis of this technique was attempted. In this analysis a large
patient population was evaluated and a standard technique was
used in addition to well-defined interpretation criteria. There
was uniform image resolution and the image quality was individually assessed and considered in the analysis of the results.
The purpose of this study was (1) to set a standard that may
become more acceptable for judging B-mode imaging techniques, and
(2) to place this modality in its proper perspective of noninvasive cerebrovascular testing.

METHODS

During the past 26 months, over 4000 patients were evaluated in
three vascular laboratories with bilateral real-time B-mode
ultrasound carotid imaging. In addition, pulse arrival time
oculoplethysmography (OPG) and carotid phonoangiography (CPA) were
performed. Bilateral contrast arteriography was available in 439
patients and unilateral arteriograms were obtained in 6 patients
for a total of 884 vessels available for x-ray correlation.

The imaging system was the Biosound ultrasound scanner, which uses an 8 MHz transducer. The Zira OPG model 100 and the Medical Electronic Devices CPA were also used. All studies were performed and interpreted without knowledge of the results of the arteriogram.

The percent stenosis of the scans and x-ray films was determined by caliper measurement and refers to the diameter reduction of the lumen relative to the most normal part of the internal carotid artery distal to the stenosis.

Arteries were classified on x-ray film and scan as Grade I (0-39% stenosis), Grade II (40-69% stenosis), and Grade III (70% or more stenosis). Noninvasive studies were evaluated as to their quality according to previously defined criteria (9). The quality of the scans was then correlated to accuracy.

Three hundred eighty-four patients had concurrent pulse arrival time OPG and CPA performed. An analysis of the correlation of the scan with the OPG and CPA was made for each grade of disease.

Resolution

The resolution of this imager is its axial resolution (along the beam axis). Axial resolution is determined by how near two interfaces may be brought together without the reflected sound waves overlapping. Since this phenomenon occurs at a distance of one-half the spatial pulse length, resolution can be determined if the spatial pulse length is known (10). The spatial pulse length (length of each "packet" of sound waves) is the product of the pulse duration time and the speed of sound in tissue. Therefore, $(0.4 \times 10^{-6}$ sec) $\times (1.54 \times 10^{6}$ mm/sec$) = 0.6$ mm. The spatial pulse length is 0.6 mm, and the calculated resolution is 0.3 mm. This 0.3-mm resolution is achievable at the optimal focal point of this transducer (2 cm) because of the 6-power magnification of the video image.

RESULTS AND DISCUSSION

No adverse effect of the application of high-frequency sound waves or the mechanical probe pressure on the carotid artery was noticed in any of the over 4000 patients studied. As indicated in Table 2, the stenosis estimated by the B-mode scanner was categorized according to its corresponding x-ray film. The asterisks represent exact correlation of the scan with the arteriogram. Three x-ray films did not adequately visualize the internal carotid and were excluded from analysis. A total of 22 scans did not visualize the carotid artery. It was also observed that as the magnitude of the disease increased, the relative percentage of nonvisualized scans also increased.

Analysis of Errors

All scan errors were tabulated and analyzed (Table 3). The majority of the errors occurred in the group in which scan and arteriogram were mismatched. A mismatch was defined as a technically good scan documenting a higher grade of disease than did the arteriogram, and in which no technical, anatomic, or interpretative error could be identified. The overwhelming majority of these scans were classified as Grade II disease with the corresponding arteriogram identifying only a Grade I lesion. Of the 49 patients in this category, 12 underwent carotid endarterectomy. In 10 instances, it was the opinion of the operating surgeon that the scan more correctly identified the disease process. In one instance the arteriogram was more accurate, and in one case it was not determined.

Table 2. Arteriogram versus scan.

| Grade | Scan | | | | |
	I	II	III	Non-vis.	Total
I	519*	57	9	12	597
II	19	96*	9	4	128
III	17	37	96*	6	156
Non-vis.	2	0	1	0	3
Total	557	190	115	22	884

The specificity of the scan was 87%. The sensitivity of the scan for Grade II disease was 75% and the sensitivity of the scan for Grade III disease 62%.

Table 3. Analysis of errors.

Type of Error	Number of Errors
Scan-Angiogram Mismatch	49
Technically Poor/Inaccurate Scan Due to Disease	47
Interpretation Error	16
Poor Scan - Cause Uncertain	14
ICA Not Visualized High Enough to See Stenosis	11
ICA/ECA Misidentification	9
Red Thrombus	9
Poor Technique	7
Artifact	4
Anatomic Variation	2
Orientation of Plaque	2
	170

Forty-seven of the errors were secondary to a technically poor scan because of significant disease. Since the sound waves cannot penetrate calcified or thick fibrotic plaque, the disease could not be precisely quantitated, resulting in an error. An interpretation error occurred in 16 instances and a poor scan occurred for reasons that cannot be determined in 14 instances. The internal carotid could not be visualized high enough because of a high bifurcation in 11 cases. The internal carotid was misidentified as the external in 9 instances, however, this occurred more frequently in the early part of the evaluation. The scan missed red thrombus or very soft plaque in 9 vessels. Since the density of clotted blood is similar to that of nonclotted blood, the interface necessary for image visualization by this technique is eliminated. Poor technique, artifact, anatomic variation and an unusual orientation of the plaque were all minor causes of errors.

Total Occlusion

The diagnosis of the totally occluded internal carotid artery has been historically poor with this technique (6,10). However, when the diagnosis was made, it could be made with confidence under certain conditions:

1. A technically good scan
2. Disease identified at the origin of the internal
   carotid
3. The absence of arterial pulsation to the internal
   carotid lesion
4. The absence of any flow distal to the internal carotid
   lesion, as determined by the integrated Doppler.

With experience, better application of the above criteria and
a much-improved Doppler ultrasound system, the ability to identify
the totally occluded vessel has significantly improved. As
demonstrated in Table 4, there was a very poor 28% sensitivity
during the first 13 months of the study and a much-improved 77%
sensitivity during the second half of the study.

Scan Quality

Tables 5 and 6 categorize scan accuracy as compared to scan
quality, and a constant trend is noted. As the quality of the
scan increases, so does the accuracy. This was found throughout
all grades of disease.

When only Grade I scans were analyzed, a 93% negative predictive value was found: however, if only those Grade I scans of
good-to-excellent quality were considered, the negative predictive
value was 98%. The majority of errors occurred in the poorer
quality scans.

Looking at the other end of the spectrum, at Grade III scans,
96 of 114 scans were proven correct for a positive predictive
value of 84%. However, if the poorer-quality scans were eliminated and only the good and fair scans examined, the positive
predictive value rose to 88%. These results show that when a

Table 4. Total occlusion

Period	Sensitivity
August 1979-August 1981	33/66 = 50%
August 1979-August 1980	10/36 = 28%
September 1980-September 1981	23/30 = 77%

Table 5. Accuracy versus quality

Quality	Correct	Incorrect	Total	Accuracy (%)
Excellent	18	0	18	100%
Good	413	48	461	90%
Fair	256	73	329	78%
Poor	24	27	51	47%
Non-vis	0	25	25	0%

vessel was severely diseased, it was difficult to obtain a scan of
good quality and this could be achieved in only 36% of the vessels
with Grade III disease. However, if a scan of good quality was
obtained and showed significant disease, it was generally accurate.

Scan Plus OPG and CPA

Five hundred and eighty-four patients had concurrent pulse arrival
time OPG and CPA studies performed with the B-mode scan. The
results showed that when the tests agree, a high level of accuracy
is obtained throughout all grades of disease (Table 7).

However, the data also show that when the scan and the OPG
disagreed, the scan was more accurate than the physiologic studies
in the less diseased vessels (Grades I and II), whereas the OPG
was more sensitive in the severely diseased vessels (Table 8).
This difference has decreased during the course of the study as
the sensitivity of the B-mode scan in diagnosing Grade III disease
has increased. The results show that these techniques are complementary and that neither should supplant the other.

Characterization of Atherosclerotic Plaque

Three types of atherosclerotic plaques were categorized by Javid
(11): (1) fatty streak, (2) fibrous plaque, (3) complicated
lesion. Direct evaluation of endarterectomy specimens and the
corresponding real-time B-mode carotid scans was possible for
fibrous plaques and complicated lesions. The correlation of
proposed B-mode findings of fatty streaks with surgical specimens

A. J. Comerota

Table 6. Quality versus accuracy by grade of disease from scan.

	Grade I				Grade II				Grade III			
	Corr.	Inc.	Tot.	Acc.	Corr.	Inc.	Tot.	Acc.	Corr.	Inc.	Tot.	Acc.
Excellent	18	0	8	100%	0	0	0	0%	0	0	0	0%
Good	306	7	313	98%	51	31	82	62%	56	10	66	85%
Fair	178	21	199	89%	40	48	88	45%	38	4	42	90%
Poor	17	8	25	68%	5	15	20	25%	2	4	6	33%
Total	501	36	537	93%	96	94	190	51%	96	18	114	84%

Table 7. Comparative diagnostic accuracy. Scan and
OPG-CPA agreement.

X-ray Grade	Correct	Incorrect	Total	Accuracy
I	341	23	364	94%
II	46	13	59	78%
III	66	15	81	81%
Total	453	51	504	90%

is difficult, since these patients are not operated upon for this
lesion alone. However, fatty streaks are frequently found
proximal to the more advanced lesions, and the intimal thickening
and subintimal fatty deposition are common observations on the
scan and in the operating room.

The real-time B-mode carotid scan shows a fatty streak as a
constant minor change of the vessel wall. This area of low-level
echoes appears as a gray band and is bound by the lumen of the
vessel and the high echoes of the remaining layers of the arterial
wall. The band is generally small in width, does not cause any
acoustic shadowing and can best be described as an area of intimal
thickening.

The real-time B-mode scan of fibrous plaques shows various
shades of gray within the lumen of the vessel. Each plaque has
relatively distinct borders and may produce a radiolucent umbra
deep to the lesion. With multiple longitudinal views and a
transverse projection of each vessel, the diameter reduction can
be calculated.

Table 8. Comparative diagnostic accuracy. Scan and
OPG/CPA disagreement

X-ray Grade	Scan Correct	OPG Correct	Total	Accuracy
I	121	33	154	79%
II	39	13	52	75%
III	19	39	58	33%
Total	179	85	264	68%

The complicated lesion is a fibrous plaque that has been anatomically altered. Its appearance on real-time B-mode scan varies depending on its calcium content. Calcified lesions appear as highly echogenic areas with acoustic shadowing deep to them. The high density of the calcified area hinders the penetration of sound waves, thus producing an ultrasonic shadow deep to them. The ulcerated, complicated lesion as shown by real-time scan appears as a plaque with an irregular surface. Distinctive craters and tail-like projections are often visualized, but an ulcerated lesion can also appear as a small interruption of the surface layer echoes. Subintimal hemorrhage has been identified as a lucent area contained within a prominent atherosclerotic plaque.

It was only after reviewing the operative specimen and the scans that the conclusion could be made by the B-mode scan. While these conclusions seem to be correct, this was a retrospective study and it remains to be seen if this technique can accurately characterize types of atherosclerotic lesions. A prospective study on cadaver vessels is about to be undertaken to answer this question. If it is indeed possible to characterize the type of atherosclerotic lesion within the vessel, then a definite advance will have been achieved.

CONCLUSIONS

Several important conclusions can be drawn from this study. The accuracy of the real-time B-mode carotid image is directly related to the quality of the image and the severity of the disease within the vessel; i.e., the grade of stenosis. It was found that as the disease increases, the quality of the scan decreases. However, it was also demonstrated that a scan of good quality has a high degree of accuracy no matter what the grade of disease.

The totally occluded carotid has not been reliably diagnosed; however, improvement in its detection has been achieved with standardized criteria, an improved Doppler system, and experience with the technique. High carotid bifurcations as well as red thrombus within the lumen may not be visualized.

A rather surprising result was that the resolution of the scan was better than that of the arteriogram in several cases with operative documentation. Therefore, when a scan of good quality shows disease not shown by arteriogram, the arteriogram is probably falsely negative.

The indirect physiologic cerebrovascular studies are complementary to the direct anatomic study of real-time carotid imaging. Experience with the direct carotid Doppler examination should significantly improve these results.

Qualitative evaluation of atherosclerotic lesions may be possible with this technique, in addition to quantitating the magnitude of the disease.

SUMMARY

Over 4000 patients in three vascular laboratories underwent a cerebrovascular examination by real-time B-mode ultrasound carotid imaging (Biosound), oculoplethysmography (OPG), and carotid phonoangiography (CPA). Four hundred thirty-nine patients underwent bilateral contrast arteriography to form the basis of this study. The X-ray films were compared to the scans and other noninvasive studies. The quality of the B-mode scans was graded according to the severity of the disease: Grade I (0-39% stenosis), Grade II (40-69% stenosis), and Grade III (70% stenosis and greater). The results of the specificity of the scan was 87%, with the sensitivity of detecting Grade II disease equal to 72% and the sensitivity for detecting Grade III disease equal to 62%. Thirty-three of 66 totally occluded vessels were correctly identified for an overall sensitivity of 50%. However, during the second half of the study, 23 of 30 totally occluded vessels were correctly identified for an improved sensitivity of 77% in detecting the totally occluded internal carotid.

The data show a direct correlation of scan quality with scan accuracy. Scans of good-to-excellent quality had 92% accuracy, whereas poor-quality scans had a 47% accuracy. Of the 49 scan-arteriogram-mismatch patients, 12 underwent carotid endarterectomy. In 10 instances the operating surgeon thought that the scan more accurately represented the disease process. When the scan was combined with the OPG/CPA and the results agreed, there was a uniformly high accuracy rate throughout all grades of disease. However, when the scan and OPG disagreed, the scan was more reliable in the Grade I and Grade II categories, whereas the OPG was more reliable in Grade III disease. The reliability of this technique can be improved with experience and the addition of a high-quality Doppler system. Characterization of the type of atherosclerotic disease may be possible with this technique; however, that remains to be evaluated in a prospective manner.

REFERENCES

1. Olinger C (1969) Ultrasonic carotid echoarteriography. AJR 106:282-295
2. Blue SK, McKinney W, Barnes R, Toole JF (1972) Ultrasonic B-mode scanning for study of extracranial vascular disease. Neurology 22:1079-1085
3. Green PS (1978) Real-time, high-resolution ultrasonic carotid arteriography system. In: Bernstein EF (ed) Noninvasive diagnostic techniques in vascular disease. CV Mosby Co, St Louis, pp 29-39
4. Mercier LA, Greenleaf JF, Evans TC, Sandor BA, Hattery RR (1978) High-resolution ultrasound arteriography: a comparison with carotid angiography. In: Bernstein EF (ed) Noninvasive diagnostic techniques in vascular disease. CV Mosby Co, St Louis, pp 231-244
5. Cooperberg PL, Robertson WD, Fry P, Sweeney V (1979) High-resolution real-time ultrasound of the carotid bifurcation. J Clin Ultrasound 7:13-17
6. Hobson RW, Silvia MD, Katocs AS, O'Donnell JA, Jamil Z, Savitsky P (1980) Pulsed Doppler and real-time B-mode echo arteriography for noninvasive imaging of the extracranial arteries. Surgery 87:286-293
7. Humber PR, Leopold GR, Wickbom IG, Bernstein EF (1980) Ultrasonic imaging of the carotid arterial system. Am J Surg 140:199-202

8. Fell G, Phillips DJ, Chikos PM, Harley JD, Thiele BL, Strandness DE Jr (1979) Ultrasonic duplex scanning for disease of the carotid artery. Circulation 64:1191-1195
9. Comerota AJ, Cranley JJ, Cook SE (1981) Real-time B-mode carotid imaging in diagnosis of cerebrovascular disease. Surgery 89:719-729
10. Foss MD Physics in diagnostic medical sonography. Florida Institute of Technology.
11. Javid H (1979) Development of carotid plaque. Am J Surg 138:224-227

DISCUSSION: ROBERT S. LEES

It is hard to make any other than general and laudatory comments about Dr. Comerota's paper and the very conservative interpretations that he has made. He has emphasized the retrospective nature of the angiographic and the limited pathologic correlations that he has found. In terms of the theme of this conference, i.e.,in terms of the quantitation and follow-up of patients with atherosclerosis, one of the remaining problems with the B-mode ultrasound scan is to determine whether it can be made quantitative and can estimate the exact residual lumen diameter of stenotic vessels. Even more important, perhaps, is its reproducibility and usefulness for follow-up of particular patients. I look forward to seeing studies on that in the future.

I would like to emphasize the theme of Dr. Comerota's paper and of some of the previous papers--the difference in accuracy of various diagnostic techniques with different degrees of disease. For instance, B-mode ultrasound, as Dr. Comerota has shown, is good for detection of stenosis of less than 50% of vessel diameter, but progressively poorer as stenosis increases, and poorer with all degrees of disease as calcification of the vessel increases. Doppler ultrasound techniques, by contrast, are generally insensitive at low degrees of stenosis, although hopefully this will change, and both sensitive and fairly accurate at high degrees of stenosis. Here, too, calcification may severely and adversely affect accuracy. The obvious conclusion is that one should use multiple diagnostic techniques that depend as far as possible on independent physical methods.

In that regard, I would like to describe briefly our use of spectral analysis of audible bruits (1-3), a technique that is highly accurate at all levels of stenosis sufficient to create a bruit (generally stenosis of between 40 and 99% by diameter). I will review, as well, our recent data on the combination of spectral bruit analysis with the ATL duplex Doppler scanner, which gives us quantitative diagnosis with a very high degree of

accuracy in a very high percent of patients (4). We combine the
accuracy of audible bruit analysis in significant stenosis with
the anatomical and flow information afforded by ultrasound
scanning. The audible bruit shown in Fig. 15 A.1 is seen on the
display of the American-Edwards Spectraview, the commercial
instrument we use for this analysis. One takes, from the display
a 40-ms segment at the peak of the bruit and analyzes it, and
gets, by fast Fourier transform (FFT) spectral analysis, a plot of
log amplitude versus log frequency. It turns out that there is a
simple relationship among the residual lumen diameter, the flow
velocity, and the break frequency. For the human carotid
bifurcation we have determined empirically from a large number of
patients (4) that flow velocity was close to constant at rest and
that by dividing 500 by the break frequency on the FFT of the
bruit, one can get an exact numerical estimate of the residual
lumen diameter. Here are displayed sound tracings of a mild
carotid stenosis and a severe stenosis. At the top of Fig. 15 A.1
is the time display of the bruit. One can learn little from this
except that the longer and louder the bruit, especially if it
extends into diastole, the more likely it is to be significant.
By contrast, on the FFT one can see that this bruit has a break
frequency of 200 Hz and is therefore from a mild stenosis of 2.5
mm diameter. The bruit from a severe carotid stenosis has a break
frequency at about 600 Hz. Thus it has a residual lumen of less
than 1 mm in diameter. One can readily obtain these data in a few
minutes time. Earlier results in a blinded prospective comparison
showed that we could predict the residual lumen to within one
millimeter of the x-ray diameter in 92% of the patients (5). The
reproducibility is excellent. At 0-6 months, as you can see,
three-quarters of the patients had a break frequency within less
than 50 Hz of the first one, at 7-12 months follow-up, two-thirds
of them did, and at 13-24 months, interestingly, still about
two-thirds had not changed. However, 2 of the 16 patients in that
group, or 12%, had a break frequency that was > 100 Hz different.

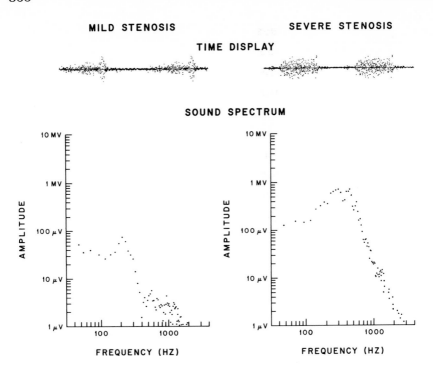

Fig. A.1 Examples of phonangiography: time display and sound spectrum from each of two patients, one with mild and the other with severe internal carotid artery (ICA) stenosis. Above, time display recorded from microphone on the neck at a location where maximal intensity of the bruit is detected by the examiner, on the left with mild and on the right with severe ICA stenosis. These records by themselves provide qualitative, but not quantitative, information. Below, spectral analysis (frequency-intensity plots) of the same bruits. Note that, in the case of mild stenosis, a sharp fall in amplitude occurs at about 200 Hz, whereas in the sound spectrum from the patient with severe ICA stenosis, the break frequency is greater than 400 Hz (corresponding to residual lumen diameters of approximately 2.5 and 1.2 cm, respectively). (From Ref. 3, reprinted with permission of Year Book Medical Publishers.)

Both of these patients had "before and after" angiograms showing progression of their disease; thus the phonoangiogram had accurately reflected disease progression. Now, we combine this technique with the duplex Doppler scan described by Baker, Barber, Strandness, and their colleagues (6-8). As you know, this gives one the ability on a sector scan of the carotid, to place the

range-gated Doppler sampling volume so as to interrogate selectively each vessel at the carotid bifurcation. When we combine these
tests, (using the duplex Doppler scan alone in patients without a
bruit) in 240 consecutive patients, 45 angiograms of 270 vessels
were performed. We were able to identify complete carotid occlusion in all of 8 vessels so affected. In the overall series we
were able to predict accurately in 97% of vessels the location of
the stenosis in either the external, internal, or common carotid
artery and the extent of the stenosis to within 1 mm. These data
support our original hypothesis that multiple diagnostic modalities that make use of different physical principles can allow one
very high accuracy, high reproducibility, and, in this case, the
ability to follow carotid stenosis to determine progression or
regression in man and, I suspect, experimental animals as well.

REFERENCES

1. Lees RS, Dewey CF Jr (1970) Phonoangiography: A new noninvasive diagnostic method for studying arterial disease.
   Proc Natl Acad Sci USA 67:935-942
2. Lees RS, Kistler JP, Miller A (1982) Quantitative carotid
   phonoangiography. In: Bernstein EF (ed) Noninvasive
   diagnostic techniques in vascular disease, 2nd ed. CV Mosby
   Co, St Louis, pp 200-207
3. Lees RS, Myers GS (1982) Noninvasive diagnosis of arterial
   disease. In: Advances in internal medicine, vol 27. Year
   Book Medical Publishers, Chicago, pp 475-509
4. Duncan GW, Gruber JO, Dewey CF Jr, Myers GS, Lees RS (1975)
   Evaluation of carotid stenosis by phonoangiography. New Engl
   J Med 293:1124-1128
5. Kistler JP, Lees RS, Friedman J, Pessin M, Mohr JP, Roberson
   GS, Ojemann RG (1978) The bruit of carotid stenosis versus
   radiated basal heart murmurs. Differentiation by phonoangiography. Circulation 57:975-981
6. Barber FE, Baker DW, Strandness DE Jr, Ofstad JM, Mahler GU.
   (1974) Duplex Scanner II: For simultaneous imaging of artery
   tissues and flow. IEEE Trans Sonics Ultrasonics 74:896
7. Baker DW (1980) Applications of pulsed Doppler techniques.
   Radiol Clin North Am 18:79-103
8. Blackshear WM Jr, Strandness DE Jr (1981) Angiographic
   imaging by ultrasound compared with indirect methods. In:
   Nicolaides AN, Yao JST (eds) Investigation of vascular disorders. Churchill Livingstone, New York, pp 165-200

16

Correlation of Morphological and Biochemical Components of Atherosclerotic Plaques

C. Richard Minick, Domenick J. Falcone, and David P. Hajjar

It is clear from preceding presentations in this symposium that existing morphologic and morphometric techniques are adequate to quantitate the extent of atherosclerotic change. Biochemical techniques have also been utilized to assess the severity of atherosclerotic change by quantitating the amount of various components in arterial segments containing lesions and, in some instances, within arterial lesions themselves. Although much progress has been made in quantitating components of atherosclerotic lesions chemically, their assessment with morphologic techniques has lagged badly. This is unfortunate; the use of morphometric techniques in evaluation of lesions is potentially useful in describing areas of change within lesions too small to characterize chemically and in understanding qualitative changes--particularly those involving spatial relations of altered cellular and extracellular components during lesion initiation, progression, and regression. An appreciation of the biochemical and subcellular changes and spatial relations of lesion components at various points in time is essential to understanding the pathogenesis of atherosclerosis. The importance of these relationships to understanding the pathogenesis of disease was clearly stated by Virchow over 100 years ago.

Supported by research grants HL-18828 from the National Heart, Lung, and Blood Institute of the National Institutes of Health, an NIH training grant HL-07423, and a grant from the Cross Foundation.

When we require cellular pathology to be the basis
of the medical viewpoint, a most concrete and quite
empirical task is at stake, in which no *a priori* or
arbitrary speculation is involved. All diseases are
in the last analysis reducible to disturbances, either
active or passive, of large or small groups of living
units, whose functional capacity is altered in accor-
dance with the state of their molecular composition and
is thus dependent on physical and chemical changes of
their contents. Physical and chemical investigation has
a very great significance in this respect, and we can do
no more than wish a prosperous development to the school
which is striving to form itself. But we should not
conceal from ourselves that the story of metabolic
interchange will be brought to a satisfactory conclusion
only when it is carried back to the primary active parts;
in other words, when it becomes possible to describe the
particular role every tissue, and every pathologically
altered part of a tissue, plays in that story. Therefore, although one may begin with the outworks, the
ultimate goal, beyond the urine and the sweat and the
various waste products of organic activity, must never
be lost from sight, nor should it be supposed that these
waste products are themselves the goal. There would
always be the danger of suffering shipwreck in a more
or less exclusively humoral pathology, if this were to
be the case (1).

Nothwithstanding the importance of this type of information,
we know of only one study in which investigators have attempted to
correlate quantitative biochemical analysis of normal arterial
wall with quantitative morphologic observations obtained by use of
modern morphometric techniques. Rather, arteries or lesions are
often investigated quantitatively with respect to biochemical
changes and at best findings are compared to qualitative or
semiquantitative morphologic observations. For reasons outlined
above, there is a great need for the development of new morphologic techniques for specific characterization of lesion components, quantitating these morphometrically, and comparing the
results to biochemical analysis of lesions.

METHODOLOGICAL CONSIDERATIONS

As currently utilized, both biochemical and morphologic techniques
have several advantages but are limited by certain assumptions and

restrictions. We believe that the two approaches to lesion analysis are complementary, and when used together they offer a perspective on atherosclerotic lesions that cannot be obtained from either technique alone. Until more specific histochemical and immunochemical techniques are available and the validity of morphometric assessment of arterial tissue is established by biochemical analysis of the same tissue, parallel chemical and morphologic analysis of lesions is clearly the best approach.

Biochemical analysis provides the capability of measuring various components from arterial lesions with precision and a high degree of specificity. This type of quantitative data is particularly useful in describing and comparing changes in various components of normal artery and of human and animal lesions during different stages of development. However, it is important to bear in mind several potential problems, since they may lead to misinterpretation of the resulting data.

Limitations of biochemical techniques involve the size of sample necessary for analysis and the precision with which investigators can separate lesion from nonlesion tissue. Thus it is commonplace to find data in which entire arterial segments involving both lesion and nonlesion areas, and intimal-medial layers of pooled arterial tissue from several animals have been analyzed. This type of analysis provides little information regarding the distribution of components between normal arterial wall and lesions or between portions of lesion areas, e.g., intima or media, cellular or extracellular. Moreover, the data are usually expressed as a function of the total arterial segment, e.g., wet weight, DNA, and total protein, suggesting that the tissue analyzed is homogeneous with respect to the distribution of lesion components analyzed. Any experienced morphologist knows that this assumption is not true, either at a gross, light microscopic, or ultrastructural level. Although on reflection we are all aware of these assumptions, there is danger that we forget them when we generalize or draw conclusions from the resulting data. Other problems arise because various materials measured in chemical analysis may not be completely removed from the wall. In instances where material cannot be completely extracted, e.g., collagen or lipoprotein, it is important to determine that the sample extracted is representative of all of the material of the arterial wall. There are also limitations in our ability to analyze some materials chemically, particularly those that occur in small quantities, and are unevenly distributed.

Additional problems concern units used to express chemical data derived from lesion analysis. Should data be expressed on the basis of DNA (cellularity), tissue protein, luminal surface area, wet weight, dry weight, or percent of weight of the arterial segment? Ideally, the morphologic features of the lesions should be carefully characterized before deciding how to express the data. Each of these denominators are dependent on assumptions which are not always true. For example, as has been pointed out by Wolinsky et al. (2), in reference to changes in connective tissue induced in the wall by experimental hypertension, it may be misleading to express data as percent weight. If various components of the arterial wall increase proportionately, e.g., lipid, collagen, or proteoglycans, and data are expressed as a percentage or normalized in other ways, it will appear that there is no difference from the normal artery although clearly the absolute amount of each material has increased. In this instance, findings are best expressed on the basis of absolute amount in defined arterial segments. It is noteworthy that the increase in thickness of aortic wall observed microscopically in hypertensive animals was important in suggesting the possibility for misinterpretation (2). The use of total protein may also lead to error, since the amounts of protein-rich components in connective tissue vary in lesion areas but not necessarily in parallel to the material being measured. Lesions may differ in cellularity. For this reason, DNA may be misleading. Moreover, surface area does not account for increased mass due to variation in intimal or medial thickness, and considerable contraction or shrinkage can occur on removal of the vessel from the animal. Finally, it is important to note that the highly quantitative data that is obtained by biochemical analysis of lesions may provide a false sense of importance with respect to its ultimate significance. Measurement of a particular component with great precision does not necessarily lead to a better understanding of its role in the pathobiology of the arterial lesion. This is especially true when the distribution of that component is poorly understood in the tissue being analyzed.

Analysis of lesions from a morphologic perspective with the use of modern morphometric techniques has several advantages. This type of analysis permits compartmentalization of lesion components and study of their spatial relations. With the use of modern morphometric techniques, e.g., point counting, planimetry, contour mapping, and various histochemical stains, it is possible to quantitate with considerable precision the portion of lesions occupied by elastic tissue, collagen, proteoglycans, calcium, cellular and extracellular neutral lipid, and express them as volume fractions. The use of digitizers and computers has made these very tedious studies feasible. Ultimately, with the use of these techniques it should be possible to precisely characterize the interaction of different cells and tissues during atherogenesis.

Unfortunately, these seemingly precise morphological measurements are plagued with their own particular problems. First, there is the problem of the specificity of the histochemical stains for collagen, elastin, proteoglycans, etc. Since the mechanism of staining and specificity of several of the stains used for analysis--e.g., collagen, elastin, and proteoglycans--is not understood, there is the danger of quantitating nonspecific changes with greater and greater precision. Second, there are few biochemical studies on the same lesions to validate the accuracy of these histochemical/morphometric techniques in indicating changes in lipid and other lesion components, although such studies are currently in progress. Third, measurements are often made on one or two sections of the lesions and it is difficult to prove that this is representative of the entire lesion; in fact, it is very likely that it is not. Four, problems of specimen preparation also need to be considered. Even though for many types of analysis, such as quantitation of luminal stenosis, it is current practice to use perfusion-fixed specimens, these procedures may introduce their own peculiar series of changes. There is surprisingly little information on the effect of perfusion fixation on the composition of the arterial wall in comparison to its normal, unfixed state. Further, there is the problem of controlling section thickness, which may be crucial for certain measurements such as cellularity. Difficulties also arise in comparing data from biochemical studies because of differences in procedures used for expressing the data, such as volume fractions used with morphometric data as compared to biochemical components usually expressed on the basis of weight. Finally, even with modern techniques using digitizers and computers, morphometry may be a time-consuming and tedious procedure.

Ultimately, quantitation of tissue components, either within normal arteries or small areas of lesion, may be possible with the use of specific stains. For example, specific antibodies coupled to a suitable marker may provide an accurate means of quantitating relative concentrations of collagen types in small areas of normal and diseased arteries. In this manner, it may be possible to measure amounts of lesion components with precision and study their relation to other materials in the vessel wall during atherogenesis. However, until this goal is achieved we believe that correlation of biochemical and morphologic changes in arteries and lesions offers the best chance of understanding lesion development.

An example from experiments in our laboratories will emphasize some of the significant advantages of a combined approach to lesion analysis. In recent years we have investigated the mechanism of lipid accumulation in arterial lesions resulting from injury, particularly the role of the endothelial barrier in lipid accretion. It is posited that arterial injury predisposes to lipid accumulation as a direct consequence of increased permeability of the wall resulting from persistent loss of endothelium. We tested this hypothesis by use of the balloon catheter injury in rabbit aorta. Unanticipated results of our initial morphometric studies indicated an increased amount of oil-red-O positive material in reendothelialized areas of the injured aorta and not in adjacent deendothelialized areas as the hypothesis suggested (see Table 1) (3).

In an attempt to more precisely characterize the type and distribution of lipid in the two areas, reendothelialized and deendothelialized segments of injured aortas were dissected and quantities of various lipid classes in the two areas were measured (4). As expected, a striking increase occurred in amounts of cholesterol and cholesteryl ester in intima of injured as compared to uninjured aortas. However, we were initially unable to demonstrate consistent differences between the quantity of total cholesterol in areas of the reendothelialized injured aorta as compared to the adjacent deendothelialized areas (compare columns I and III, Table 2), even though our initial morphometric findings indicated striking differences. In fact, it appeared from this analysis that the initial morphometric findings were misleading.

After further consideration of the discrepancy in the morphologic and chemical data it became apparent that we had not considered an important assumption of the chemical analysis,

Table 1. Intimal lipid accumulation in reendothelialized (REA) and deendothelialized (DEA) areas in injured aortas of rabbits fed a cholesterol-supplemented diet

	Distribution of grades of lipid accumulation (No. [%])			
	None	Slight	Moderate	Marked
REA N = 44	0 (0%)	(%)	18 (41%)	26 (59%)
DEA N = 44	8 (18%)	17 (39%)	19 (43%)	(0%)

Source: From Ref. 3, with permission of the American Journal of Pathology.

Table 2. Cholesterol content of reendothelialized (REA) and deendothelialized (DEA) injured rabbit aorta

	REA	REA (Corrected)	DEA
Thoracic Aorta	11.6 ± 1.3[a]	28.8 ± 9.1	7.1 ± 1.2
Abdominal Aorta	9.6 ± 1.5	20.9 ± 4.2	11.5 ± 2.4

[a] μg total cholesterol/mg wet wt.; Mean ± SE.
Source: Falcone, Hajjar, and Minick, unpublished observations (1980).

namely that of sample homogeneity. In our analysis, we had compared the intima-media of an entire reendothelialized island with an adjacent deendodthelialized area. However, our previous morphologic observations demonstrated that the reendothelialized island was heterogeneous. It included a central grey zone with little or no intima or stainable lipid (nonlesion area), and a peripheral white zone with appreciable intima (a lesion area). As might be expected, the oil-red-O positive material was almost entirely within the intima of the peripheral white zone with very little material in the media of the adjacent grey zone or the white zone. Since we had homogenized the entire reendothelialized island, there was considerable dilution of the lipid-rich white area of the reendothelialized islands by the uninvolved grey zone, compared to the adjacent deendothelialized area, which is more homogeneous. In an attempt to account for this dilutional effect, we measured the grey and white surface areas of thoracic and abdominal aortas and corrected specimen weights accordingly. As indicated in Table 2, these corrected data suggested that our initial impression was valid, i.e., that there was approximately three times as much cholesterol present in reendothelialized areas of thoracic and abdominal aortas. Quantitation of lipid in white areas of reendothelialized islands and comparison with the deendothelialized areas confirmed these estimates (Table 3) (4). Differences between actual cholesterol content of tissues (Table 3) and those predicted by the corrected data (Table 2) can be

Table 3. Cholesterol content of reendothelialized (REA) and
deendothelialized (DEA) rabbit aorta

	REA	DEA
Thoracic Aorta	4.65 ± 1.28[a]	$1.62 \pm .64$
Abdominal Aorta	6.21 ± 1.11	$2.87 \pm .61$

[a]µg total cholesterol/mg wet wt. Mean ± SE.
Source: Modified from Falcone et al. (4), with permission of
the American Journal of Pathology

explained by different feeding regimens and serum cholesterol
levels in the two experiments.

Thus, after taking into account the heterogeneity of the sample,
results of chemical analysis of total cholesterol in the more
homogeneous lesion area of the tissue sample clearly supported our
initial morphologic observation that white areas of the reendothelialized injured aorta contained significantly more lipid than did
adjacent deendothelialized aorta. It is important to emphasize
that in the absence of the original morphologic observations we
might have reached an erroneous conclusion from the chemical data.
The analogy between this experience and many studies in which
investigators have analyzed the chemical changes in entire arterial
segments including lesion areas and nonlesion areas are obvious.

There are other situations in which similar considerations may
be important. It is clear from existing morphologic data that
increased proteoglycan in lesions is often focally distributed
within the deeper portion of the intima. Chemical analysis of
glycosaminoglycans (GAGs) in vessels with lesions has often given
inconsistent and conflicting results. One of the reasons may
relate to the highly selective localization of the increased GAGs
within the intima of specific stages of developing lesions. The
quantity of GAGs may be greatly underestimated or not appreciated
in an analysis of entire vascular segments which may contain
lesion areas of various types as well as nonlesion areas and/or
full thickness specimens of the arterial wall in which there may
be considerable dilution of intima by media.

We have also used tissue obtained from animal experiments previously described to correlate lipid assessed biochemically with the amount of oil-red-O staining measured morphometrically in intima and media of aorta (4). In general, our results indicated a poor correlation with oil-red-O staining and the amount of lipid measured chemically, e.g., total cholesterol, cholesteryl ester, or triglyceride. The results are of interest because they illustrate another problem inherent in lesion evaluation with morphometric analysis. Our analysis revealed that total cholesterol correlated relatively well with oil-red-O staining at low concentrations of total cholesterol (4 µg/mg wet wt.) but not at higher concentration. Thus, as might be expected, the morphometric measurements became insensitive at high concentrations because of inability to perceive differences in intensity of staining.

LITERATURE REVIEW

To the best of our knowledge, there are no experiments in which the same arterial lesions have been analyzed by both chemical and morphologic analysis with use of modern quantitative morphometric techniques. Studies incorporating both a chemical and morphologic analysis within arterial segments as assessments of the severity of atherosclerotic change have been made in similar lesions but seldom the same lesion. Since lipid accumulation is one principle feature of the atherosclerotic lesion, the biochemical analysis in many of these studies has been directed toward quantitating the amount of lipid accumulating within the arterial wall as an index of lesion severity. Other investigators have attempted to correlate biochemical changes with the type of arterial lesion in order to learn more about lesion development.

An example of the first type of study are recently reported experiments of Alexander and Clarkson comparing the amount of atherosclerosis in vasectomized and sham-operated nonhuman primates, *Macaca fascicularis*, fed a lipid-rich diet (5). The degree of atherosclerotic change was evaluated chemically as the quantity of free and esterified cholesterol in one half of the aorta and assessed morphologically in the other half. Total, free, and esterified cholesterol were expressed on the basis of wet weight or surface area involved. Extent of change evaluated morphologically was expressed as the percent of surface involved, on a scale of 0-4+, or in the instance of the coronary lesions, on the basis of the percent luminal stenosis. Comparison of the chemical and morphologic data in this study indicates a reasonably good correlation between the morphologic assessment of atherosclerosis and the extent of atherosclerosis determined chemically by evaluating cholesterol content. For example, the conclusions were similar when the thoracic and abdominal aorta, iliacofemoral artery, and carotid artery were compared. Both the morphologic and biochemical studies indicated that changes in the thoracic aorta could not be shown to be different in the two treatment groups, and that significant differences in the extent of atherosclerosis were present in the other arteries.

However, it is noteworthy that there are potential pitfalls with the use of one biochemical component as a sole measure of lesion severity. Morphologic observation from human disease and animal lesions indicates large variation in the character of fibrous plaques. Fibrous plaques may differ considerably with respect to the quantity of lipid even though they all partially or fully occlude arteries. It is possible to construct hypothetical situations where the quantity of lipid would be less in chronic, advanced, experimentally-induced atherosclerosis than in early, evolving lesions. This potential problem can best be avoided with the use of morphologic observations of the same lesions, as in the experiments of Alexander and Clarkson (5).

Perhaps one of the principal stimuli for the combined use of quantitative morphometric data and biochemical data has been assessment of the effect of various types of intervention on the regression of atherosclerosis. Here, changes induced in costly long-term animal experiments may be relatively small, and it is important to develop sensitive and accurate methods of assessing severity and character of lesions in order to determine if a specific form of intervention, e.g., diet modification, has had an effect. Examples of this use of correlative biochemical and morphologic analysis are the recently reported studies of Daoud et al. (6) and Fritz et al. (7), on regression of atherosclerosis that was induced by balloon catheter injury and feeding of lipid-rich diets. Following an induction period in which swine with injured aortas were fed an atherogenic diet, animals were fed a relatively lipid-poor mash diet and sacrificed at 6 weeks, 5 months, or 14 months. After 5 and 14 months of regression, results indicated a significant decrease in aortic sudanophilia as assessed grossly on the luminal surface, and decreases in the amount of necrosis and the number of foam cells, even though the extent of intimal thickening as determined by the intimal/medial ratio was not significantly changed (6). In addition, there were qualitative changes not reflected in the semi-quantitative morphologic assessment of the data. These included a change in the type of grossly visible lesions with more fibrous and fewer fatty lesions, increased calcium deposition, and increased thickness of fibrous caps. Although trends in the biochemical data appear to correlate with morphologic changes in lesions, many of the biochemical changes were not significant, probably because of the small numbers of animals at each time period (7).

With respect to the morphologic measurements, it is important to note that the use of intimal/medial ratios may be misleading. These measurements assume that the media remains constant. It is obvious from the study of human atherosclerosis and advanced lesions in animals that the media is often considerably thinned underlying intimal plaques. In this instance, the intimal/medial ratio will overestimate intimal thickness. Therefore, the burden is on the investigator to prove that the media is normal with respect to controls.

In the second type of study, other investigators have attempted to correlate structural and chemical changes in order to better understand lesion pathogenesis. Experiments of Peters and deDuve (8) and Shio and coworkers (9) have furnished morphologic and histochemical evidence to indicate that some vacuoles in foam cells were lysosomal in origin. These initial studies were interpreted to suggest that cholesteryl ester accumulated within lysosomes as a result of a deficiency of acid cholesteryl ester hydrolase, and that the cellular accumulation of lipids in lesions was an example of a lysosomal storage disease. Additional experiments correlated histocytochemical observations at the ultrastructural level with findings of cytochemical studies to localize cholesterol and cholesteryl esters within the cytoplasma of foam cells isolated from lesion areas. Results indicated that lysosomes of foam cells contained both free and ester cholesterol and that lipid droplets were almost entirely cholesteryl ester (10). One possible interpretation of these findings is that cholesterol storage in cells is not necessarily a lysosomal storage disease as previously suggested, since sufficient acid cholesteryl ester hydrolase was present in the lysosome to hydrolyze cholesteryl ester.

In an attempt to better understand the interaction of serum lipids and particularly lipoprotein in the arterial wall, other investigators have attempted to correlate biochemical and physiochemical measurements of lipid in the arterial wall with the lesion type, as determined morphologically, e.g., fatty streaks or fibrous plaque. Smith et al. (11) described the accumulation of perifibrous lipid in the normal intima with age and compared the qualitative and quantitative characteristics of this lipid with that seen in fatty-streak lesions. Cholesteryl esters of perifibrous lipid in normal intima were similar to those in serum containing approximately 20% oleic acid and 40% linoleic acid, suggesting that they were derived from increased filtration of lipid from the serum. In contrast, cholesteryl esters in fatty streaks were primarily cholesteryl oleate, a form of cholesteryl ester that is believed to be synthesized by the foam cell. This suggests that the lipids derived from the plasma, now localized in fatty-streak lesions, may be modified by the presence of foam cells (11).

Insull and Bartsch made similar observations in normal intima and media and fatty streaks, and they attempted to correlate lipid patterns in normal intima and normal media with those in fatty streaks (12). Other investigators have compared the physical state of lipid in various arterial lesions with the morphology of the lesion, fatty streak, fibrous plaque, or normal intima. Normal intima was found to have lipid in a lamellar or membranous state. Fatty-streak lipid was present in two phases, membrane lipid and oily droplets. In the fibrous plaque, three phases were present with addition of a crystalline phase of cholesterol. An "intermediate" type of plaque between the fibrous plaque and fatty streak was also identified which contained three phases of lipid (13, 14). On the basis of these studies it was suggested that at least some fatty streaks may progress to fibrous plaques, since intermediate lesions were identified. It was also suggested that the presence of large quantities of oil droplets and crystalline phase in fibrous plaques may correlate with the difficulty in removing these types of lipids and inducing regression of this type of advanced plaque.

In other studies, Smith and coworkers were able to demonstrate that much of the lipid accumulating in normal intima, gelatinous lesions, and early fibrous plaques appeared to be associated with low-density lipoproteins and that the quantity of lipoprotein increased in fibrous plaques as compared to normal intima (15). These investigators also established that the increased lipoprotein was present in two forms. One type could be solubilized in buffer extracts. Another type, so-called bound lipoprotein, could be released from the wall only after digestion with various proteolytic enzymes, including collagenase, trypsin, and plasmin. The portion of bound lipoprotein in the atheromatous portion of fibrous plaques was considerably greater than that found in the gelatinous lesions and in normal intima. On the basis of these studies it was suggested by these investigators that lipoprotein in the lesion was bound to fibrin (16), which has also been shown to be present in plaques. In similar studies, Hoff and coworkers

also found that the amount of buffer-extractable apo-B (apolipoprotein-B) was greatest in normal intima and least in fibrous
plaques, whereas tightly bound apo-B extracted with Triton was in
highest concentration in fibrous plaques (17). The percent of
lipoprotein extracted by buffer and Triton correlated with the
total cross-sectional area that was fibrotic or necrotic. Findings were substantiated by subsequent experiments in which the
fibrotic and necrotic areas of the plaque were isolated by microdissection and the apo-B content of buffer and Triton-extractable
fractions measured separately (18).

The ultimate goal of analysis of lesion components is to
combine the advantages of both approaches of lesion analysis,
i.e., the potential for interrelating various lesion components
spatially, quantitating very small amounts of material that are
optimized morphologically, and the potential for measuring components with great precision biochemically. Although these types of
studies have been carried out with great precision in other organ
systems, e.g., the liver (19), there is little published data on
their use in normal or atherosclerotic arterial tissue. In a
recently published study, Glagov et al. have compared morphologic
and chemical data from rabbit aortas with respect to connective
tissue components of arterial tissues (20). Table 4 summarizes
some of the essential findings of these experiments.

This study is unique in that the investigators attempted to
correlate the connective tissue quantitated morphometrically with
that analyzed biochemically in the arterial sample. Morphometric
studies involved contour mapping and determination of volume
fractions for each component in sections of pressure fixed and
unfixed rabbit aorta. Adjacent areas of unfixed aorta were used
for chemical analysis. There are several problems with these
types of studies that were identified and discussed by the
investigators. Histologic sections taken from the center of
tissue samples used for chemical analysis may not always be
representative of the distribution of material within the sample.
Further, tissue samples for chemical analysis were made only on

Table 4. Comparison of sterologic and chemical determinations

	Volume Fractions[a]		Chemical Analysis[b]
	Undistended	Distended	
Elastin (E)	37.9 ± 5.5%	5.2 ± 2.4%	45.6
Collagen (C)	8.8 ± 2.4%	16.2 ± 2.4%	3.1
E/C[c]	4.31	3.42	3.48
Nuclei	4.11 ± 0.43%	7.8 ± 1.17%	4.57[d]
Cellularity[e]	10.1 ± 0.4	19.1 ± 0.6	

[a]Determination on proximal thoracic aorta.
[b]mg/100 mg wet weight.
[c]Ratio of mean value of elastin and collagen.
[d]DNA (μg/mg).
[e]Nuclei/1000 μm^2.
Source: From Glagov et al. (20) with permission.

undistended specimens, while these morphometric analyses were made on both distended and undistended fixed specimens. The effect of pressure fixing specimens on the normal interrelationships of arterial components is not completely understood. Further problems relate to the fact that morphometric assessment of several components, particularly nuclei, may depend on section thickness. In addition, chemical data were expressed on the basis of wet weight, since tissues for morphometry were processed in such a manner that wet volume was maintained throughout. Expressing such chemical data on the basis of wet weight can be a source of inaccuracy. Notwithstanding all of these problems it is of considerable interest that ratios of volume fractions for collagen and elastin agreed quite closely with ratios of chemical data.

One of the major purposes of this report is to point out the considerable advantages of correlation of biochemical and morphologic data in the analysis of atherosclerotic lesions. It is also our intent to encourage the development of new approaches to lesion analysis with the use of modern morphometric, histochemical, and immunohistochemical techniques. Finally, we wish to emphasize that we believe that it is essential to our understanding of atherogenesis to relate new information regarding cellular, subcellular, and extracellular lesion components to the intact atherosclerotic plaque.

> Contemplations of nature and of bodies in their simple form break up and distract the understanding, while contemplations of nature and bodies in their composition and configuration overpower and dissolve the understanding... for that school is so busy with the particle that it hardly attends to the structure, while the others are so lost in admiration of the structure that they do not penetrate to the simplicity of nature.

> Francis Bacon

REFERENCES

1. Rather LJ (transl) (1958) Disease, life and man. Selected essays by Rudolf Virchow.   Stanford University Press, Stanford, CA
2. Wolinsky H (1970) Response of the rat aortic wall to hypertension: importance of comparing absolute amounts of wall components. Atherosclerosis 11:251-255
3. Minick CR, Stemerman MB, Insull W Jr (1979) Role of endothelium and hypercholesterolemia in intimal thickening and lipid accumulation. Am J Pathol 95:131-158
4. Falcone DJ, Hajjar DP, Minick CR (1980) Enhancement of cholesterol and cholesteryl ester accumulation in re-endothelialized aorta. Am J Pathol 99:81-104
5. Alexander NJ, Clarkson TB (1978) Vasectomy increases the severity of diet-induced atherosclerosis in *Macaca fascicularis*. Science 201:538-540
6. Daoud AS, Jarmolych J, Augustyn JM, Fritz KE (1981) Sequential morphologic studies of regression of advanced atherosclerosis. Arch Pathol Lab Med 105:233-239
7. Fritz KE, Augustyn JM, Jarmolych J, Daoud AS (1981) Sequential study of biochemical changes during regression of swine aortic atherosclerotic lesions. Arch Pathol Lab Med 105:240-246
8. Peters TJ, deDuve C (1979) Lysosomes of the arterial wall. II. Subcellular fractionation of aortic cells from rabbits with experimental atheroma. Exp Mol Pathol 20:228-250
9. Shio H, Haley NJ, Fowler S (1978) Characterization of lipid-laden aortic cells from cholesterol fed rabbits. II. Morphometric analysis of lipid-filled lysosomes and lipid droplets in aortic cell populations. Lab Invest 39:390-397
10. Shio H, Haley NJ, Fowler S (1979) Characterization of lipid-laden aortic cells from cholesterol fed rabbits. III. Intracellular localization of cholesterol and cholesteryl ester. Lab Invest 41:160-167

11. Smith EB, Evans PH, Dounham MD (1967) Lipid in the aortic intima. The correlation of morphological and chemical characteristics. J Atheroscler Res 7:171-186

12. Insull W Jr, Bartsch GE (1966) Cholesterol, triglyceride, and phospholipid content of intima, media, and atherosclerotic fatty streak in human thoracic aorta. J Clin Invest 45:513-522

13. Small DM, Shipley GG (1979) The physical state of lipids helps to explain lipid deposition and lesion reversal in atherosclerosis. Science 185:222-229

14. Katz SS, Shipley GG, Small DM (1976) Physical chemistry of the lipids of human atherosclerotic lesions. Demonstration of a lesion intermediate between fatty streaks and advanced plaques. J Clin Invest 58:200-211

15. Smith EB (1974) The relationship between plasma and tissue lipids in human atherosclerosis. Adv Lipid Res 12:1-49

16. Smith EB, Massie TB, Alexander KM (1976) Release of an immobilized lipoprotein fraction from atherosclerotic lesions by incubation with plasmin. Atherosclerosis 25:71-84

17. Hoff HF, Heideman CL, Gaubatz JW, Scott DW, Gotto AM Jr (1978) Detergent extraction of tightly-bound apo-B from extracts of normal aortic intima and plaques. Exp Mol Pathol 28:290-300

18. Hoff HF, Heideman CL, Gaubatz JW, Scott DW, Titus JL, Gotto AM Jr (1978) Correlation of apolipoprotein-B retained with the structure of atherosclerotic plaques from human aortas. Lab Invest 38:560-567

19. Bolender RP (1978) Correlation of morphometry and sterology with biochemical analysis of cell fractions. Int Rev Cytol 55:247-289

20. Glagov S, Grande J, Vesselinovitch D, Zarins CK (1981) Quantitation of cells and fiber in histologic sections of arterial walls: Advantages of contour tracing on a digitized plate. In: McDonald TF, Chandler AB (eds) Connective tissues in arterial and pulmonary disease. Springer-Verlag, New York, pp 57-93

DISCUSSION: WILLIAM INSULL, JR.

I would like to look at this kind of data from a longer distance and try to develop a perspective for it. Dr. Minick has summarized quite succinctly, with a number of examples, the power of the biochemical approach to analysis of atherosclerotic lesions, an area that has received a lot of intensive work over the last decade or so. However, in the context of our present conference I would like to point out that the biochemical probe we are talking about is quite different from any of the other measures of atherosclerotic lesions that we have discussed before, because it is more sensitive than the standard examination we usually refer to, mainly the conventional pathological techniques of histology. The biochemical probe enables the investigator to go into the tissue in much more detail and to look at specific structures in parts of the tissue, and actually in parts of cells, so that we have a probe here whose power for microprobing is exceedingly strong.

However, the full power of the probe requires that we be able to correlate its findings with conventional morphology. This is not strong at the present time. The power of the biochemical analyses is that it can tell us about the tissues' or cells' specific kinds of lipid molecules, proteins, apolipoproteins, the components of connective tissue, elastin, collagen, the various kinds of elastin, the various kinds of collagen. Those analyses have not yet been brought to bear systemically upon the fine morphology of the cells and, in turn, upon the kinds of cells that go into the tissues. When that is done we will be in a strong position to achieve understanding the pathogenesis of the disease, and this has been the main motivation for these kinds of studies.

Today we are concerned more about the use of these tools for clinical diagnosis and for assessment of clinical treatment and preventive measures. Because of the relative lag and practical difficulties in the application of the biochemical methods we are not able to bring these to bear into the clinical situation as much as we would like. Obviously the need is for more comprehensive development and application of these biochemical probes to define the morphological changes, and thus rationally link morphological changes to atherogenesis.

17

Multicenter Trial for Assessment of B-Mode Ultrasound Imaging

JAMES F. TOOLE AND ALAN BERSON

Vascular disease, specifically atherosclerosis, continues to be one of the major causes of morbidity and mortality in this country. In 1973, the National Heart and Lung Advisory Council emphasized the need for developing noninvasive techniques for its detection. Subsequently, this need was incorporated as a part of the National Plan of the Institute. In 1975, the first solicitation for such instrument development was released, followed in 1977, and again in 1980 by competitive renewals for expansion of this program. In 1980 the Division of Heart and Vascular Diseases, in response to advances made in noninvasive instrument development, solicited proposals for assessment of ultrasonic B-mode imaging vis-à-vis arteriography and pathology for detection and quantification of atherosclerotic lesions in human and nonhuman primate carotid and iliofemoral arteries. In 1981 this resulted in the award of seven contracts to establish one animal center, five clinical centers and a coordination center (Table 1).

We recognize that validation studies of ultrasound B-mode imaging are essential for patient care and research. If validated, this method will be very useful for diagnostic studies in

This study is supported by National Heart, Lung and Blood Institute grants HV 12916 and HV 12904.

Table 1. Centers for assessment of ultrasonic B-mode imaging.

Principal Investigator	Field of Interest	Institution
M. Gene Bond, Ph.D.	Comparative medicine pathology	Bowman Gray School of Medicine
Barry Goldberg, M.D.	Radiology	Jefferson Medical College
Jeffrey Raines, Ph.D.	Clinical physiology	Miami Heart Institute
Daniel O'Leary, M.D.	Neurology Radiology	New England Deaconess Hospital
James DeWeese, M.D.	Vascular surgery	University of Rochester
James F. Toole, M.D.	Neurology	Bowman Gray School of Medicine
Fred A. Bryan, Ph.D.	Data management	Research Triangle Institute

symptomatic patients, screening of high-risk, asymptomatic populations, evaluation of therapeutic interventions designed to populations, evaluation of therapeutic interventions designed to retard the development of reverse atherosclerosis, and in studying longitudinally the course of the disease in human beings and experimental animals.

The goal of this three-year study is to determine the accuracy and reliability of B-mode ultrasound imaging for detecting and quantifying atherosclerotic lesions in human beings and in animal models.

The objectives of the clinical and animal centers are to collect data which will be used to determine the sensitivity, specificity, accuracy, and repeatability of B-mode imaging relative to arteriography and anatomic pathology for detection of atherosclerosis in carotid and iliofemoral arteries.

Each clinical center will recruit approximately 200 patients per year who are scheduled for arteriography because of suspected atherosclerotic lesions. In many, a surgical specimen or postmortem examination will be available for correlation. The animal center will develop a colony of atherosclerotic *M. fascicularis* monkeys using known pathogenetic factors of hypercholesterolemia and hypertension. Carotid and iliofemoral arteries as well as abdominal aortas will be evaluated by arteriography and ultrasound B-mode imaging as atherosclerosis progresses and just prior to sacrifice. The last images will be compared with the pressure-fixed pathology specimens for determination of sensitivity, specificity, accuracy, and predictability of B-mode imaging in diagnosis of atherosclerosis.

Because large variations are suspected to occur in interpretations of arteriograms and B-mode images, randomized studies will determine inter- and intraobserver variability for both B-mode and arteriography. Arteriograms will be interpreted by individuals who are unaware of the patients' clinical history and B-mode imaging data. Conversely, B-mode image interpretation will be done by individuals who do not have knowledge of either arteriographic or clinical history data. In order to accomplish this, images will be distributed randomly among institutions.

Functional studies will also be performed; specifically, for carotid arteries phonoangiography, oculoplethysmography, and Doppler flow, and for iliofemoral arteries, pulse volume recordings, and treadmill test. A spin-off of this trial may be the accumulation of a cohort of symptomatic patients who have been evaluated by standardization history, functional studies, B-mode ultrasound, and arteriography who can be followed longitudinally to determine the natural history of the disease and/or the effects of remedial intervention.

These data will permit the assessment of intra- and interobserver variability for both arteriography and B-mode imaging as well as differences between arteriography and B-scan images relative to size and location of lesions, including differences in performance of instrumentation.

Data regarding the imaging procedures will be used for evaluation of the utility of imaging procedures as a screening device prior to arteriography. There will also be a determination of the ease of application of the procedure, length of time required for a procedure, and level of training necessary for personnel.

Histories and physical findings including age, sex, height, weight, vascular symptoms (e.g., transient ischemic attacks, stroke, claudication), risk factors, presence or absence of pulses, bruits, and neurologic and peripheral vascular findings will be collected. These data together with results of arteriography, imaging procedures, flow data, examination of specimens resulting from surgery, or autopsy, will be forwarded to the data coordinating center.

In addition longitudinal studies of atheromatosis of the arterial system opposite that treated surgically will be performed, allowing a comparative study of natural history of atheromatosis.

Plasma levels of high-density lipoproteins/cholesterol, low-density lipoproteins/cholesterol, total cholesterol, and total triglyceride concentrations will be gathered for (1) corroborative evidence of arterial disease in validating ultrasonic B-mode imaging, (2) obtaining a statistical relationship between lipid levels and peripheral arterial disease, and (3) consideration of therapeutic intervention of elevated lipid levels.

The time frames for performing the work required by the contract are:
1. Six months for development of protocols and assembling teams
2. Three months for pilot studies during which the system will be tested
3. Eighteen months for data collection
4. A final six months for data analysis and preparation of collaborative publications

PROGRESS

There have been five meetings for preparation of protocol and evaluation forms. These meetings also served to develop mutual understanding and a team relationship since before this there had been no on-going dialogue aimed at determining the true role of this modality. One must keep in mind that there has already been enormous individual commitment of time, effort, and money to this project, the results of which we suspect will have great implication for health care delivery.

The members have already developed and agreed upon:

1. Patient selection criteria, informed consent, and reporting forms
2. Procedures for imaging arteries ultrasonically and arteriographically and methods for measuring lesion sizes and locations
3. Designs for determining repeatability of interpretation of arteriograms and ultrasound images
4. Procedures for obtaining pathology data from surgical specimens

The pilot study phase was initiated in February 1982, and 16 patients have been randomized. A Data Review Board has been established (Table 2) to serve as an independent advisory group for all phases of the program.

The wide geographic distribution and the many disciplines involved should suggest that this study is a careful attempt to create a multidisciplinary group of clinical and basic scientists who will evaluate the sensitivity, specificity, and accuracy of this new modality, as well as provide perceptions of its proper place in the health care delivery system. Represented within centers are cardiologists, internists, vascular surgeons, neuro-surgeons, ultrasonographers, radiologists, neurologists, neuro-radiologists, pathologists, veterinarians, physiologists, and biostatisticians.

B-mode ultrasound imaging is potentially a powerful clinical and research tool for determining the extent and severity of atherosclerosis in arteries that can be imaged. We hope it will prove to be useful for tracking lesion progression or regression.

Table 2. Members of the data review board.

DISCUSSION: ROBERT W. BARNES

This multicenter trial for assessment of B-mode ultrasound imaging represents a new era for biomedical research, namely, an attempt at rigorous scientific appraisal of the validity of the diagnostic accuracy of a rapidly evolving technology and, in addition, a systematic application of this instrument to further elucidate the natural history of clinical and preclinical stages of atherosclerosis. It is important to differentiate these two functions of noninvasive or less invasive techniques. Most previous investigations of noninvasive techniques have been directed at detection of atherosclerotic-lesions; at identification of carotid disease in the case of real-time B-mode imaging. However, in more than a decade of development of this instrument, there have been few reports, other than anecdotal case descriptions, comparing high-resolution images with arteriography. However, studies such as that described in this workshop by Comerota (see Chap. 15) as well as previous reports such as that by Hobson et al. (1) give us pause as to the clinical diagnostic value of B-mode imaging alone. Both of these studies suggest that with more advanced lesions the ability to distinguish severe stenosis from total occlusion is poor. This is a limitation which gravely restricts the clinical applicability of this instrument alone.

The combination of Doppler ultrasonic flow interrogation with B-mode scanning in the so-called duplex scanners may greatly increase the value of this instrument in arriving at clinical decisions about the presence of operable carotid occlusive disease. Fortunately, some of the instruments used in this multicenter trial have duplex capability and it will be important to evaluate the relative contribution of the B-mode and the Doppler components in arriving at a vascular diagnosis. Prior studies would suggest that high-resolution B-mode scanning would have its greatest role in detecting or excluding minor nonobstructive or ulcerated plaques, while Doppler ultrasonic velocity detection would confirm the presence or absence of operable stenosis or inoperable occlusion in more advanced disease. One would hope that the combination of these technologies would permit accurate prediction of those systematic patients with ulcerated plaque or stenosis who would benefit from arteriography and carotid endarterectomy, while excluding from angiography those patients with normal or occluded arteries who are not operative candidates.

The second, and perhaps more important, area for future application and investigation of this and other recent technology is in the further definition of the natural history of athero-sclerotic disease and its modification by medical or surgical intervention. However, no matter what our idealistic intentions are in terms of applying these tools to longitudinal or epidemio-logic surveys of disease progression or regression, the blunt facts are that these instruments, particularly B-mode scanners are proliferating for the expressed purpose of screening asymp-tomatic or atypically symptomatic patients for the presence of carotid disease. Once such disease is visualized, the patient often undergoes subsequent arteriography and experiences the greatest of all forms of plaque mobility, namely its surgical removal - all for a preclinical disease whose natural history is unknown. This dilemma has assumed increasing importance in recommendations for future planning of NIH and other funding agencies, namely that the newer technologies not only be validat-ed but also be applied in careful longitudinal epidemiologic or follow-up studies to detect disease progression or regression both in terms of lesion change and with respect to clinical outcomes.

Recently separate prospective studies by us and the groups at Wisconsin and Seattle have suggested that patients with detected asymptomatic carotid occlusive disease are not at greater risk of perioperative stroke during major cardiovascular operations, but our studies do show these patients do have an increased incidence of late postoperative neurologic deficits. Most important, these patients are at significantly greater risk of perioperative or late death due to myocardial infarction. A future prospective Veterans Administration multicenter randomized trial has been designed to assess the efficacy of prophylactic carotid endarterectomy in patients with asymptomatic carotid artery disease detected by noninvasive techniques. We have recently been funded to carry out technology transfer in affiliated family practice centers in Virginia. This technology will be used to screen for asymptomatic carotid artery atherosclerosis in high-risk patients who will be treated medically.

In conclusion, the next decade will witness increased efforts to take existing and evolving technology into carefully controlled trials of clinical diagnostic validation as well as longitudinal assessment of lesion change and clinical outcome.

REFERENCE

1. Hobson RW, Silvia MD, Katocs AS, O'Donnell JA, Jamil Z, Savitsky P (1980) Pulsed Doppler and real-time B-mode echo arteriography for noninvasive imaging of the extracranial arteries. Surgery 87:286-293.

Part 3

Critical Review of Measurements of Change in Atherosclerosis Progression and Regression

Introduction

ASSAAD S. DAOUD AND WILLIAM P. NEWMAN III

In this session, atherosclerosis in human and experimental subjects is reviewed. In his presentation on the pathobiology of atherosclerosis, Dr. Daoud reviews the various functions of the cellular elements of the arterial wall, the interaction between these cells and the extracellular substances and how these functions and interactions relate to the atherosclerotic process during both the regression and progression phases. He particularly emphasizes the role of calcium deposition and macrophage functions on regression. As to the role of calcium accumulation, he presents data from his laboratory suggesting that continued accumulation of calcium may be responsible for the retardation or lack of regression. He also discusses the postulated mechanisms of calcification, stressing the role of an apatite-nucleating proteolipid extracted by Ennever from the atherosclerotic aorta, and also found by Dr. Daoud's group to be present in the normal and atherosclerotic swine aortas. As to the possible role of macrophages in regression, he hypothesizes that macrophages play a role in the removal of necrotic debris by either phagocytosis or hydrolytic enzyme digestion. In favor of this hypothesis, he presents data showing close physical association between macrophages and necrosis, and increase in hydrolytic enzymatic activities in the atherosclerotic lesions, and the ability of lesion macrophages to phagocytize yeasts.

Finally, Dr. Daoud stresses the desirability, whenever possible, of using combined approaches, such as morphologic, biochemical, and clinical, in the study of progression and regression of atherosclerosis.

Dr. Bond presents results of progression and regression of atherosclerosis in animals. Morphometric evaluation techniques using pressure-fixed artery preparations from monkeys in which atherosclerotic lesions had been induced are presented. He gives evidence that atherosclerosis can and in some animals does increase coronary artery size. This finding is very important in that an interpretation of atherosclerosis regression based solely on lumen characteristics may be complicated because of arterial dilatation. The substantiation of this finding in humans is needed, especially as more clinical studies are being reported. Dr. Bond also reports on validation trials to assess the accuracy of B-mode ultrasound imaging for measuring artery size in nonhuman primates. Using an advanced ultrasound imaging system designed specifically to evaluate arteries in small animals, this group has been able to measure and compare abdominal aortic lumen diameters and wall thicknesses derived from B-mode images with direct measurements made from pressure-fixed pathology specimens.

Dr. Newman presents information about our knowledge of the progression of atherosclerosis from the early lesions, known to begin in childhood, to the more advanced and complicated lesions of adulthood, frequently associated with clinical events including myocardial infarction, cerebral infarction, and gangrene of the extremities. He also reviews current evidence for atherosclerosis regression in humans and in addition presents data suggesting a decrease in atherosclerotic involvement of the coronary arteries in the young New Orleans population.

Dr. Kennedy reports on the Coronary Artery Surgery Study (CASS). The CASS registry consists of 24,959 patients who had selective coronary arteriography, including 780 patients who were randomized for medical or surgical therapy. Eight hundred and seventy films were read at special quality control laboratories and at the participating site. The results show that readers have an average absolute difference of 5-10% in the interpretation of coronary artery narrowing. In a small angiographic interpretation experiment it was found that the intrareader variability was approximately one half of the interreader variability in the interpretation of percent stenosis. To minimize this variability in reading of angiograms, Dr. Kennedy stresses the importance of side-by-side double projector interpretations of films by two angiographers, and the use of calibration devices including digitizing tablets and digital calibers. Because of anticipated changes in equipment over an extended time period, he recommends the use of control cases in assessing a regression or new therapy.

Dr. Mustard discusses the role of thrombosis in the development of early and advanced atherosclerotic lesions and the relationship of atherosclerosis to clinical complications. In the early lesion, injury to the endothelium is associated with platelet accumulation on the damaged surface. This platelet accumulation leads to the release of substances that cause migration and proliferation of smooth muscle cells in the intima. In the advanced lesion, thrombi formed at the site of injury may become organized, contributing to further wall thickening. Advanced lesions may cause clinical complications by showering the microcirculation with emboli or by occluding a main vessel. He further cites evidence that withdrawal of the injurious stimulus leads to regression of the lesions. He also discusses the difficulties in quantitating endothelial injury including the measurement of the products formed or released by platelets, or products formed as a result of blood coagulation.

Dr. Mock critically reviews the status of clinical studies including epidemiologic population studies, controlled intervention studies with defined clinical endpoints--myocardial infarcts, both fatal and nonfatal, and sudden deaths--clinical angiographic studies with data on the progression of coronary atherosclerosis, and several controlled intervention studies with angiographic endpoints with information on progression, stabilization, and regression of atherosclerotic lesions. Additionally, limitations inherent in angiographic interpretation are discussed. He concludes with a discussion of the NHLBI Ultrasound B-mode Assessment Program, a multicenter validation study evaluating this important noninvasive technique. Methods used in this multicenter, multidisciplinary effort are applicable to other noninvasive techniques that may become available for evaluation of the vascular system.

Dr. Hall's presentation deals with the various statistical problems of which investigators should be aware. These include experimental design, sample size, p values, standard errors, standard deviations, and significance. He gives several examples from published data illustrating that the quality of statistical practice, particularly at the most basic and fundamental levels, should be improved.

18

Pathobiology of Atherosclerosis

Assaad S. Daoud, Katherine E. Fritz, and John Jarmolych

The normal arterial wall is an ordered structure in which the principal cellular components, smooth muscle cells, and endothelial cells, are arranged in a predictable relationship to each other and to the extracellular substances, most of which are collagen, elastin, and glycosaminoglycans. The development of an atherosclerotic lesion disturbs normal spatial relationships by altering both the cellular and extracellular composition. The cellular changes involve most notably an increase in smooth muscle cells (SMC) and the appearance of numerous "foam cells," lipid-filled cells of unidentifiable origin, as well as macrophages (1). Also documented are increases in such extracellular substances as total and esterified cholesterol, phospholipid, elastin (2) and calcium (3). These changes are accompanied by areas of necrosis (1). During the regression process the numbers of foam cells and macrophages decrease (1,4), as does lipid concentration (5-7), including total and esterified cholesterol (3,7-9). Depending on the regression regimen employed, calcium concentration may decrease (5,6,8) or increase (3), while collagen concentration has similarly been reported to increase (8) or decrease (9). A decrease in the amount of necrosis is a relatively early phenomenon (1).

Supported by the Medical Research Service of the Veterans Administration and by NIHL grant #210038

In the early phase of the process the alteration is limited to the intima, but eventually it extends to involve the media and even the adventitia. While there is general agreement that the elevated lesion, with a necrotic lipid-rich core or "gruel" is the hallmark of the atheroma, there is no agreement as to the characterization of the earlier intimal changes which lead to the development of this lesion. It is still debatable if the flat, yellow lesion designated "fatty streak," which is characterized by an abnormal accumulation of intra- and extracellular lipid, is a precursor of the atheroma, or whether the latter arises independently. More controversial is the role of the focal fibromuscular intimal thickening (cushion or intimal cell mass), which shows no abnormal lipid deposition, in the genesis of the atherosclerotic lesion.

The lack of definitive characterization of the early lesion led to multiple hypotheses as to its pathogenesis. Among the leading theories offered to explain the pathogenesis of atherosclerosis are the "lipid infiltration" theory, the "thrombogenic" theory, the "injury and repair" theory, and the "monoclonal" theory. In this communication we will not attempt to validate any hypothesis or to propose new ones. Instead, we will review briefly the various functions of the cells in the atheroma and interactions between these cells and the extracellular substances. In the final analysis, it is these interrelationships that will determine the fate of the lesion: whether it will continue to increase in size, or perhaps remain stable in dimensions but undergo qualitative changes, or, under favorable conditions, regress. Recent reviews (10-12) have discussed many of these interrelationships in considerable detail. Phenomena related to thrombosis are discussed by Dr. Mustard in Chap. 22. However, we will focus on two of the components that, from our own work, may play a pivotal role in the regression process: calcium, for which we postulate a negative influence; and macrophages, which we are assuming to be beneficial.

LITERATURE REVIEW

Function of Lesion Cells

Let us first look at some of the functions that have been described
for the most prevalent cell of the arterial wall, the smooth muscle
cell. Perhaps the most important is the ability to contract (13).
However, at least in vitro, the ability of SMC to contract at a
given time is in inverse ratio to their secretory and replicative
activity (10,14).

    SMC also migrate. In in vivo studies the SMC "trapped" in the
fenestra of the internal elastic lamina of the aorta, with one
part in the intima while the other is in the media, is not an uncommon sight. In vitro studies using explants, which support the
mobility of the SMC, include work from our laboratory in which
SMC in free-floating explants have moved from the interior to the
outside to form a peripheral growth (15), and from that of Wissler
and coworkers (16), in which the extent of migration of SMC from
a substrate-attached explant is the basis for assessment of the
effect of hyperlipidemic (HL) sera on growth patterns. In fact,
it is this property of SMC which is exploited in "classical"
methods of establishing SMC cell cultures (10). The reversible
tendency of porcine aortic SMC, in essentially monolayer cultures,
to form nodular structures (17,18) shows that the ability of the
SMC to migrate is not lost when they are separated from the
arterial wall or wall fragment, with their structural integrity.
This is further underscored by studies on the capacity of SMC to
fill an experimentally-derived culture "wound" (19,20). The
extent to which this movement can be ascribed to chemotactic
factors of whatever origin is of considerable interest.

    SMC have the ability to modify their own external environment
by synthesis of such extracellular components as collagen, elastin,
and glycosaminoglycans (GAG) (21-25). In addition they secrete
hydrolytic enzymes, such as β-glucuronidase, cholesteryl ester
hydrolase (26), collagenase (27), and cathepsin D (28), each of

which will presumably play a role in the degradation of the extracellular matrix. They may even influence the activity of these enzymes, as by secreting an inhibitor of collagenase (29).

They can partially determine their internal composition by regulation of uptake of a number of substances via specific receptors, for example, low-density lipoprotein (LDL) (30), heparin (31) and platelet-derived growth factor (PDGF) (10). The specific binding of LDL initiates a cascade of effects that, except in the presence of large excesses of LDL, controls the synthesis of cholesterol and the accumulation of intracellular cholesteryl ester (30). The cell can influence the influx of cholesterol via control of the synthesis of LDL receptors (32). Pinocytosis is also involved in the internalization of some substances, and its rate can be enhanced by exposure to PDGF (33). Finally, under some conditions SMC have been shown to be phagocytic (34,35). In addition to these diverse functions, the proliferative activity of the SMC is a major contributing factor to pathogenesis of the lesion. Proliferation of SMC of normal arterial wall occurs at a very slow rate, whether measured autoradiographically or biochemically (36), whereas the proliferation of SMC in the early lesions is greatly enhanced (3), probably in response to exposure to a variety of mitogens.

The documented functions of the other major cell of the normal artery, the endothelial cell (EC), are even more extensive. A primary function obviously is to serve as a barrier between the arterial wall and the blood being transported. As an obvious corollary, if they serve as a barrier for some blood components, they must necessarily provide for transport of necessary substances from the blood. The exact mode of transport depends to a considerable degree on the size of the substance in question (37). Various proteins such as ferritin are apparently transported in vesicles. Even small hemepeptides are apparently transported via vesicles or chains of vesicles which form transendothelial channels (38).

Another important function of EC is migration, being especially crucial in the repair of a denuded surface (19). The control of migration is separable from that of multiplication (20,39). The presence of a growth factor is not required for migration (12). Another related function is that of spreading, which has been studied especially in vitro (40).

EC have been shown to synthesize and secrete a number of substances, among them a growth factor stimulating SMC growth (41), and another (heparin-like) inhibiting SMC growth (42). They contribute to their extracellular milieu by the secretion of collagen (Types I (43), III (44,45), V (45,46)), elastic fibers (46), and fibronectin (47), and are involved in the coagulation process through their synthesis of Factor VIII (48) and PGI_2 (49). Further, they can affect their environment by the secretion of hydrolytic enzymes (28). Under certain injurious conditions they have been shown to produce Fc and C3b receptors (50). The internal environment, and with it a number of processes, is modulated by uptake of a number of substances via specific receptors, among them LDL (30,51,52), chylomicrons (52), fibroblast growth factor (53), platelet factor IV (54), β-thromboglobulin (55), and chemotactic agents (56).

With the addition of macrophages to the cell population, as in a lesion, the number of potential functions of the cells is greatly enhanced. The many functions of macrophages related to the immune response will not be considered here, although the possibility of an immune component in the lesion should not be ignored (57-59). Their very presence in the lesion attests to their ability to migrate, as has been documented (60-62). Perhaps equal in importance is their phagocytic capacity. As one of the two "professional phagocytic" cell types, their involvement in the resolution of inflammation and bacterial infection is well established (63). Actively phagocytizing cells with many of the characteristics of macrophages have been recovered in suspension from atherosclerotic lesions (64,65). Macrophages have been shown to phagocytize even calcium in mineral form, as well as collagenous matrix (66). Both pinocytosis and phagocytosis are increased when macrophages are in the activated state (67). To some extent,

they control their own shape and mobility by their secretion of
factor B, a complement-associated protein, a cleavage product of
which is a potent spreading factor (67). They exercise some
measure of control over their milieu via control of the synthesis
of collagen and GAG (68), and by their production of proteinases
that degrade elastin (69,70), glycoproteins, and collagen (69,71).
In addition, they secrete an impressive array of other substances:
complement components (72), acid hydrolases (72,73), lysozyme
(73), plasminogen activator (74), peroxidase, superoxide dismutase
(10), reactive O_2 metabolities (67), enzyme inhibitors, and chemotactic factors (10). Of special interest is their secretion of
two substances, a growth factor stimulating proliferation of both
SMC and EC (75,76), and fibronectin, a protein involved in cell
adhesion and in non-immune opsonization of particles for phagocytosis (77-79). Like the other two cell types, the macrophage also
excercises limited control of its cholesterol metabolism by uptake
of LDL via specific receptors (80).

Interactions Among Arterial Components

This chronicling of some of the functions of the cells of the
artery wall serves to emphasize the complexity of the factors involved in atherogenesis. But to these cellular functions must be
added interactions among these cells. For instance, in addition
to the stimulation of SMC proliferation by EC and macrophages via
growth factor, in vitro EC enhancement of the production of GAG,
especially hyaluronic acid and chondroitin sulfate, by SMC has
been demonstrated (81). There are numerous interactions between
the cells and the extracellular substance. For instance, there
is evidence that heparin serves to bind lipoprotein lipase to EC
(82). On the other hand, heparin apparently decreases SMC proliferation (83). Within limits, an increase in extracellular LDL
concentration inhibits the synthesis of LDL receptors and thus
helps minimize the accumulation of cholesteryl esters in SMC (30)
and macrophages (84). Such an LDL increase also stimulates the

proliferation of SMC (85) and depresses the phagocytic activity of macrophages (86,87).

The synthesis of cholesteryl ester by macrophages (88) is stimulated by β-very-low-density lipoproteins. Evidence from in vitro studies that HDL, or at least some apoprotein components, when combined with phospholipid, may play a role in the removal of cellular lipids, especially cholesterol (89). Ca^{2+} ion is required for the binding of LDL to its specific receptors; heparin promotes the release of LDL from the receptor (30). Both heparin and heparan sulfate activate lipoprotein lipase (90). Heparin, in combination with fibronectin, facilitates phagocytosis by macrophages (91). Another GAG, hyaluronic acid, has been identified as a macrophage agglutinating factor (92). The presence of glycoproteins in the in vitro extracellular matrix inhibits elastolysis by macrophages (93).

If we add to the above the interactions among extracellular components, the complexities increase. The GAG become especially prominent with their reactions with β- and pre-β-lipoprotein (94-98), where the types of GAG present may be definitive. The sulfated GAG tend to form insoluble complexes with β- and pre-β-lipoprotein, with heparin having the greatest affinity. The differing affinities of various GAG for collagen or elastin have been documented, with chondroitin sulfate and dermatan sulfate binding to collagen, and heparan sulfate to elastin (99). A relation to changes in permeability and fibrinolytic activity has been suggested for changes in GAG content at different stages of atherogenesis (100). In addition, the type of GAG present will influence their interactions with fibronectin, since the latter has been shown to bind to hyaluronic acid and heparin but not to chondroitin sulfate (101). Elastin apparently plays a role in the accumulation of both lipid (102) and calcium (103), and there is some evidence that cholesterol accumulation may influence collagen synthesis (104) and the accumulation of calcium (105).

There are important interactions between extracellular components and the coagulation process, notably involving heparin and calcium (90,106-108) and collagen (109). For example, heparin retards the rate of thrombin formation and potentiates the action of antithrombin III; Ca^{2+} ion is involved in this reaction. Heparin also reversibly binds and neutralizes complement.

Calcium and Regression

Our interest in calcium in regression was enhanced and focused by a recent experiment in which we studied sequentially a number of morphological and biochemical changes occurring in swine aortic and coronary atherosclerotic lesions in the course of a 14-mos regression regimen (1,3). The lesions in the abdominal aorta, by far the most severe we have ever elicited, resulted from a combination of a single balloon catheter injury and 6 mos feeding of an atherogenic diet containing 1.8% cholesterol, with total fat (including lard and peanut oil) of 33.8%, and sodium cholate. The lesions of the coronary arteries were induced by the diet only. At the end of the induction period the aortic lesions morphologically showed minimal calcium deposition. Biochemically, in dissected lesion tissue, a mean concentration of 9.1 µg/mg dry wt represented a two- to three-fold increase in calcium concentration as compared to non-lesion areas. After 6 weeks of the regression regimen, calcium concentration of the lesion tissue had increased six-fold, and by 5 mos had reached a mean level of 87 µg/mg dry wt. The mean lesion concentration at the end of the 14-mos regression period was 129 µg/mg dry wt. This remarkable and significant elevation of tissue calcium had occurred in the absence of any increase in calcium concentration in the adjacent non-lesion tissue over that of comparable tissue from mash-fed controls. Morphologically, this increased calcium concentration was expressed in such large accumulations in lesion tissue that decalcification prior to sectioning was required after 5 mos and 14 mos of regression. A most important finding, as shown by morphometric analysis, was that these lesions did not decrease in size throughout the 14-mos regression period. This was in contrast to a previously shown

significant decrease in the size of less severe but still complicated, calcified lesions during a similar regression regimen (110).

Calcium in the coronary arteries of the same animals in the
sequential study was estimated morphometrically. Calcium deposition involved a mean of 0.098 mm^2 or 6% of the area of the lesions
of the combined baseline and 6-weeks arteries, and 0.082 mm^2 or
13% of the area of the late regression (5- and 14-mos) lesions.
There was no significant decrease in the actual area of calcification during the late stages of regression; the slight increase
in the mean percent lesion area involved in calcification reflects
the fact that were was a significant reduction in the mean lesion
area at this time.

These results raised many questions. Was the difference in
reaction of the size of the lesion in response to the regression
regimen due to: (1) the difference in arterial beds; (2) differences in the mode of induction (diet only vs diet plus injury);
(3) differences in severity of the lesions (the coronary lesions
were less severe than those of the aorta); (4) differences in the
extent of cholesterol accumulation; or (5) perhaps to the continued and severe accumulation of calcium, as in the aortic lesions,
in contrast to no increased accumulation, as seen in the coronaries? Perhaps the most provocative finding was the more than
thirty-fold elevation of calcium concentration of the lesions over
that of the adjacent non-lesion tissue in the 5- and 14-mos regression animals. To what can one attribute this accumulation?
There was no significant elevation of serum calcium throughout the
entire experiment. The postulated mechanism for calcium accumulation via preferential affinity to elastin followed by binding to
collagen and/or polar proteoglycans (103) does not appear to be
able, by itself, to account for this extent of calcium accumulation, since the amount of (newly synthesized) elastin in the
lesion morphologically appears to be less than the total elastin
present in the normal aortic wall. One can invoke a variety of
possible mechanisms which might explain this phenomenon. One

which is of great interest to us is the possibility that the lesions contain greater amounts of an apatite-nucleating proteolipid, extracted by Ennever from such calcified tissue as bone (111), dental calculus (112), calcifying bacteria (113), and most pertinently, from human calcified aorta (114). Since we have shown, by energy-dispersive spectral analysis (EDSA) and line profile analysis, in at least the larger calcium deposits from these lesions, that the major constituents are calcium and phosphorus, we know that the component's requisite for apatite formation are: (1) present in the artery and (2) concentrated in the lesions. Further, by selected-area electron diffraction we have obtained diffraction patterns comparable to those of apatite, which has been reported to be a major form of calcification in human (115,116) and rat aorta (117). Thus, it is pertinent to ask whether there is more of the nucleating proteolipid present in: (1) lesions as compared to adjacent non-lesion areas, and (2) in highly calcified as opposed to less calcified lesions. If so, what controls its synthesis or accumulation? An alternative question which may be equally important is whether the proteolipid extractable from calcifying lesions may be qualitatively different from that of non-lesion tissue. Does it differ in its apoprotein composition, in the phospholipid moiety, or perhaps in configuration? These are questions which are relatively straightforward and we are currently involved in experiments designed to provide at least partial answers to them. Another question, relating to the control of apatite nucleation in lesions, perhaps more difficult to approach, is what substances may be present which inhibit apatite nucleation and/or growth? In the complex milieu of the lesion perhaps one of the normally present consitutents--a particular GAG?--serves this function. Or alternatively, an unidentified protein or lipid component might be involved. These are problems which should be addressed.

However, there is another important aspect to the problem of calcification and its role in either the atherogenesis or the regression process. This is the definition of the effects that accumulated calcium, as a mineral, has on the many cellular functions and interactions of the arterial wall. One might expect, based on the large excess of calcium present, to encounter problems normally associated with excess calcium, among them an increased contractability of both SMC (118) and EC (119), and inhibition of some enzymes such as cathepsin B1 (120), inorganic pyrophosphatase (121), phosphorylase a (122), piruvate kinase (123), and superoxide dismutase (124). But it should be noted that it is by no means certain that an excess of available calcium ion exists, even in the presence of large amounts of mineral calcium. The affinity of calcium for a growing apatite crystal is so great that, following nucleation, there may exist focal micro- or macro-areas of actual Ca^{2+} ion deficiency. The potential effects of this situation are many, depending, in fact, on the molarity of Ca^{2+} ion actually present. Thus, such Ca^{2+} ion-requiring reactions as platelet aggregation and release reaction (125), Ca- and Mg-dependent ATPase activity, protein secretion (126), chemotaxis (127), lipomobilization (128), synthesis and/or hydrolysis of connective tissue proteins (70,71), and the binding of LDL and VLDL to GAG may or may not be affected at any one time. Clearly, however, the definition of whether or not a Ca^{2+} ion deficiency exists, and, if so, which processes are affected, poses a difficult, yet potentially very rewarding, challenge.

For the same reasons, the importance and prevalence in aortic tissue of another calcium-associated protein, atherocalcin (129), now considered to be osteocalcin (130-131), should be investigated. This protein presumably binds calcium via its component of γ-carboxyglutamic acid, an amino acid with an affinity for calcium (132). Osteocalcin is extractable from lesions, together with the calcium component, into ethylenediamine tetraacetic acid (EDTA) (129), and can be assayed by radioimmunoassay. Efforts to establish the importance of osteocalcin in the arterial calcification process, primarily by quantitative assessment, are under way in various laboratories, including ours. Once this has been established, and assuming a greater prevalence in calcified lesions as opposed to adjacent non-lesion tissue, the fundamental question of what controls its accumulation becomes paramount. Also, the same questions as to the effect(s) of the calcium binding to osteocalcin, discussed above, must be considered. Is a focal deficiency of Ca^{2+} ion created, or is there an excess of available Ca^{2+} ion?

Simultaneously with biochemical study of the apatite-nucleating proteolipid and/or osteocalcin in attempting to understand the mechanisms producing, and consequences of, arterial calcification, it is imperative that detailed comprehensive morphological studies of the sequence of events leading to or abrogating the dense calcification seen in our 14-mos regression animals be performed. This implies sequential studies during both progression and regression utilizing histochemical staining (von Kossa and alizarin red) on the light microscopic level, and numerous approaches on the ultrastructural level. For example, transmission electron microscopic (TEM) study of electron-dense structures, examined before, and reexamined after EDTA or ethyleneglycol-bis (β-amino-ethyl ether) N,N^1-tetraacetic acid (EGTA) treatment, are crucial to any sequential study. The addition of energy dispersive spectral analysis (EDSA), with line profile analysis, together with scanning transmission electron microscopy (STEM) provides fundamental information as to composition of the variety of intra- and extracellular electron dense structures present. And finally, use of selected area electron diffraction will be most helpful in providing confirmation of crystalline structure at various stages of both the biochemical and morphological studies.

The addition of calcium antagonists, such as ethane-1-hydroxy-1, 1-diphosphonate or lanthanum, to such coordinated studies, as planned in our laboratory, can potentially result in an enhancement or identification of the mechanisms or factors affected by calcium accumulation in the arterial wall.

Macrophages in Regression

Our interest in the role of macrophages in the regression process
is also an outgrowth of the same sequential study of the regression process described above. The occurrence and localization of
macrophages in this experiment are of interest temporally and
spatially. As to the first, while there were a number of ultrastructurally identifiable macrophages in the lesions at the end of
the induction period, their presence became a much more predominant feature in the lesions of the 6-week regression animals,
when, as noted previously, the serum cholesterol levels had returned approximately to normal. Subsequently, as the regression
regimen was prolonged, there were relatively few macrophages. In
any discussion of macrophages it is important to note that, in the
lesions seen immediately following the induction period (baseline),
a major cellular component was the foam cell. Identification of
the precursor(s) of foam cells is difficult, at best, but a body
of evidence points to a macrophage origin for many of these cells
(4,60), suggesting an even greater macrophage involvement in these
baseline lesions than might have been deduced from the numbers of
identifiable macrophages. The increase in macrophages noted in
the 6-week regression lesions was concomitant with a decrease in
the number of foam cells, raising the question of a possible foam
cell origin for some of the "classical" macrophages, via a lipid
depletion process. Whether or not this "transformation" had taken
place, by the later phases of regression there was a decrease in
numbers of both foam cells and macrophages, which was paralleled
by a decrease in the size of necrotic areas in the lesions.

Spatially, the majority of macrophages was to be found in
physical association with areas of necrosis and/or calcification.
That macrophages may play a role in the resolution of necrosis is
consistent with their role as "professional phagocytes," but their
function as regards mineral deposits is less clearly understood.
However, the evidence that they will engulf mineralized calcium
(66) suggests: (1) that their presence in close apposition to

areas of calcification in this experiment may not have been simply fortuitous, and (2) that they may have some mechanism for removing such deposits, either by some form of biochemical degradation or by physically scavenging and removing it to another milieu for further processing. On the other hand, their demonstrated decrease in numbers even as the calcium concentration increased perhaps argues either against a major role for macrophages in calcium removal, or for some control pathway being overwhelmed by the influx of calcium.

The possible effects of a large complement of macrophages on either the exacerbation or the resolution of a lesion are many. By referring even to the abbreviated list of junctions given above, we can suggest that: (1) they may have been the source of some of the growth factors responsible for the replication of SMC and EC; (2) they may have been a major contributor to the pool of acid hydrolases and neutral proteinase whose elevated activities have been shown to be present in lesions; (3) they may have enhanced their own capacity for phagocytosis of lesion debris by their secretion of fibronectin; or (4) they may have, via phagocytosis, played a major part in "cleaning up" the necrotic areas of the lesions, which had virtually disappeared after 14-mos regression. Did the macrophages contribute actively to the documented decrease in lipid concentration by physical removal of phagocytized debris as suggested by Gerrity and others (133), and/or by intra- or extracellular degradation by their complement of hydrolytic enzymes? Or did they, via "leakage" or secretion of their hydro- lytic enzymes, as has been shown to accompany the act of phagocy- tosis (72), contribute to the extension of the necrotic areas? These and other questions deserve to be investigated, and in many instances will require very innovative approaches.

Viewed from another perspective one can ask: if, on balance, the contribution of macrophages to the regression process is positive, how could this contribution be maximized? Here one turns to the body of information on "activation" of macrophages and its results for suggestions. Activation is generally accepted to include an enhanced spreading and oxygen consumption and increased levels of hydrolytic enzyme activities and of phagocytic activity. However, these diverse processes vary in their response to a given method of activation, as, for instance, stimulation by endocytosis of *E. coli* endotoxin, which resulted in a three-fold increase in acid-phosphatase activity at the same time there was no change in cathepsin D activity (134). Different modes of stimulation also selectively stimulate certain responses. For instance, stimulation by thioglycolate does not result in the appearance of tumoricidal capability, while agents such as complete Freund's adjuvant, *Corynebacterium parvum* or pyran copolymer will induce this response (135). In spite of some of the above-mentioned differences in response, the production of a non-specific enhanced reactivity, as a result of a specific immune stimulus has been well documented (135-137). Included in the enhanced activities are the levels of hydrolytic enzymes and generalized phagocytic capability.

The efficacy of BCG immunization in increasing survival of patients with early lung cancer or acute myelogenous leukemia must rest on such a premise (138-139). Based on this approach to enhancement of macrophage phagocytic and/or hydrolytic enzymatic activity, it is reasonable to make a direct attempt at influencing the regression process by creating and maintaining, in non-immune animals, a hyperimmune state toward a specific antigen, such as BCG. Since the endpoint in such a trial is only assessable at sacrifice, it is impossible to monitor changes in the state of lesion macrophages that may be occurring in the course of the regression regimen. But it is possible to monitor certain pertinent parameters on a "non-destructive" basis. For instance, skin testing with Old Tuberculin at intervals would confirm the existence of hyperimmunity. Perhaps most helpful in judging the effect of the immunization on macrophage function would be periodic harvesting of peritoneal macrophages and measuring their phagocytic potential and the activity of representative hydrolytic enzymes. It is possible, by taking suitable precautions, to recover a large number of macrophages from the peritoneal cavity repeatedly, thus making it feasible to follow changes in these activities that may be occurring in at least one representative component of the reticuloendothelial system.

DISCUSSION

From the above summary it is obvious that the atherosclerotic process is a complex one. While there is much known about the function of the various cellular elements of the lesion and the interactions between these cells and the various extracellular elements, as well as between these and components of the blood, understanding of the sequence of events leading to the formation of an atheroma is still speculative at best. For some, the lipoproteins, especially LDL, are the initiating factors. In favor of this assumption are: (1) the fact that lipids are major constituents of the atheroma, especially in its necrotic center, and (2) the development of premature atherosclerosis in patients having marked hypercholesterolemia. In addition, LDL, which is the major class of lipoproteins associated with atherosclerosis, appears to cause several manifestations of the disease. LDL may cause injury to the endothelium (140-142), which will disturb the endothelial barrier and lead to abnormal accumulation of lipoproteins in the intima. A special category of LDL obtained from hyperlipemic monkeys is reported to be a mitogen for SMC (10,143) and finally both SMC and macrophages possess surface membrane receptors for binding LDL (30,80), which is important in the development of foam cells. The major weakness of this hypothesis has been the occasional occurrence of severe atherosclerosis at an early age in the absence of hypercholesterolemia. Other investigators believe that endothelial injury is the primary cause of atherogenesis. As was mentioned above, injury to the endothelium, by disrupting the endothelial barrier, provides avenues through which plasma lipoproteins may enter more readily, and this concept adds support to the role of LDL in atherogenesis. However, probably the most interesting aspect of this theory is related to the interaction between damaged endothelium and platelets. Recently researchers have discovered that endothelial injury, with resultant sticking of platelets to the damaged intimal surface followed by the release reaction, is an important contributor to the development of experimental atherosclerosis. These studies are an outgrowth of the work of Mustard and coworkers (144,145). Ross and Vogel (146) discovered that a platelet component, presumably released at the site of endothelial injury, is a mitogen for SMC. Finally, EC themselves are able to secrete a factor which causes SMC proliferation (12). While this injury hypothesis is the most popular one at present, there has not been convincing evidence that areas of spontaneous denudation occurs. However, as stated by Schwartz (12), lack of convincing evidence for spontaneous denudation makes it worthwhile to consider the possible role of non-denuding injuries in atherosclerosis.

Finally, an innovative hypothesis proposed by Benditt and coworkers (147) suggests that the initiation of the atherosclerotic lesion resides in the smooth muscle cells that undergo somatic mutation. Benditt found that many foci of SMC from atheromas of black women, who were heterozygous for the isoenzymes of glucose-6-phosphate dehydrogenase (G-6-PD), usually showed only one form of this enzyme, which suggested that this collection of cells was monoclonal. Similar findings are reported in benign tumors of SMC. While the findings of Benditt have been confirmed by others, recent work by Thomas (148,149) tends to support a "natural selection" mechanism to explain the origin of these "monotypic" cells rather than a somatic mutation.

Given the complex spectrum of functions and interactions of the arterial wall cited above, the ideal approach to studying the sequence of changes occurring in various arterial wall components during the progression and regression regimens in experimentally produced animal atherosclerosis would be to study, simultaneously, as many important phenomena as technically feasible. Obviously, no one can approach studying the "whole elephant" in such a multi-faceted disease process. One must, of course, be selective in choosing the question of major emphasis. But in addition one should define, to the degree possible, which other factors or interactions may impinge upon, or be influenced by, the area of major focus in order to identify relationships that might be susceptible to concomitant study. Also, in order to learn the most from a given experiment, it is most productive to combine approaches, whenever possible, such as using both morphological and biochemical methods. In expansion of this concept, using as an example the studies on calcification presented above, from a morphological point of view, the combination of light and transmission electron microscopy with scanning electron micros-copy, EDSA, and electron diffraction should yield much more useful information than any one or two of these techniques above. Bio-chemically, one would hope to combine quantitation of the proteolipid nucleator with, at the least, analysis of the amount and type of lipid present in, and the calcium concentration of, the same tissue. The total picture resulting from such a study, combining a number of technical approaches, might be expected to (1) help put the importance of calcification in perspective and (2) suggest other, related areas to investigate in greater depth.

Finally, in designing experiments to elucidate a sequence of events during progression and regression it is imperative that the same, consistent protocol be used for each time period studied. Inherent animal variation is so great that, for mean-ingful results, it is imperative not to add any other components of variability via less than rigorous control of procedures and techniques. Changing--even optimizing--techniques employed in sequential studies can render the affected parameters not comparable.

REFERENCES

1. Daoud AS, Jarmolych J, Augustyn JM, Fritz KE (1981)
   Sequential morphologic studies of regression of advanced
   atherosclerosis. Arch Path Lab Med 105:233-239
2. Clarkson TB, Lehner NDM, Wagner WD, St Clair RW, Bond MG,
   Bullock BC (1979) A study of atherosclerosis regression in
   Macaca mulatta. I. Design of experiment and lesion induction. Exp Mol Pathol 30:360-385
3. Fritz KE, Augustyn JM, Jarmolych J, Daoud AS (1981) Sequential study of biochemical changes during regression of swine
   aortic atherosclerotic lesions. Arch Path Lab Med 105:
   240-246
4. Stary HC (1979) Regression of atherosclerosis in primates.
   Virchows Arch [Pathol Anat] 383:117-134
5. Wagner WD, Clarkson TB, Foster J (1977) Contrasting effects
   of ethane-1-hydroxy-1, 1-diphosphonate (EHDP) on the regression of two types of dietary-induced atherosclerosis.
   Atherosclerosis 27:419-435
6. Hollander W, Paddock J, Nagraj S, Colombo M, Kirkpatrick B
   (1979) Effects of anticalcifying and antifrobrotic drugs on
   pre-established atherosclerosis in the rabbit. Atherosclerosis 33:111-123
7. Armstrong ML, Megan MB (1972) Lipid depletion in atheromatous coronary arteries in rhesus monkeys after regression
   diets. Circ Res 30:675-680
8. Wagner WD, St Clair RW, Clarkson TB (1980) A study of
   atherosclerosis regression in *Macaca mulatta*: II. Chemical
   changes in arteries from animals with atherosclerosis induced
   for 19 months then regressed for 24 months at plasma cholesterol concentration of 300 or 200 mg/dl. Exp Mol Pathol
   32:162-174
9. Wissler RW, Vesselinovitch D (1977) Regression of atherosclerosis in experimental animals and man. Mod Concepts
   Cardiovasc Dis 46:27-32
10. Ross R (1981) Atherosclerosis: a problem of the biology of
    arterial wall cells and their interactions with blood compo-
    nents. Arteriosclerosis 1:293-311
11. Wissler RW (1980) Principles of the pathogenesis of athero-
    sclerosis. In: Braunwall E (ed) Heart disease: a textbook
    of cardiovascular medicine. WB Sanders Co, Philadelphia,
    pp 1221-1245
12. Schwartz SM, Gajdusek CM, Selden SC III (1981) Vascular wall
    growth control: the role of the endothelium. Arterioscle-
    rosis 1:107-126
13. Ives HE, Schultz GS, Galardy RE, Jamieson JD (1978) Prepara-
    tion of functional smooth muscle cells from the rabbit aorta.
    J Exp Med 148:1400-1413
14. Chamley-Campbell JH, Campbell GR, Ross R (1981) Phenotype-
    dependent response of cultural aortic smooth muscle cells to
    serum mitogens. J Cell Biol 89:379-383

15. Daoud AS, Fritz KE, Jarmolych J, Augustyn JM (1973) Use of aortic medial explants in the study of atherosclerosis. Exp Mol Pathol 18:177-189

16. Fischer-Dzoga K, Wissler RW (1976) Stimulation of proliferation in stationary primary cultures of monkey aortic smooth muscle cells. Part 2. Effect of varying concentrations of hyperlipemic serum and low density lipoproteins of varying dietary fat origins. Atherosclerosis 24:515-525

17. Brennen MJ, Fritz KE, Millis AJT (1980) Density-dependent nodulation of smooth muscle cell cultures. J Cell Biol 87:59a (abstract)

18. Gimbrone MK, Cotran RL (1975) Human vascular smooth muscle in culture. Lab Invest 33:16-27

19. Gottlieb AI, Spector W (1981) Migration into an in vitro experimental wound. A comparison of porcine aortic endothelial and smooth muscle cells and the effect of culture irradiation. Am J Pathol 103:271-282

20. Thorgeirsson G, Robertson AL Jr, Cowan DH (1979) Migration of human vascular endothelial and smooth muscle cells. Lab Invest 41:51-62

21. Daoud AS, Fritz KE, Jarmolych J, Augustyn JM, Mawhinney TM (1977) Production of glycosaminoglycans, collagen and elastic tissue by aortic medial explants. In: Manning GW, Haust MD (eds) Atherosclerosis, metabolic and clinical aspects. Plenum Publishing Corp, New York, pp 928-933

22. Wight TN, Ross R (1975) Proteoglycans in primate arteries. II. Synthesis and secretion of glycosaminoglycans by arterial smooth muscle cells in culture. J Cell Biol 67:675-686

23. Wight TN (1980) Differences in the synthesis and secretion of sulfated glycosaminoglycans by aorta explant monolayers cultured from atherosclerosis-susceptible and resistant pigeons. Am J Pathol 101:127-142

24. Larjava H, Saarni H, Tammi M, Penttinen R, Ronnemaa T (1980) Cortisol decreases the synthesis of hyaluronic acid by human aortic smooth muscle cells in culture. Atherosclerosis 35: 135-143

25. McCullagh KA, Balian G (1975) Collagen characterization and cell transformation in human atherosclerosis. Nature 258: 73-75

26. Fritz KE, Daoud AS, Jarmolych J (1981) Cholesteryl ester hydrolase and β-glucuronidase activities in swine aortic lesions. Fed Proc 40:351

27. Fritz KE, Daoud AS, Jarmolych J (to be published) Collagenolytic activity in swine aortic atherosclerotic lesions. Fed Proc (abstract)

28. Hayes LW, Goguen CA, Stevens AL, Magargal WW, Slakey LL (1979) Enzyme activities in endothelial cells and smooth muscle cells from swine aorta. Proc Natl Acad Sci USA 76:2532-2535

29. Kerwar SS, Nolan JC, Ridge SC, Oronsky AL, Slakey LL (1980) Properties of a collagenase inhibitor partially purified from

cultures of smooth muscle cells. Biochim Biophys Acta 632:183-191
30. Goldstein JL, Brown NS (1977) The low density lipoprotein pathway and its relation to atherosclerosis. Annu Rev Biochem 46:897-930
31. Karnovsky MJ (1981) Endothelial-vascular smooth muscle cell interactions. Am J Pathol 105:200-206 (Rous-Whipple Award Lecture)
32. Bierman EL, Albers J (1977) Regulation of low density lipoprotein receptor activity by cultured human arterial smooth muscle cells. Biochim Biophys Acta 488:152-160
33. Davies PF, Ross R (1978) Mediation of pinocytosis in cultured arterial smooth muscle and endothelial cells by platelet-derived growth factor. J Cell Biol 79:663-671
34. Simpson CF (1977) Phagocytosis by aortic modified smooth muscle cells. Artery 3:210-217
35. Garfield RE, Chacka S, Blose S (1975) Phagocytosis by muscle cells. Lab Invest 33:418-427
36. Thomas WA, Florentin RA, Nam SC, Jones RM, Lee KT (1968) Preproliferative phase of atherosclerosis in swine fed cholesterol. Arch Path Lab Med 86:621-643
37. Huttner I, Boutet M, More RH (1973) Studies on protein passage through arterial endothelium. Lab Invest 28:672-677
38. Simionescu N, Simionescu M, Palade GE (1975) Permeability of muscle capillaries to small hemepeptides. Evidence for the existence of patent transendothelial channels. J Cell Biol 64:586-607
39. Sholley MM, Gimbrone MA, Cotran RS (1977) Cellular migration and replication in endothelial regeneration. A study using irradiated endothelial cultures. Lab Invest 36:18-25
40. Gold LI, Pearlstein E (1980) Fibronectin-collagen binding and requirement during cellular adhesion. Biochem J 186:551-559
41. Gajdusek CM, DiCorleto P, Ross R, Schwartz SM (1980) An endothelial-cell-derived growth factor. J Cell Biol 85:467-472
42. Castellot JJ Jr, Addonizio ML, Rosenberg R, Karnovsky MJ (1981) Cultured endothelial cells produce a heparin-like inhibitor of smooth muscle cell growth. J Cell Biol 90:372-379
43. Cotta-Pereira G, Sage H, Bornstein P, Ross R, Schwartz SM (1980) Studies of morphologically atypical ("Sprouting") cultures of bovine aortic endothelial cells. Growth characteristics and connecting tissue protein synthesis. J Cell Physiol 102:183-191
44. Sage H, Crouch E, Bornstein P (1979) Collagen synthesis by bovine aortic endothelial cells in culture. Biochemistry 18:5433-5442
45. Sage H, Pritzl P, Bornstein P (1981) Characterization of cell matrix associated collagens synthesized by aortic endothelial cells in culture. Biochemistry 20:436-442

46. Jaffe EA, Minick CR, Adelman B, Becker CG, Nachman R (1976) Synthesis of basement membrane collagen by cultured human endothelial cells. J Exp Med 144:209-225

47. Saba TM, Jaffe EA (1980) Plasma fibronectin (opsonic glyco-protein): Its synthesis by vascular endothelial cells and role in cardio-pulmonary integrity after trauma as related to reticuloendothelial function. Am J Med 68: 577-594

48. Jaffe EA, Hoyer LW, Nachman RL (1973) Synthesis of anti-hemophilic factor antigen by cultured human endothelial cells. J Clin Invest 52:2757-2764

49. Jaffe EA, Weksler BR (1979) Recovery of endothelial cell prostacylin production after inhibition and low doses of aspirin. J Clin Invest 63:532-535

50. Ryan US, Schultz DR, Ryan JW (1981) Fc and C3b receptors on pulmonary endothelial cells: induction by injury. Science 214:557-558

51. Vlodavsky I, Fielding PE, Fielding CJ, Gospodarowicz D (1978) Role of contact inhibition in the regulation of receptor-mediated uptake of low density lipoprotein in cultured vascular endothelial cells. Proc Natl Acad Sci 75:356-360

52. Fielding CJ, Vlodavsky I, Fielding PE, Gospodarowicz D (1979) Characteristics of chylomicron binding and lipid uptake by endothelial cells in culture. J Biol Chem 254: 8861-8868

53. Gospodarowicz D, Brown KD, Birdwell CR, Zetter BR (1978) Control of proliferation of human vascular endothelial cells. Characterization of the response of human umbilical vein endothelial cells to fibroblast growth factor, epidermal growth factor and thrombin. J Cell Biol 77: 774-788

54. Busch C, Dawes DS, Wasteson P, Wasteson A. (1979) Binding of platelet factor N to cultured endothelial cells. Thromb Haemost 42:43

55. Hope W, Martin TJ, Chesterman CN, Morgan FJ (1979) Human β-thromboglobulin inhibits PGI_2 production and binds to a special site in bovine aortic endothelial cells. Nature 282:210-212

56. Hoover RL, Folger R, Haering WA, Ware BR, Karnovsky MJ (1980) Adhesion of leukocytes to endothelium: roles of divalent cations, surface charge, chemotactic agents and substrate. J. Cell Sci 45:73-86

57. Hollander W, Columbo MA, Kramsch DM, Kirkpatrick B (1974) Immunological aspects of atherosclerosis. Adv Cardiol 13:192-207

58. Lamberson HV Jr, Fritz KE (1974) Immunological enhancement of atherogenesis in rabbits. Arch Pathol 98:9-16

59. Hardin NJ, Minick R, Murphy GE (1973) Experimental induction of athero-arteriosclerosis by the synergy of allergic injury to arteries and lipid-rich diet. Am J Pathol 73: 301-325

60. Gerrity RG (1981) The role of monocyte in atherogenesis: I. Transition of blood borne monocytes into foam cells in fatty lesions. Am J Pathol 103:181-190

61. Gerrity RG (1981) The role of monocyte in atherogenesis: II. Migration of foam cells from atherosclerotic lesions. Am J Pathol 103:191-200
62. Issekutz TB, Issekutz AC, Movat HC (1981) The in vivo quantitation and kinetics of monocyte migration into acute inflammatory tissue. Am J Pathol 103:47-55
63. Steinman RM, Cohn ZA (1974) The metabolism and physiology of the mononuclear phagocytes. In: Zweifach BW, Grant L, McClusky RT (eds) The inflammatory process. Academic Press, New York, San Francisco, London, pp 449-510
64. Schaffner T, Taylor K, Bartucci EJ, Fisher-Dzoga K, Beeson JH, Glagov S, Wissler RW (1980) Arterial foam cells with distinctive immunomorphologic and histochemical features of macrophages. Am J Pathol 100:57-80
65. Fritz KE, Daoud AS, Jarmolych J. Unpublished data.
66. Rifkin BR, Baker RL, Somerman MJ, Pointon SE, Coleman SJ, Au WYW (1980) Osteoid resorption by mononuclear cells in vitro. Cell Tissue Res 210:493-500
67. Cohn ZA (1978) The activation of mononuclear phagocytes; fact, fancy and future. J Immunol 121:813-816
68. Kulonen E, Potila M (1980) Macrophages and the synthesis of connective tissue components. Acta Path Microbiol Scand (C) 88:7-13
69. Werb Z, Banda MJ, Jones PA (1980) Degradation of connective tissue matrices by macrophages. I. Proteolysis of elastin, glycoproteins and collagen by proteinases isolated from macrophage. J Exp Med 152:1340-1357
70. Werb Z, Gordon S (1975) Elastase secretion by stimulated macrophages. Characterization and regulation. J Exp Med 142:361-377
71. Werb Z, Gordon S (1975) Secretion of a specific collagenase by stimulated macrophages. J Exp Med 142:346-360
72. Unane ER (1976) Secretory function of mononuclear phagocytes. Am J Pathol 83:396-417
73. Cohn ZA, Wiener E (1963) The particulate hydrolases of macrophages. I. Comparative enzymology, isolation and properties. J Exp Med 118:991-1008
74. Unkeless JC, Gordon S, Reich E (1974) Secretion of plasminogen activator by stimulated macrophages. J Exp Med 139:834-850
75. Martin BM, Gimbrone MA Jr, Unanue ER, Cotran RS (1981) Stimulation of nonlymphoid mesenchymal cell proliferation by a macrophage-derived growth factor. J Immunol 126: 1510-1515
76. Glenn KC, Ross R (1981) Human monocyte-derived growth factor(s) for mesenchymal cells: activation of secretion by endotoxin and concanavalin A (CON A). Cell 25:603-615
77. Villiger B, Kelley DG, Engleman W, Kuhn C III, McDonald JA (1981) Human alveolar macrophage fibronectin: synthesis, secretion and ultrastructural localization during gelatin-coated latex particle binding. J Cell Biol 90:711-720

78. Alitalo K, Hovi T, Vaheri A (1980) Fibronectin is produced by human macrophages. J Exp Med 151:602-613

79. Johansson S, Rubin K, Hook M, Ahlgren T, Seljelid R (1979) In Vitro biosynthesis of cold insoluble globulin (fibronectin) by mouse peritoneal macrophages. FEBS Letters 105:213-216

80. Schechter I, Fogelman AM, Haberland ME, Seager J, Hokom M, Edwards PA (1981) The metabolism of native and malondialdehyde altered low-density lipoproteins by human monocyte-macrophages. J Lipid Res 22:863-871

81. Merrilees MJ, Scott L (1981) Interaction of aortic endothelial and smooth muscle cells in culture. Effect on glycosaminoglycan levels. Atherosclerosis 39:147-161

82. Olivecrona T, Bengtsson G, Marklund SE, Lindahl U, Hook M (1977) Heparin-lipoprotein lipase interactions. Fed Proc 36:60-65

83. Clowes AW, Karnovsky MJ (1977) Suppression by heparin of smooth muscle cell proliferation in injured arteries. Nature 265:625-626

84. Traber MG, Kayden HJ (1980) Low density lipoprotein receptor activity in human monocyte-derived macrophages and its relation to atheromatous lesions. Proc Natl Acad Sci 77: 5466-5470

85. Fischer-Dzoga K (1979) Cellular proliferation, cellular death and atherosclerosis. Artery 5:222-236

86. Feo F, Canuto RA, Torrielli MV, Garcea R, Dianzani MU (1976) Effect of a cholesterol-rich diet on cholesterol content and phagocytic activity of rat macrophages. Agents and Actions 6:135-142

87. Klurfeld DM, Allison MJ, Gerszten E, Dalton HP (1979) Alterations of host defenses paralleling cholesterol-induced atherogenesis. II. Immunologic studies of rabbits. J Med 10:49-64

88. Mahley RW, Innerarity TL, Brown MS, Ho YK, Goldstein JL (1980) Cholesteryl ester synthesis in macrophages: stimulation by β-very low density lipoproteins from cholesterol-fed animals of several species. J Lipid Res 21:970-980

89. Jackson RL, Stein O, Gotto AN, Stein Y (1975) A comparative study on the removal of cellular lipids from Lundschutz ascites cells by human plasma apolipoproteins. J Biol Chem 250:7204-7209

90. Wight TN (1980) Vessel proteoglycans and thrombogenesis. In: Spaet H (ed) Progress in hemostasis and thrombosis, 5th edn. Greene and Stratton, New York, 1980, pp 1-39

91. Van de Water L III, Schroeder S, Crenshaw EB III, Hynes RO (1981) Phagocytosis of gelatin-latex particles by a murine macrophage line is dependent on fibronectin and heparin. J Cell Biol 90:32-39

92. Love SH, Shannon BT, Myrvik QN, Lynn WS (1979) Characterization of macrophage agglutinating factor as a hyaluronic acid-protein complex. J Reticuloendothel Soc 25:269-282

93. Jones PA, Werb Z (1980) Degradation of connective tissue matrices by macrophages. II. Influence of matrix composition on proteolysis of glycoproteins, elastin, and collagen by macrophages in culture. J Exp Med 152:1527-1536

94. Berenson GS, Radhakrishnamurthy B, Dalferes ER Jr, Srinwasan SR (1971) Carbohydrate macromolecules and atherosclerosis. Hum Pathol 2:57-79

95. Stevens RL, Colombo M, Gonzales JJ, Hollander W, Schmid K (1976) The glycosaminoglycans of the human artery and their changes in atherosclerosis. J Clin Invest 58:470-481

96. Avila EM, Lopez F, Camejo G (1978) Properties of low density lipoprotein related to its interaction with arterial wall components: in vitro and in vivo studies. Artery 4:36-60

97. Biheri-Varga M, (1978) Influence of serum high density lipoproteins on the low density lipoprotein-aortic glycosaminoglycan interactions. Artery 4:504-511

98. Iverius PH (1977) Possible role of glycosaminoglycans in the genesis of atherosclerosis. In: Atherogenesis initiating factors. Ciba Symposium 12. Elsevier, North Holland, Amsterdam 7:185-196

99. Radhakrishnamurthy B, Ruiz HA Jr, Berenson GS (1977) Isolation and characterization of proteoglycans from bovine aorta. J Biol Chem 252:4831-4841

100. Klynstra FB, Böttcher CJF, Van Melsen JA, Van der Laan EJ (1967) Distribution and composition of acid mucopolysaccharides in normal and atherosclerotic human aortas. J Atheroscler Res 7:301-309

101. Yamada KM, Kennedy DW, Kimata K, Pratt RM (1980) Characteristics of fibronectin interactions with glycosaminoglycans and identification of active proteolytic fragments. J Biol Chem 255:6055-6063

102. Kramsch DM, Franzblau C, Hollander W (1971) The protein and lipid composition of arterial elastin and its relationship to lipid accumulation in the atherosclerotic plaque. J Clin Invest 50:1666-1677

103. Keeley FW, Partridge SM (1974) Aminoacid composition and calcification of human aortic elastin. Atherosclerosis 19:287-296

104. Modrak JB, Langner RO (1980) Possible relationship of cholesterol accumulation and collagen synthesis in rabbit aortic tissues. Atherosclerosis 37:211-218

105. Kramsch DM, Chan CT, Aspen AJ, Wells H (1978) Prevention therapy of induced atherosclerosis in rabbits and monkeys regardless of serum cholesterol levels. In: Haust WH, Wissler RW, Lehman R (eds) International symposium: state of prevention and therapy in human arteriosclerosis and in animal models. Westdeutscher Verlag, Oppladen, pp 153-172

106. Perlin AS (1977) NMR spectroscopy of heparin. Fed Proc 36:106-109

107. Stivala SS (1977) Physicochemical properties of heparin and its interaction with Cu (II) and calcium in relation to acticoagulation. Fed Proc 36:83-88

108. Engelberg H (1977) Probably physiologic functions of heparin. Fed Proc 36:70-72

109. Stemerman MB (1975) Vascular intimal components: precursors of thrombosis. In: Spaet TH (ed) Hemostasis and thrombosis. Grune and Stratton Inc, New York, pp 1-47

110. Daoud AS, Jarmolych J, Augustyn JM, Fritz KE, Singh JK, Lee KT (1976) Regression of advanced atherosclerosis in swine. Arch Pathol Lab Med 100:372-379

111. Ennever J, Vogel JJ, Levy BM (1974) Lipid and bone matrix calcification in vitro. Proc Soc Exp Biol Med 145:1386-1388

112. Ennever J, Vogel JJ, Riggan LJ, Paoloski SB (1977) Proteolipid and calculus matrix calcification in vitro. J Dent Res 56:140-142

113. Ennever J, Vogel JJ, Rider LJ, Boyan-Salyers B (1976) Nucleation of microbiologic calcification by proteolipid. Proc Soc Exp Biol Med 152:147-150

114. Ennever J, Vogel JJ, Riggan LJ (1980) Calcification by proteolipid from atherosclerotic aorta. Atherosclerosis 35:209-213

115. Schmid K, McSharry WO, Pameijer CH, Binette JP (1980) Chemical and physicochemical studies on the mineral deposits of the human atherosclerotic aorta. Atherosclerosis 37: 199-210

116. Kim KM (1976) Calcification of matrix vesicles in human aortic valve and aortic media. Fed Proc 35:156-162

117. Martin GR, Schiffmann E, Bladen HA, Nylen M (1963) Chemical and morphological studies of the in vitro calcification of aorta. J Cell Biol 16:243-252

118. Andersson R (1973) Role of cyclic AMP and CA^{++}, mechanical and metabolic events in isometrically contracting vascular smooth muscle. Acta Physiol Scand 87:84-95

119. Numano F, Watanabe Y, Takano K, Takano T, Arita M, Numano F, Maezawa H, Shimamoto T, Adachi K (1976) Microassay of cyclic nucleotides in vessel wall. I cyclic AMP. Exp Mol Pathol 25:172-181

120. Burleigh MC, Barrett AJ, Lazarus GS (1974) Cathepsin B1. A lysosomal enzyme that degrades native collagen. Biochem J 137:387-398

121. Butler LG (1971) Yeast and other inorganic pyrophosphatases. In: Boyer PD (ed) The enzymes, vol IV, 3rd edn. Academic Press, New York, pp 529-541

122. Graves DJ, Wang JH (1972) α-Glucan phosphorylases. In: Boyer PD (ed) The enzymes, vol VII, 3rd edn. Academic Press, New York, pp 435-482

123. Kayne FJ (1973) Pyruvate kinase. In: Boyer PD (ed) The enzymes, vol VIII, 3rd edn. Academic Press, New York, pp 353-382

124. Winterbourne CC, Hawkins RE, Brian M, Carrell RW (1975) The estimation of red cell superoxide dismutase activity. J Lab Clin Med 85:337-341

125. Packham MA, Cazenave JP, Kinlough-Rathbone RL, Mustard JF

(1978)   Drug effects on platelet adherence to collagen and damaged vessel walls.   Adv Exp Med Biol 109:253-276

126. Hellman B, Sehlin J, Taljedal IB (1976)   Calcium and secretion: distinction between 2 pools of glucose-sensitive calcium in pancreatic islets.   Science 194:1421-1423

127. Boucek MM, Snyderman R (1976)   Calcium influx requirement for human neutrophil chemotoxis inhibition by lanthanum chloride. Science 193:905-907

128. Fassina G (1978)   Mechanisms of lipomobilization.   Adv Exp Med Biol 109:209-223

129. Levy RJ, Lian JB, Gallop P (1979)   Atherocalcin, a γ-carboxyglutamic acid containing protein from atherosclerotic plaque. Biochem Biophys Res Commun 91:41-49

130. Levy RJ, Gundberg CM (1981)   The presence of the bone specific protein, osteocalcin, in calcified atherosclerotic plaque and mineralized heart valves.   Circulation 64, Suppl IV:44

131. Deyl Z, Macek K, Vancikova O, Adam M (1979)   The presence of γ-carboxyglutamic acid-containing protein in atheromatous aortae.   Biochim Biophys Acta 581:307-315

132. Lian JB, Prien EL Jr, Glimcher MJ, Gallop PM (1977)   The presence of protein-bound γ-carboxyglutamic acid in calcium-containing renal calculi.   J Clin Invest 59:1151-1157

133. Gerrity RG (1981)   Migration of foam cells from atherosclerotic lesions. Am J Pathol 103:191-200

134. Morland B, Morland J (1978)   Selective induction of lysosomal enzyme activities in mouse peritoneal macrophages.   J Reticuloendothel Soc 23:469-477

135. Hibbs JR Jr (1976)   The macrophage as a tumoricidal effector cell; a review of in vivo and in vitro studies on the mechanism of the activitated macrophage nonspecific cytotoxic reaction.   In: Fink MA (ed) The macrophage in neoplasia. Academic Press, New York, pp 83-111

136. MacKaness GB (1967)   The relationship of delayed hypersensitivity to acquired cellular resistance.   Br Med Bull 23:52-54

137. Murray M, Morrison WI (1979)   Nonspecific induction of increased resistance in mice to Trypanosoma congolense and Trypanosoma brucei by immuno stimulants.   Parasitology 79: 349-366

138. Whittaker JA, Slater AJ (1977)   The immunotherapy of acute myelogenous leukaemia using intravenous BCG.   Br J Haematol 35:263-273

139. McKneally MF, Maver C, Kausel HW, Alley RD (1976)   Regional immunotherapy with intrapleural BCG for lung cancer.   Surgical considerations. J Thorac Cardiovasc Surg 72:333-338

140. Ross R, Glomset J (1973)   Atherosclerosis and the arterial smooth muscle cell.   Science 180:1332-1339

141. Ross R, Glomset J (1976) The pathogenesis of atherosclerosis.   N Engl J Med 295:369-377

142. Ross R, Harker L (1976) Hyperlipidemia and atherosclerosis. Science 193:1094-1100

143. Fischer-Dzoga K, Fraser R, Wissler RW (1976) Stimulation of proliferation in stationary primary cultures of monkey and rabbit aortic smooth muscle cells: 1. Effects of lipoprotein fractions of hyperlipemic serum and lymph. Exp Mol Pathol 24:346-359
144. Mustard JF, Glynn MF, Jorgensen L, Nishizawa EE, Packham MA, Rowsell HC (1968) Recent advances in platelets, blood coagulation factors and thrombosis. In: Miras LJ, Howard AN, Paoletti R (eds) Progress in biochemical pharmacology, vol 4. Plenum, New York, pp 508-532
145. Mustard JF, Packham MA, Rowsell HC, Jorgensen L (1968) The role of thrombogenic factors in atherosclerosis. Ann NY Acad Sci 149:848-859
146. Ross R, Vogel A (1978) The platelet-derived growth factor. Cell 14:203-210
147. Benditt EP, Benditt JM (1973) Evidence for a monoclonal origin of human atherosclerotic plaques. Proc Natl Acad Sci 70:1753-1756
148. Thomas WA, Reiner JM, Florentin RA, Janakidevi K, Lee KT (1977) Arterial smooth muscle cells in atherogenesis: births, deaths and clonal phenomena. In: Schlettler G, Goto G, Hata Y, Klose G (eds) Atherosclerosis IV. Springer-Verlag, New York, pp 16-23
149. Thomas WA, Janakidevi K, Florentin RA, Reiner JM (1978) The reversibility of the human atherosclerotic plaque. In: Hauss WH, Wissler RW, Lehman R (eds) International symposium: state of prevention and therapy in human arteriosclerosis and in animal models. Westdeutscher Verlag, Opladen, pp 73-80

DISCUSSION: MARK L. ARMSTRONG

This overview of cell and matrix changes in the arterial wall sums up the array of sequences that accompanies and largely determines atherosclerotic and regressive states. Previous presentations have simplified this discussant's role of putting this important paper in perspective. For example, Dr. St. Clair's discussion of Chapter Five provides a convenient preview. The workshop has also emphasized issues of quantitation. Pathobiologic changes within the wall may present problems as to their quantitative expression. Dr. Minick emphasized the importance of the way in which data should be expressed.

The choice of terms to emphasize in expressing structural or chemical data is a recurrent problem of quantitation. The problem happens when the arterial mass changes during the interval(s) of observation. Thus, given internal mass change, chemical data expressed in terms of arterial mass (e.g., weight^{-1}, protein^{-1}, DNA^{-1}) may not register true differences, and it may be helpful to express the data per unit of artery (cm length^{-1}, surface area^{-1}) as well as per unit of mass.

Table A.1 illustrates aspects of the problem. Marked loss of coronary cholesterol had occurred in regression. Residual cholesterol, relative to that found in atherosclerosis, was 35% per unit weight and 20% per centimeter length of artery. Intimal tissue was lost in regression, and expression of the cholesterol per unit length of artery reflects this, with residual cholesterol only 57% of what it was when calculated by unit weight. Suppose, however,

Table A.1.   Coronary arterial cholesterol.

Units	Atherosclerosis (AS)	Regression (R)	R/AS
μg/mg	51	18	0.35
μg/cm length artery	239	48	0.20
mg/extramural coronary artery	55	1	0.20

that the residual cholesterol was also diluted during regression because of animal growth with larger arteries. Expression of the data per total arterial tissue within anatomically defined boundaries (e.g., extramural coronary arteries^{-1}) is a way of correcting for growth, or of showing that it is not a factor (Table A.1) in changes expressed as unit length or unit area of artery. The choice of denominators is highly relevant to the quantitative description of pathobiologic structural and chemical changes.

Dr. Daoud's paper is a detailed survey of the pathobiology of atherosclerosis. I would note two important aspects of his presentation. One is that he offers what must still be considered a novel view of arterial calcification. The evidence is good that vesicles normally subserve calcification of cartilage, and it will be of great interest to see to what extent dystrophic calcification in atherosclerotic arteries is dependent on a similar process. The other notable point in this splendid summary of the pathobiology of atherosclerosis is a hypothesis that atherosclerotic lesions may be improved by amplifying phagocyte responses of the macrophage in the host. Here we have the macrophage depicted as a potential friend rather than a foe in the process of atherogenesis, and Dr. Daoud and his colleagues are to be commended for setting out to explore this arresting concept.

19

Animal Studies of Atherosclerosis Progression and Regression

M. Gene Bond, Janet K. Sawyer, Bill C. Bullock, Ralph W. Barnes, and Marshall R. Ball

Atherosclerosis continues to be the leading cause of mortality and morbidity in the United States and in several other countries. This disease has an insidious onset early in life, is progressive in extent and severity, and usually remains clinically silent until the fourth or fifth decade of life. The natural history of this disease is such that the onset of symptoms is associated with the presence of severe lesions characterized on the basis of significant stenosis, ulceration, or thrombosis.

Atherosclerosis per se, although clinically manifested primarily in the fourth through seventh decades, is not a disease of older individuals exclusively. Numerous autopsy studies have documented the presence of anatomically significant lesions in people who have died accidently at a relatively early age.

Recognition, diagnosis, and treatment of individuals, before they develop clinical signs and symptoms of atherosclerosis, is a laudable goal. A more important and more formidable goal, however,

The authors wish to express their gratitude to Mrs. Marie Plyler, Ms. Nancy Julian, and Ms. Lea Nading for assistance in preparation of histological material, to Ms. Hermina Trillo, Ms. Diana Swaim, and Mrs. Jean Gardin for assistance in the pathology laboratory, and to Mrs. Lonnie Ellis, Mrs. Shirley Pegram, and Mrs. Linda Trust for assistance in manuscript preparation. This work was supported in part by NIH contracts HV 72925, HV 12902, HV 12916, and SCOR-A grant HL 14164.

is the potential monitoring of atherosclerosis in specific
segments of the cardiovascular system in individual subjects.
Methods that would allow this kind of evaluation could generate
new information on the natural history of the disease, and could
potentially provide valuable data on suspected risk factors as
well as allow monitoring of changes in the arterial lumen and
wall in response to therapeutic or surgical intervention.

The continuing development and testing of sophisticated
instrumentation, particularly digital subtraction methods used
in arteriography, Doppler, and B-mode ultrasound, and nuclear
magnetic resonance that is aimed at revealing anatomical or
biochemical characteristics of arteries, are at present the
promising methods that may allow realization of these goals.
As mentioned by several speakers in this Workshop, however,
instrumentation, as well as the methods of interrogation and
interpretation, must be carefully evaluated for accuracy, reliability, validity, and predictability.

B-mode ultrasound instrumentation and the methods of arterial
interrogation have developed rapidly during the last decade, and
are now being used with increasing frequency in clinical settings. Recently completed studies of atherosclerotic carotid
arteries interrogated with B-mode instruments have been very
promising, particularly in patients who have severe disease (see
Chap. 15). Other studies of symptomatic patients include the US
multicenter trial for assessment of B-mode ultrasound imaging,
which is presently underway at five clinical centers (see Chap.
17). The overall goal of this study is to determine the sensitivity, specificity, and reproducibility of B-mode ultrasound
images in diagnosing atherosclerosis in symptomatic patients.
Comparison of data derived from arteriographs will be made with
B-mode images. Particularly important in this study, however,
will be the comparison of clinically derived information with the
pathology of endarterectomy specimens from the carotid arteries.

There are certain questions, particularly in determining the
validity, reliability, and predictability of noninvasive instru-

mentation in diagnosing and monitoring lesions in asymptomatic
subjects that are difficult to approach in clinical settings.
These questions are primarily concerned with having direct and
continuous access to subjects for noninvasive and invasive
studies, control of risk factor exposure, and perhaps most
importantly, the availability of arteries prepared under the
exacting requirements that would allow valid and reliable comparisons of images with the artery per se.

Animal models of atherosclerosis have been used extensively
in studies of atherogenesis and atherosclerosis progression and
regression.   An excellent comprehensive review of currently
available animal models, including rabbits, birds, swine, dogs,
and nonhuman primates, will be published in 1983 (1).

Nonhuman primates have been studied particularly intensively
as animal models for atherosclerosis during the past two decades.
The study of these types of models presents several advantages
for asking critical questions that cannot be tested easily in
human subjects, and that are related to atherogenesis and atherosclerosis progression and regression.   These advantages include
control of both dosage and duration of either single- or
multiple-risk-factor exposure, the potential to study synergistic
effects of multiple-risk-factor exposure, the opportunity to
examine the arteries invasively and noninvasively, and the
opportunity to examine in detail both gross and microscopic
preparations that have been prepared by pressure fixation.
Because atherosclerosis can be induced in these models by dietary
methods, they may provide the opportunity to determine
reliability, validity, and predictability of various clinical
methods for detecting and describing atherosclerotic lesions, and
in monitoring changes occurring during atherosclerosis
progression and regression.

Morphologically and chemically, the atherosclerotic lesions
of nonhuman primates are similar in many ways to those present
in human beings in terms of localization of the early lesions,
predilective sites for plaque development near bifurcations,

and tissue characteristics of plaques--including necrosis and accumulations of smooth muscle cells, fibroblast-like cells, macrophages, lipid, and mineralization (2-5). Lesions in these animal models also tend to occur in similar arterial segments as found in human beings, i.e., carotid arteries (including the carotid bifurcation), epicardial coronary arteries, abdominal aorta, iliac, and femoral arteries. Nonhuman primates, when exposed to the potent risk factor of hypercholesterolemia, developed severe atherosclerosis (6) and also have been noted to develop coronary artery thrombosis, myocardial ischemia, and myocardial infarcts that closely resemble those observed in people (7-10).

Nonhuman primates have also been used to determine the potential for atherosclerosis regression. In the majority of these experiments, atherosclerosis was induced in rhesus monkeys (*Macaca mulatta*) (11-26) or cynomolgus monkeys (*Macaca fascicularis, Macaca irus*) (27-35) by feeding high-fat, high-cholesterol diets for periods ranging from weeks to years, followed by varying periods of time during which total plasma cholesterol concentration was reduced by diet and/or drug inter-vention. In general, most studies have shown that there are beneficial effects of arterial wall morphology when total plasma cholesterol concentrations are reduced. However, the extent of this change is dependent on the species of animal, the dosage and time period used to induce atherosclerosis, the specific arterial site being examined and importantly, the severity of lesions induced during the progression phase.

ATHEROSCLEROSIS PROGRESSION

We have examined and compared coronary artery atherosclerosis among three types of male macaques, *Macaca fascicularis* (Malayan type), *Macaca fascicularis* (Philippine type) and *Macaca nemestrina* (36). Animals were three to five years of age at the time of acquisition. Test animals (n = 6 per group) of each type

were fed an atherogenic diet containing 1.0 mg cholesterol/Kcal
with approximately 42% of calories from lard for a period of 36
months. Control animals (n = 6 per group) were fed the same
diet, but without the added cholesterol for the same period of
time. Test and control animals from each type of macaque were
housed in similar environments.

At the time of necropsy, the heart and coronary arteries were
pressure-perfusion-fixed in situ with barium gel mass at 100 mmHg
pressure. Five sequential tissue blocks, each measuring 3 mm in
length, were trimmed from the proximal extent of the left anteri-
or descending, left circumflex, and right coronary arteries. A
single tissue block was taken from the midregion of the left main
coronary artery. Two 6-μm-thick tissue slices were taken from
each block and stained with Verhoeff van Gieson stain and hematoxylin and eosin stain. The cross-sectional area of intima
(plaque), area enclosed within the internal elastic lamina (IEL),
and lumen area were measured directly or indirectly from projected microscopic images using a sonic digitizer interfaced with
a minicomputer.

The group characteristics of the animals and the description
of the severity of coronary artery atherosclerosis are presented
in Tables 1 and 2, respectively.

Two test *Macaca fascicularis* (Malayan type) died during the
course of the experiment, and at autopsy were found to have
severe coronary artery atherosclerosis and myocardial infarcts
(7). The only other loss in this animal colony was a control
Macaca fascicularis (Philippine type) monkey that died from
causes unrelated to arterial disease. Feeding the test diet
resulted in high total plasma cholesterol concentrations among
the three groups of test animals studied. At the end of the
experimental period, no significant differences in body weight
or heart weight were observed between test and control animals
for any type of monkey (Table 1).

Test animals in each group developed considerable, but
variable amounts of plaque (intimal area) as shown in Table 2.

Control animals developed a few small lesions. The most important change noted, however, was in the area enclosed within the
IEL. In normal animals the tissue within the IEL is small and
consists of a thin endothelial layer and a few layers of subendothelial cells and connective tissue. For each type of monkey,
mean IEL area in the test animals was considerably larger than
that of the control group, by a factor of four for the *Macaca
fascicularis* (Philippine type) and by a factor of eight for
Macaca nemestrina. The overall effect of this arterial enlargement on cross-sectional lumen area in *Macaca fascicularis*
(Philippine type) and in *Macaca nemestrina* was that even in the
presence of severe atherosclerosis, the mean lumen area was
larger in test animals than in control animals. Only in *Macaca
fascicularis* (Malayan type) was mean lumen area smaller in test
animals than in control animals. There was considerable variability within animals from each test group in extent of arterial
enlargement when compared to the respective control groups. In
the test *Macaca fascicularis* (Malayan type) monkeys only one of
the four animals had a lumen area that was larger than that of
controls. Coronary artery lumen areas were smaller in the two

Table 1. Comparative study of atherosclerosis in macaques.
Total plasma cholesterol concentrations, body weight, and
heart weight.

	N	Plasma Cholesterol Concentration (mg/dl)	Body Weight (kg)	Heart Weight (gm)
M. fascicularis (Malaya)				
Test	4	799 ± 85	5.4 ± 0.7	25.5 ± 5.7
Control	6	210 ± 47	5.9 ± 1.0	21.7 ± 6.0
M. fascicularis (Philippine)				
Test	6	683 ± 124	5.5 ± 0.9	21.2 ± 2.9
Control	5	176 ± 41	6.8 ± 0.6	23.5 ± 3.2
M. nemestrina				
Test	6	841 ± 167	7.7 ± 0.9	46.0 ± 10.1
Control	6	162 ± 67	9.4 ± 1.2	48.6 ± 9.2

Note: All values are mean ± SD.

Table 2.   Comparative study of atherosclerosis in macaques.
Coronary artery atherosclerosis.

	Intimal Area (mm^2)	IEL Area (mm^2)	Lumen Area (mm^2)
M. fascicularis (Malaya)			
Test	1.84 ± 1.2	2.24 ± 1.5	0.40 ± 0.4
Control	0.02 ± 0.02	0.52 ± 0.2	0.50 ± 0.2
M. fascicularis (Philippine)			
Test	1.62 ± 1.0	2.94 ± 2.2	1.32 ± 1.2
Control	0.01 ± 0.01	0.74 ± 0.2	0.74 ± 0.2
M. nemestrina			
Test	5.27 ± 3.7	8.15 ± 4.2	2.88 ± 2.14
Control	0.04 ± 0.04	0.73 ± 0.1	0.70 ± 0.15

Note: All values are mean ± SD from 16 cross sections from
coronary arteries of each animal.

animals from this group that died with myocardial infarcts and in
the other three animals that finished the experiment than were
those of the control group.   In *Macaca fascicularis* (Philippine
type) monkeys, 4/6 (67%) had cross-sectional lumen areas that
were very close to the mean lumen area found in controls.   The
remaining 2/6 (33%) of test animals, had cross-sectional lumen
areas much greater than those of controls.   Test *Macaca nemestrina*
animals responded in an entirely different manner.   Of the
animals in this group 2/6 (33%) had lumen areas that were similar
to controls.   The remaining 4/6 (67%) of animals had lumen
diameters that were considerably larger than controls, even
though severe atherosclerosis was present.   Subsequent morphometric analysis of the area enclosed within the external elastic
lamina showed high correlation with the data derived from the IEL
area in test *Macaca nemestrina*.

Arterial enlargement unquestionably occurred in the coronary
arteries of animals in this study, but there was considerable
inter- and intraspecies variability, i.e., some animals, for
whatever reason(s), had the capability to increase overall artery
size as plaque developed, and did so in such a way that mean
cross-sectional lumen area was not compromised.   The conditions
and mechanisms by which this arterial dilatation occurred were

unclear, but in this experiment they did not appear to be related to age, body weight, or heart weight. Blood pressure and exercise levels were not measured during these experiments, but could have influenced artery size.

Due to the potential importance of these observations to investigators who study atherosclerosis using animal models, and because arterial enlargement, for whatever reason(s), is known to occur in human beings, we designed a time course study of atherosclerosis progression in *Macaca fascicularis* (Malayan type). Young adult male animals were divided into five test groups, which were fed a diet containing 1 mg cholesterol/Kcal with 42% of calories supplied by butter for either 6-, 12-, 18-, 24-, or 30-month periods. Control animals were fed a basal monkey chow diet for either 18, 24, or 30 months.

At the time of necropsy, anesthetized animals were exsanguinated through the posterior vena cava and the cardiovascular system was flushed briefly with a buffered phosphate solution. The carotid arteries bilaterally and the coronary arteries were pressure fixed in situ at 100 mmHg pressure. Intravascular pressure was monitored by a cannula placed within the left ventricle. The coronary arteries were sampled as described previously. The carotid arteries were sampled as follows: 3 tissue blocks measuring approximately 3 mm in length were trimmed from the right and left carotid artery. Sites were chosen in such a way that they were equidistant from each other, and sampled the exact mid-regions of the proximal, middle, and distal segments of common carotid arteries. A single tissue block was also taken from the carotid bifurcation bilaterally.

As part of the experimental design we performed carotid arteriographic studies using aortic arch injections on each animal immediately before sacrifice. We also attempted to evaluate carotid arteries noninvasively using a 5 MHz real-time B-mode imaging system, designed and developed by one of our group (Dr. Ralph W. Barnes). Although we were able to visualize the arteries using this instrument, the small size of the vessels (lumen diameter of 2-3 mm), combined with the axial resolution of the instrument (approximately 0.5 mm), limited our ability to define and measure lumen diameter and wall thickness accurately.

The size characteristics of coronary artery atherosclerosis for animals fed the atherogenic diet for 6, 18, and 30 months, and for the control animals sacrificed at 18 and 30 months are presented in Table 3. There was an almost linear increase in intimal area throughout the 30-month test period. At the end of 18 months induction, the amount of atherosclerosis present was as great as the total lumen area in the 30-month control group. IEL area also increased during the progression phase with mean values being considerably larger at 18 and 30 months when compared to controls. As we had observed in the previously described experiment on *Macaca fascicularis* (Malayan type), there was considerable variability in the extent to which arteries increased in size. Lumen area among test groups did not decrease inversely as intimal area increased.

Arterial size characteristics of progressing common carotid artery atherosclerosis are presented in Table 4. Atherosclerosis in these arteries also progressed in a linear fashion; however, significant arterial dilatation did not occur until animals had consumed the atherogenic diet for 18 months. Again, by examining the standard deviation of animals progressed for 18 and 30 months

Table 3. Progression of coronary artery atherosclerosis: *Macaca fascicularis* (Malayan).

Group	N	Intimal Area (mm^2)	IEL Area (mm^2)	Lumen Area (mm^2)
Progression				
6 mos	8	0.22 ± 0.25	0.81 ± 0.36	0.60 ± 0.27
18 mos	8	0.93 ± 0.45	1.59 ± 0.66	0.66 ± 0.31
30 mos	5	1.57 ± 0.35	3.02 ± 0.94	1.45 ± 0.71
Control				
18 mos	5	0.01 ± 0.01	0.71 ± 0.12	0.70 ± 0.12
30 mos	5	0.02 ± 0.03	0.95 ± 0.22	0.92 ± 0.23

Note: All values are mean ± SD for 16 cross sections of coronary arteries.

there was considerable variation among animals in terms of arterial enlargement. The evaluation of in vivo arteriographic lumen diameters also indicates that, at least through the early stages of atherosclerosis progression, lumen diameters do not decrease even though plaques become larger.

The results of these experiments suggest that basic assumptions concerning the effect of lesion progression on lumen size must be carefully reevaluated, especially if lumen measurements or ratios based on lumen characteristics are used as indicators of atherosclerosis progression or regression.

As part of a concentrated effort at the Bowman Gray School of Medicine, pathologists, neurologists, radiologists, and sonographers are presently attempting to determine the reliability, validity, and predictability of B-mode imaging in diagnosing and monitoring changes in arteries of *Macaca fascicularis* monkeys. Currently, we are using a 10 MHz, real-time, B-mode imaging system that has been designed specifically to evaluate arteries in small nonhuman primates (Horizons Research Laboratories Inc). Using this instrument on anesthetized monkeys, ranging in weight from 2.5 to 3.5 kg, we have been able to clearly visualize the distal abdominal aorta and proximal common iliac arteries.

Table 4. Progression of carotid artery atherosclerosis:
Macaca fascicularis (Malayan)

Group	N	Intimal Area (mm^2)	IEL Area (mm^2)	X-ray Lumen Diameter (mm)
Progression				
6 mos	8	0.29 ± 0.2	2.58 ± 0.2	2.4 ± 0.1
18 mos	8	0.99 ± 0.2	3.25 ± 0.3	2.4 ± 0.1
30 mos	5	1.51 ± 0.6	3.20 ± 1.0	2.0 ± 0.2
Control				
18 mos	5	0.0 ± 0.0	2.14 ± 0.2	2.2 ± 0.1
30 mos	5	0.02 ± 0.0	2.42 ± 0.3	2.3 ± 0.1

Note: All values are mean ± SD for 16 cross sections of coronary arteries.

During the past several months we have had the opportunity to evaluate, using B-mode imaging, the abdominal aortas from 10 *Macaca fascicularis* monkeys, which were then sacrificed. Lumen diameter measurements and arterial wall thicknesses were determined at a preselected site 10.0 mm superior to the tip of the flow divider at the aortic bifurcation. Measurements of arterial wall characteristics in these animals were made directly from images on a video display as close to peak systole as possible. The animals were sacrificed within 72 h of the B-mode examination, and the abdominal aorta perfusion fixed in situ with 10% neutral buffered formalin at systolic pressure. Barium gel mass was then infused into the artery and allowed to solidify. The site and angles of B-mode interrogation were marked directly on the gross specimens in vivo and the arteries were transected at that site. Direct measurements were made from cross sections of the gross aorta using a 7X magnified micrometer retical graduated in 0.1 mm increments. Measurements from the pathology specimens were made without the knowledge of the results of the B-mode interrogation. The results of this study are presented in Table 5.

Although the number of animals evaluated in this experiment was small (n = 10), the data comparing B-mode measurements with direct measurements from the gross artery suggest that on a group mean basis, ultrasound is accurate in determining both lumen diameter and artery wall thickness. In each case, however, the variability in lumen diameter and artery wall thickness from measurements of pathology specimens is greater than that determined from the B-mode images. These data, at present, must be considered tentative due to (1) the small number of animals evaluated and (2) the relative lack of atherosclerosis in the aortas of this small colony. Nevertheless, the correlation of the data derived from B-mode images with those from the pathology specimens is encouraging.

In summary, animal models offer distinct advantages for studying the progression and regression of atherosclerosis. In

Table 5. Comparison of abdominal aorta lumen diameter and wall
thickness between B-mode image and gross pathological specimen

	Lumen Diameter (mm)	Near Wall Thickness (mm)	Far Wall Thickness (mm)
B-Mode	3.2 ± 0.3	0.51 ± 0.1	0.54 ± 0.1
Pathology	3.4 ± 0.8	0.53 ± 0.2	0.51 ± 0.2

Note: All values are expressed as mean ± SD; n = 10 animals.

addition, they are appropriate models in which to examine the
accuracy, reliability, validity, and predictability of newly
developed diagnostic modalities. Arterial enlargement, whether
due to influence of the atherosclerotic plaque per se or to
growth or exercise of the animal, is a complicating factor in
monitoring changes during atherosclerosis progression or regression. Application of traditional methods for diagnosing atherosclerosis, combined with more newly developed techniques may
allow us in the near future to detect and modify atherosclerosis
progression in asymptomatic subjects.

REFERENCES

1. St Clair RW (to be published) Atherosclerosis regression in
   animal models: current concepts of cellular and biochemical
   mechanisms.
2. Armstrong ML (1976) Atherosclerosis in rhesus and cynomolgus
   monkeys. Primates Med 9:16-44
3. Clarkson TB, Hamm TE, Bullock BC, Lehner NDM (1976) Atherosclerosis in Old World monkeys. Primates Med 9:66-89
4. Clarkson TB, Lehner NDM, Bullock BC, Lofland HB, Wagner WD
   (1976) Atherosclerosis in New World monkeys. Primates Med
   9:90-144
5. Wissler RW, Vesselinovitch D (1977) Atherosclerosis in
   nonhuman primates. In: Brandly CA, Cornelius CE, (eds)
   Advances in veterinary science and comparative medicine.
   Academic Press, New York, pp 351-420
6. Clarkson TB, Lehner NDM, Wagner WD, St Clair RW, Bond MG,
   Bullock BC (1979) A study of atherosclerosis regression in
   Macaca mulatta. I. Design of experiment and lesion induction. Exp Mol Pathol 30:360-385
7. Bond MG, Bullock BC, Bellinger DA, Hamm TE (1980) Myocardial
   infarction in a large colony of nonhuman primates with
   coronary artery atherosclerosis. Am J Pathol 101:675-693

8. Kramsch DM, Hollander W (1968) Occlusive atherosclerotic disease of the coronary arteries in monkey (*Macaca irus*) induced by diet. Exp Mol Pathol 9:1-22

9. Taylor CB, Cox GE, Counts M, Yogi N (1959) Fatal myocardial infarction in the rhesus monkey with diet-induced hypercholesterolemia. Am J Pathol 356:674 (abstract)

10. Taylor CB, Patton DE, Cox GE (1963) Atherosclerosis in rhesus monkeys. VI. Fatal myocardial infarction in a monkey fed fat and cholesterol. Arch Pathol 76:404-412

11. Armstrong ML, Megan MB (1972) Lipid depletion in atheromatous coronary arteries in rhesus monkeys after regression diets. Circ Res 30:675-680

12. Armstrong ML, Warner ED, Connor WE (1970) Regression of coronary atheromatosis in rhesus monkeys. Circ Res 27:59-67

13. Clarkson TB, Bond MG, Bullock BC, Marzetta C (1981) A study of atherosclerosis regression in *Macaca mulatta*. IV. Changes in coronary arteries from animals with atherosclerosis induced for 19 months and then regressed for 24 or 48 months at plasma cholesterol concentrations of 300 or 200 mg/dl. Exp Mol Pathol 34:345-368

14. DePalma RG, Bellon EM, Koletsky S, Schneider DL (1979) Atherosclerotic plaque regression in rhesus monkeys induced by bile acid sequestrant. Exp Mol Pathol 31:423-439

15. DePalma RG, Klein L, Bellon EM, Koletsky S (1980) Regression of atherosclerotic plaques in rhesus monkeys. Angiographic, morphologic, and angiochemical changes. Arch Surg 115: 1268-1278

16. Eggen DA, Strong JP, Newman WP III, Catsulis C, Malcom GT, Kokatnur MG (1974) Regression of diet-induced fatty streaks in rhesus monkeys. Lab Invest 32:294-301

17. Kokatnur MG, Malcom GT, Eggen DA, Strong JP (1975) Depletion of aortic free and ester cholesterol by dietary means in rhesus monkeys with fatty streaks. Atherosclerosis 21:195-203

18. Stary HC (1978) The origin in atherosclerotic lesions of extracellular lipid and debris and their elimination during regression. In: Hauss WH, Wissler RW (eds) State of prevention and therapy in human atherosclerosis and in animal models. Westdeutscher Verlag, Opladen, pp 39-53

19. Stary HC, Strong JP (1976) The fine structure of nonatherosclerotic intimal thickening, of developing, and of regressing atherosclerotic lesions at the bifurcation of the left coronary artery. Adv Exp Med Biol 67:89-108

20. Strong JP, Eggen DA, Stary HC (1976) Reversibility of fatty streaks in rhesus monkeys. Primates Med 9:300-320

21. Tucker CF, Catsulis C, Strong JP, Eggen DA (1971) Regression of early cholesterol-induced aortic lesions in rhesus monkeys. Am J Pathol 65:493-514

22. Vesselinovitch D, Wissler RW, Hughes R, Borensztajn J (1976) Reversal of advanced atherosclerosis in rhesus monkeys. Part I. Light-microscopic studies. Atherosclerosis 23:155-176

23. Wagner WD, St Clair RW, Clarkson TB (1980) A study of atherosclerosis regression in *Macaca mulatta*. II. Chemical changes in arteries from animals with atherosclerosis induced for 19 months then regressed for 24 months at plasma cholesterol concentrations of 300 or 200 mg/dl. Exp Mol Pathol 32:162-174

24. Wagner WD, St Clair RW, Clarkson TB, Connor Jr (1980) A study of atherosclerosis regression in *Macaca mulatta*. III. Chemical changes in arteries from animals with atherosclerosis induced for 19 months and regressed for 48 months at plasma cholesterol concentrations of 300 or 200 mg/dl. Am J Pathol 100:633-650

25. Weber G, Fabbrini P, Resi L, Jones R, Vesselinovitch D, Wissler RW (1977) Regression of arteriosclerotic lesions in rhesus monkey aortas after regression diet. Scanning and transmission electron microscope observations of the endothelium. Atherosclerosis 26:535-547

26. Wissler RW, Vesselinovitch D (1976) Studies of regression of advanced atherosclerosis in experimental animals and man. Ann NY Acad Sci 275:363-378

27. Armstrong ML, Megan MB (1974) Responses of two macaque species to atherogenic diet and its withdrawal. In: Schettler G, Weizel A (eds) Atherosclerosis III. Proceedings of the third international symposium on atherosclerosis, Springer-Verlag New York Inc, New York, pp 336-338

28. Armstrong ML, Megan MB (1975) Arterial fibrous proteins in cynomolgus monkeys after atherogenic and regression diets. Circ Res 36:256-261

29. Berenson GS, Radhakrishnamurthy B, Srinivasan SR, Dalferes ER Jr, Malinow MR (1981) Chemical changes in the arterial wall during regression of atherosclerosis in monkeys. Artery 9:44-58

30. Hollander W, Kirkpatrick B, Paddock J, Colombo M, Magraj S, Prusty S (1979) Studies on the progression and regression of coronary and peripheral atherosclerosis in the cynomolgus monkeys. I. Effects of dipyridamole and aspirin. Exp Mol Pathol 30:55-73

31. Malinow MR, McLaughlin P, McNulty WP, Haito HK, Lewis LA (1978) Treatment of established atherosclerosis during cholesterol feeding in monkeys. Atherosclerosis 31:185-193

32. Malinow MR, McLaughlin P, Naito HK, Lewis LA, McNulty WP (1978) Effect of alfalfa meal on shrinkage (regression) of atherosclerotic plaques during cholesterol feeding in monkeys. Atherosclerosis 30:27-43

33. Malinow MR, McLaughlin P, Papworth L, Naito HK, Lewis L, McNulty WP (1975) A model for therapeutic interventions on established coronary atherosclerosis in nonhuman primates. Adv Exp Med Biol 67:3-31

34. Srinivasan SR, Patton D, Radhakrishnamurthy B, Foster TA, Malinow MR, McLaughlin P, Berenson GS (1980) Lipid changes in atherosclerotic aortas of *Macaca fascicularis* after various regression regimens. Atherosclerosis 37:591-601

35. Zarins CK, Bomberger RA, Taylor KE, Glagov S (1980) Artery
    stenosis inhibits regression of diet-induced atherosclerosis.
    Surgery 88:86-92
36. Bond MG, Adams MR, Kaduck JM, Bullock BC (1981) Effects of
    atherosclerosis on coronary artery size: Implications for
    myocardial infarction. Fed Proc 40:773 (abstract)

DISCUSSION: WILLIAM HOLLANDER

Our findings in the coronary arteries are similar to those described by Dr. Bond.   I would like to briefly review our
observations.

Both during the induction and regression of atherosclerosis
in the cynomolgus monkey, vessel size increased without a significant reduction in luminal area.   When the lesion exceeded
a critical size, vessel size did not change and, as a result,
the luminal area of the vessel decreased.   On the basis of these
findings we would like to suggest that the enlargement of the
coronary arteries during the course of atherosclerosis represents
a compensatory response to luminal narrowing caused by the atherosclerotic plaque.   The continued growth of the lesion leads
to the exhaustion of this compensatory response, and as a result
the lumen narrows and reduces the blood flow to the myocardium.
This concept was supported by the in vivo coronary angiographic
and blood flow studies, which showed significant correlations
with the luminal area of the involved coronary arteries but not
with the size of the lesion of these vessels.

The coronary arteriogram showed normal and patent coronary
arteries in the absence of severe atherosclerotic disease and
luminal narrowing.   However, when the coronary disease had become
far advanced with luminal narrowing, as revealed by the morphological and morphometric findings at necropsy, the coronary
arteriogram became abnormal and showed filling defects consistent
with the presence of obstructive coronary disease.   Thus, the
coronary arteriogram was found to be useful for determining the
caliber of the coronary lumen but was of limited value in assessing the severity of the atherosclerosis unless the disease
was far advanced.

The capacity of the coronary arteries to enlarge in response
to atherosclerosis appears to play an important role in determining the course of coronary artery disease.   Although the
primary stimulus for the vessel enlargement is not known, it

likely arises from a disturbance of blood flow through the involved vessel or from the pathological process occurring in the
vessel wall. There are a number of factors that are known to
affect vessel and lumen size and these include: (1) the normal
physiological process of growth and development; (2) the level
of blood pressure; (3) the quantity, velocity, and type (laminar
vs turbulent flow) of blood flow through the artery; (4) the
activity of the sympathetic nerves and (5) the action of vasoactive hormones on the vessel wall such as the prostaglandins,
catecholamines, angiotensin, and bradykinin. There also are a
number of "growth factors" that may influence vessel size. These
factors have been implicated in the pathogenesis of atherosclerosis and have been shown to be derived from the endothelial
cells, platelets, and macrophages.

20

Human Studies of Progression and Regression

WILLIAM P. NEWMAN III

The importance of atherosclerosis is directly related to its disease-producing potential. Abundant evidence exists that the arterial lesions of atherosclerosis are pathogenetically related to coronary artery occlusion and myocardial infarction, cerebral infarction, and ischemic damage to other organs. Some uncertainty exists about the interrelationships of the different steps of the atherosclerotic process--which are known to begin in childhood but which do not become clinically manifest until later life.

Most of the material that I will be reviewing involves studies of arterial specimens that were opened longitudinally and stained grossly with Sudan IV for demonstration of lipid. The following working definitions are offered for different types of atherosclerotic lesions detected grossly in specimens prepared in this manner. Such a classification may imply a pathogenetic sequence, but it may also be used as a descriptive classification regardless of the ideas of pathogenetic interrelationships among the lesion types.

A fatty streak is a fatty intimal lesion that is stained distinctly by Sudan IV and shows no other underlying change.

This research was supported in part by grant HL-08974 from the National Heart, Lung, and Blood Institute, National Institutes of Health, U.S. Public Health Service. The author is indebted to Evelyn Dorsey for typing the manuscript.

Fatty streaks are flat or only slightly elevated and do not significantly narrow the lumina of blood vessels.

A fibrous plaque is a firm elevated intimal lesion, which in the fresh state is gray white, glistening, and translucent. The surface of the lesion may be sudanophilic, but usually is not. Human fibrous plaques characteristically contain fat. Often a thick fibrous connective tissue cap containing varying amounts of lipid covers a more concentrated "core" of lipid. If a lesion also contains hemorrhage, thrombosis, ulceration, or calcification, that lesion is classified according to one of the next two categories.

This classification of lesions based on gross examination does not permit distinction between those plaques with and without a core of degenerated or necrotic lipid-rich debris. Those plaques with necrotic foci and ulceration of the surface would of course be classified as complicated lesions. The plaques with necrotic centers and intact intimal surface ("atheroma" according to some classifications) would be classified as fibrous plaques. Microscopic examination is usually necessary to distinguish various subtypes of fibrous plaques.

A complicated lesion is an intimal plaque in which there is hemorrhage, ulceration, or thrombosis with or without calcium.

A calcified lesion is an intimal plaque in which insoluble mineral salts of calcium are visible or palpable without overlying hemorrhage, ulceration, or thrombosis.

The term *raised atherosclerotic lesion* is used to indicate the sum of fibrous plaques, complicated lesions, and calcified lesions.

HISTORY

Concern with the very early lesions of aortic atherosclerosis is by no means new. In 1911, Klotz and Manning (1) introduced their study of the aortas from 90 cases between 1 and 73 years of age with this statement: "It is quite useless to argue the questions concerning the development of intimal scleroses if we study and

discuss the late stages of the disease alone...If we wish to gain
a true insight into the complex question of arteriosclerosis we
must attempt to follow the lesion from its earliest beginning."
These authors found a high incidence of fatty streaks (which they
considered the earliest lesions of arteriosclerosis) without using
any gross staining technique.

Saltykow (2) in 1915, in attempting to differentiate normal
developmental and degenerative changes in the aorta, concluded
"the so-called fatty changes in the arteries of childhood and
youth, especially in the aorta, are nothing else but the beginning of atherosclerosis."

Mönckeberg (3) in 1921 reported aortic findings in war dead,
and found 5 of 14 cases (36%) under 20 years of age with "atheromatosis" of the aortic intima. The percentages increased in the
older age groups, i.e., 76% from the 20- to 25-year-old groups;
80%, 30-35 years of age and 100% in 16 cases of 35-40 years of
age. These and the observations of Aschoff (4) reveal that
pathologists were aware of the presence of fatty streaks in the
aortas of young persons early in the twentieth century.

Zinserling (5) in 1925 examined 320 aortas from children up
to 15 years of age after gross staining with Sudan III. He graded
these specimens into five groups on the basis of extent of surface
involved, and found that gross staining not only enhanced the
detection of lesions in the younger ages, but also increased the
estimation of the extent of intimal surface involved by fatty
streaks. He found that sudanophilic deposits were present in
some cases before the age of 4 years, and that there was a steady
increase in lesion severity with age. When he analyzed the data
on aortic lesions with respect to cause of death and the state
of nutrition, he could find no single cause of death that was
associated with significantly more extensive or advanced lesions.
There was no difference between well-nourished individuals and
those severely emaciated as a result of starvation during the
postwar famine.

Zeek (6) in 1930 made an exhaustive and critical review of the literature pertaining to juvenile arteriosclerosis, defined as "lesions believed to begin in the intima with lipoid degeneration" and concluded that arteriosclerosis may occur at any age. Most of the cases reviewed in that study had a history of renal disease and many had elevated blood pressure. These cases were those in which lesions were easily visible even without gross staining of arterial specimens using fat stains.

THE INTERNATIONAL ATHEROSCLEROSIS PROJECT (IAP)

The principal findings of this extensive investigation have been published in detail (7). The project was a collaborative effort by a group of pathologists who examined 23,000 aortas and coronary arteries collected from autopsied persons in 14 countries. The arterial specimens were collected at autopsy, opened longitudinally, fixed in a flattened position, packed in plastic bags, shipped to a central laboratory, and were subsequently stained with Sudan IV under standardized conditions.

The coded specimens were evaluated by a team of pathologists who visually estimated the percentage of the surface covered by different types of lesions. Periodic checks of reproducibility and reliability of the grading procedure were conducted to control inter- and intraobserver variability.

Racial and geographic comparisons among these populations have also been reported (8). The extent of surface involvement with fatty streaks and raised lesions varied among location-race groups at all ages. Variation was greater for raised lesions than for fatty streaks. Involvement by raised lesions was most extensive in the New Orleans and Oslo groups.

Geographic and ethnic differences in average extent of coronary atherosclerosis were large. On the average, cases from populations such as New Orleans and Oslo had about three times as much intimal surface involvement with raised lesions as did those from Guatemala and the Durban (South Africa) Bantu. Mortality rates from coronary

heart disease (CHD) are not available for all of these populations, but where such data are available, the measures of atherosclerotic lesions rank the populations in much the same order as
do the mortality rates.

When the 19 location-race groups were ranked by extent of
lesions in coronary arteries alone, in the aorta alone, in each
sex alone, and in each decade alone, a substantially similar rank
was obtained. The IAP investigators concluded that populations
with more extensive lesions in the aorta tended to have more
lesions in the coronaries and that those populations with more
extensive lesions in men also tended to have more extensive
lesions in women at the same age.

TOPOGRAPHIC DISTRIBUTION

The topographic distribution of atherosclerotic lesions was
reviewed by Duff and McMillan (9) in their classic seminar on the
pathology of atherosclerosis in 1951 and by Glagov and Ozoa (10).
Schwartz and Mitchell (11) described selective involvement of some
arteries and areas of location of arterial plaque in their necropsy survey. Early studies were generally consistent in the finding
that lesions occurred earliest and most extensively in the aorta.
Lesions that developed later and less extensively in the coronary
and cerebral arteries, and the renal, mesenteric, and pulmonary
arteries were the least susceptible to the development of atherosclerotic lesions.

The IAP studies led to the following conclusions concerning
atherosclerosis in the aorta and the coronary, carotid, vertebral,
and intracranial arteries. The severity of atherosclerosis in one
artery does not predict the severity in another artery for an
individual case. On a cross-cultural basis, however, the average
predilection for raised lesions to occur in one artery is correlated with the predilection within another artery. The location-
race groups in the IAP are ranked in approximately the same order,
regardless of whether the ranking is based on raised lesions in

one of the three major coronary arteries, the thoracic aorta, the abdominal aorta, or the cerebral arteries. This finding is consistent with the ideal that environmental conditions predominantly determine the severity of atherosclerosis in a population, despite large differences in susceptibility to lesions among individuals or among different anatomic loci within the arteries of each person (7).

DISTRIBUTION OF LESIONS WITHIN ARTERIAL SYSTEMS

Aortic Atherosclerosis

Holman et al. (12) in 1958 examined aortas from 526 necropsied individuals between 1 and 40 years of age obtained at a large general hospital and a medicolegal laboratory in New Orleans. These specimens were examined before and after gross staining with Sudan IV, and the extent of fatty streaks, fibrous plaques, and complicated lesions was estimated for each aorta in terms of percentage of intimal surface affected by each type of lesion. Gross Sudan staining increased the ability to detect fatty streaks, and thus increased both the incidence and extent of these lesions, particularly in the younger age groups.

All patients 3 years of age or older had at least minimal sudanophilic intimal deposits. Minimal lesions were found so frequently that some question was raised as to the significance of gross Sudan staining, i.e., whether it actually indicated an early lesion of atherosclerosis. Histologic sections were examined with this particular question in mind, and in every instance there were histologic alterations in the intima corresponding to the macroscopic sudanophilia. These alterations consisted of both intracellular and extracellular globules of lipid (as indicated by the application of Sudan IV), and a slight increase in interstitial mucinous material. The intima in these early lesions was not always elevated, and there was little cellular reaction.

The percentage of surface area involved increased slowly until the 6- to 10-year-old age group at which time the extent of lesions began to increase precipitously in the black population. In the 11- to 15-year-old age group, the extent of fatty streaks began to rise in the white population, but did not reach a peak as high as that present in the black population. The patterns in the black male and female were very much alike, with more severe involvement in females than in males at some ages. White females were consistently the group least affected.

Fibrous plaques began to appear in the second decade but did not increase appreciably until the fourth decade. They paralleled the development of fatty streaks, but lagged about 15 years, and the relative degree of involvement in whites and blacks was reversed when compared to fatty streaks. By 40 years of age, only about 20% of the area covered by fatty streaks had been converted into fibrous plaques. Additional lesion complications were rarely seen in this series.

The aortic ring was the first region of the aorta to develop fatty streaks, but it was the descending thoracic and particularly the abdominal portions that gave the distinctive pattern of increasing lesions between 5 and 20 years of age. Fibrous plaques also developed most extensively in the abdominal segment.

Topographic analyses have yielded differing opinions concerning the interrelationships of aortic fatty streaks and fibrous plaques. Holman and colleagues (12) indicated that there was sufficient fatty change to serve as a basis for all fibrous plaques encountered at later ages and concluded that the conversion of fatty streaks to fibrous plaques in the aorta required at least 15 years. Mitchell and Schwartz (11,13), after their study of topographic distribution of lesions, concluded that aortic fatty streaks should not be considered precursors of fibrous plaques.

These discrepancies and the growing controversy concerning the relationships of fatty streaks to fibrous plaques (14) led to additional systematic approaches to topography of lesions in other arterial segments.

Coronary Atherosclerosis

Montenegro and Eggen (15) analyzed the axial distribution of
atherosclerosis in the coronary arteries in detail for fatty
streaks, fibrous plaques, and complicated lesions in 2964 human
coronary artery specimens from Durban, Guatemala, New Orleans,
Santiago, and Sao Paulo. The presence or absence of each type
of lesion was recorded for each 1-cm segment of the three main
coronary artery branches from autopsied persons aged 10 to 69
years. Prevalence of each type of lesion by axial segment was
examined for consistency of pattern among geographic location,
race, sex, and age groups.

In the left coronary artery, prevalence of all lesion types
was greatest near the bifurcation. A marked decrease in prevalence of lesions occurred as one moved distally from the bifurcation along both the circumflex and the anterior descending branches.

The maximum prevalence of lesions in the right coronary artery
was in the region just distal to the orifice, but this maximum was
lower than that at the bifurcation of the left coronary. This
decrease in disease prevalence distally was much less pronounced
in the right coronary artery than in either branch of the left
coronary artery. There was an indication of a second, but lower,
peak in prevalence of lesions at about 8-10 cm from the orifice
of the right coronary artery.

This pattern of distribution along the axis of each artery was
similar between sexes and among location, race, and age groups.
The patterns were also similar for fatty streaks and fibrous or
complicated lesions. This finding lends support to the hypothesis
that there is a close pathogenetic association between fatty
streak and the more advanced lesions.

Carotid and Vertebral Atherosclerosis

Solberg and Eggen (16) examined the axial distribution of fatty
streaks, fibrous plaques, calcified lesions, and complicated
lesions in the carotid and vertebral arteries of 961 autopsied

patients, aged 25-69 years, from Guatemala and Oslo, Norway. The common carotid and internal carotid arteries were each divided into five equal segments and the vertebral arteries into seven equal segments. The presence or absence of each type of lesion was assessed for each segment by visual examination of the Sudan-stained artery, or of a soft x-ray radiograph of the artery (for calcified lesions). Prevalence of each type of lesion in each segment was computed for 10-year age groups by geographic location and sex for both right and left paired arteries.

The pattern of axial distribution was characteristic for each of the three major arteries. Lesions were most prevalent near the bifurcation of the common carotid and in the distal segment of the internal carotid artery. At any age the prevalence of lesions in a given segment of the carotid artery decreased successively in the proximal direction from these maxima. The trend with age and the distribution from segment to segment indicated that the athero-sclerotic process begins at the bifurcation and in the siphon region of the internal carotid artery and progresses proximally from there along the common or the internal carotid artery.

These patterns of axial distribution in the carotid and verte-bral arteries were consistent for both left and right arteries, in all age groups, in both sexes, and in both geographic locations. Since the patterns were also similar for all types of lesions, these authors suggest that their data support the hypothesis that fatty streaks are precursors of fibrous plaques and more advanced lesions.

RISK FACTORS AND ATHEROSCLEROSIS

Epidemiologic investigation of living populations has disclosed characteristics that are associated with increased risk of devel-oping CHD. The relationship of some of these risk factors for CHD to the atherosclerotic lesions has been reviewed (17) and these findings are summarized based largely on material from the IAP and on autopsy material studied in New Orleans.

Of all risk factors age has the strongest and most consistent association with lesions. The average extent of atherosclerosis increased with age in each subgroup of all the populations of IAP (18).

In a supplemental IAP study, ethnically similar groups in geographically distinct locations with vastly different ways of life were compared (19). When grouping the 19 location-race groups into five arbitary categories, atherosclerotic involvement in the white populations was high in New Orleans, Louisiana, and Oslo, Norway, medium in São Paulo, Brazil, and medium-low in Puerto Rico, Costa Rica, and Santiago, Chile. Atherosclerosis in the black population was medium-high in New Orleans, medium-low in Jamaica and Puerto Rico, and low in São Paulo and Durban. A strong gradient in the amount of coronary atherosclerosis existed both among black populations from New Orleans, Puerto Rico, Jamaica, São Paulo, and Durban and among the white populations from New Orleans, Oslo, Puerto Rico, São Paulo, Santiago, and Costa Rica. Thus environmental background seemed more important than racial background in determining the extent of coronary atherosclerosis.

Coronary atherosclerosis is generally considered to be more extensive in men than in women (19). The average extent of coronary lesions in men and women from the IAP and the ratio of lesions in men and women supported this view for the white populations; however, this sex difference was less striking or absent in the black populations. There was little or no sex difference in aortic atherosclerosis. Thus, the differences in atherosclerosis between sexes are not consistent.

Racial differences were examined in three locations in the IAP that have both black and white populations, i.e., New Orleans, Puerto Rico, and São Paulo (19). The black groups in these geographic locations have somewhat fewer extensive lesions than the white groups, particularly in the men. Any genetic or racial effect, however, is confounded with socioeconomic differences between races in any one geographic location.

The relationship of atherosclerosis, as measured in the IAP to serum cholesterol concentrations and diet has been reported by Scrimshaw and Guzmán (20). Rank order correlation of lesions with serum cholesterol concentration and with percent of calories from fat was statistically significant.

Data from the IAP confirm many studies that have reported aggravation or acceleration of atherosclerotic lesions in persons with hypertension and diabetes (21). Raised lesions in the coronary arteries were greater in the known hypertensive persons than in those without hypertension in all of these populations. Similar results were obtained when lesions in persons with and without diabetes were compared. Thus, hypertension and diabetes accelerate the natural progression of atherosclerosis in all populations.

Strong and coworkers have examined the mean extent of coronary raised lesions in relation to cigarette smoking in autopsied New Orleans white and black men (22,23). The average extent of raised atherosclerotic lesions was greater in the heavy smokers than in the nonsmokers within each 10-year age group. Studies by Auerbach et al. (24,25) have also indicated that advanced coronary atherosclerosis is much more prevalent in heavy smokers than in nonsmokers and that there is regular progression in severity of atherosclerotic lesions with increasing rate of smoking. Thus, the propensity for heavy cigarette smokers to develop CHD can, at least in part, be attributed to atherosclerotic lesions in the arterial wall. The effect of cigarette smoking on CHD is not limited to the terminal occlusive episode.

An intriguing finding is the wide variation in the extent of lesions among individuals in the most homogenous subgroups (26). Even after selecting cases according to race, sex, age, disease, and level of cigarette consumption, there is much variability in the extent of atherosclerosis. This variability should be investigated intensively by epidemiologic, pathologic, genetic, and other methods, for this unexplained variability indicates the existence of undiscovered etiologic agents or risk factors.

464   W. P. Newman III

In the more recent past, prospective studies have been initiated with careful documentation of serum lipid levels and, in some
instances, of dietary patterns, and with standardized evaluation
of atherosclerotic lesions at autopsy. Tentative results concerning antecedent risk factors and extent of atherosclerotic
lesions at autopsy have been reported (27-31). These studies for
the first time show, on a case-related basis, significant positive
relationships between the extent of atherosclerosis as measured at
autopsy and serum lipid values, cigarette smoking, and blood
pressure carefully measured during life (32).

REGRESSION OF HUMAN ATHEROSCLEROSIS

Can human lesions regress? Can therapy and modification of risk
factors in patients arrest or retard the progression of atherosclerosis or will lesions actually regress with improvement in
luminal characteristics--increased diameter and decreased lesion
size? The autopsy, an endpoint or terminal study, cannot assess
these changes. Serial measurements utilizing methods to evaluate
the condition of the arterial wall and lumen must be done in a
systematic manner to confirm or disprove the presence of possible
regression changes. Methods for evaluating changes over time and
the problems inherent with the various methods have been described
in detail in this workshop.

There is evidence that in some individuals atherosclerotic
lesions may regress and studies have been and are being reported.
Aschoff (4) reported decreased aortic atherosclerotic lesions in
individuals who had been on very meager or semistarvation diets
after World War I. Vartiainen (33) reported similar findings in
malnourished individuals autopsied after World War II. The above
reports are primarily impressions, without adequate controls.
Patients dying of cancer, a "wasting disease," were reported by
Wilens (34) in 1947 to have less coronary and aortic atherosclerosis than those dying with little or no weight loss. The choice

of controls is not clear and may have included individuals dying of atherosclerotic related complications.

Zelis (35) in 1970, in a study of six patients with peripheral vascular disease who were treated 3-6 months with dietary modification and clofibrate, found plethysmographic improvement in peripheral circulation. This finding suggests improvement in arterial lumen status, but the actual vessel characteristics are not documented.

Buchwald and coworkers (36) have reported serial coronary arteriographic findings in 22 patients treated with partial ileal bypass for hyperlipidemia. Progression of coronary artery narrowing has been documented in 5 patients, no progression in 12, questionable improvement in 2, and improvement in luminal dimensions in 3 patients. Additional information from this study will be forthcoming.

Barndt and coworkers (37) reported angiographic improvement of the femoral arteries in 9 of 25 individuals with hyperlipidemia treated with diet and in some instances drug therapy. The sequential femoral arteriograms were evaluated both visually and with a computer-controlled image-dissecting technique by Crawford and coworkers (38). The methods were developed and tested to reduce observer bias in interpreting change over time. Correlation between methods was good.

Other studies including the work of DePalma et al. (39) and Blankenhorn (40), who have paid close attention to methodologic detail so that sequential studies are as nearly equal as possible in technique, have found improvement in lumen size in femoral and coronary arteries of some patients. Many had no appreciable change or stabilization of vascular disease.

With increased sophistication in methods available to evaluate lesions, with meticulous attention to details to insure comparability, and with methods developed to reduce observer bias, additional evidence should be forthcoming supporting or refuting the hypotheses that human lesions can regress or at least remain stable. The papers of Dr. Mock and Dr. Blankenhorn in this volume will further address this important issue.

SECULAR TRENDS

In the IAP study, 1960-1964, 25- to 44-year-old white men had more extensive raised coronary artery lesions on the average than did young black men. In a population study of atherosclerosis and coronary heart disease conducted from 1968-1978 in New Orleans, the previously detected difference between the races in raised coronary artery lesions was not present.

Fig. 1 depicts graphically the data for the basal cases, the cause-of-death category from which coronary heart disease deaths and deaths from diseases known to be associated with atherosclerosis have been excluded. There was no consistent or appreciable difference in blacks between the two time periods, whereas in whites in each age subgroup there was less extensive raised lesion involvement in the second time period, indicating a secular trend with a decrease in raised lesions in young white men.

The evidence for this secular trend has been reported (41) and presently specimens from both studies are being retrieved, blindly coded, and interspersed, so that a fair evaluation can be made. Whether decreased arterial lesions are preceding or paralleling reported declines in coronary heart disease death rates can be answered in this ongoing study.

Inferences concerning the living population derived from observations based on dead persons or on autopsy data must be made with care, because collection of cases is subject to uncontrolled selection factors operating at various phases of the collection process. Nevertheless, autopsied cases are a valuable source of information about atherosclerotic lesions.

The problems of autopsy selection have received extensive attention from investigators at our institution for over 20 years and have been analyzed and reported in detail (42-45). We are continually attempting to identify bias among subsets of the deceased population.

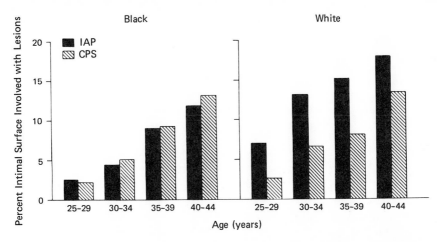

Fig. 1. Percent intimal surface area of coronary arteries involved with raised lesions, basal cases, International Athero- sclerosis Project (IAP) and Community Pathology Study (CPS), by race and 5-year age group.

SUMMARY

Many methods have been used to evaluate and estimate the extent and severity of human atherosclerosis, both clinically and at autopsy. With increasing sophistication in the clinical evaluation of atherosclerosis, including arteriography, B-mode ultrasound imaging and Doppler ultrasound, correlation with pathologists' autopsy findings will be needed. Improved techniques, pressure perfusion fixation, and measurement methods, including the use of digitizers for more accurate and reproducible measurement, will be important in these correlations. There still exists a need for information for the understanding of the underlying processes. Voids in our knowledge about the basic processes involved in atherogenesis and in atherosclerosis progression and regression may be answered in part by continued surveillance of arterial disease as it exists in populations. Methods that are best for measuring fatty streaks, fibrous plaques, and calcified lesions may not be the most suitable for measuring stenosis and occlusion. Methods for assessing "severity" may not be suited for evaluating the extent of individual types of lesions.

The type of measurement--whether based on gross, microscopic, ultrastructural, or chemical methods or clinical evaluation, will depend on the level of precision and accuracy needed to answer the questions formulated.

REFERENCES

1. Klotz O, Manning MF (1911) Fatty streaks in the intima of arteries. J Pathol 16:211-220
2. Saltykow S (1915) Jugendliche und beginnende Atherosklerose. KorrespBl schweizer 45:1057-1089
3. Mönckeberg JG (1921) Das Gefäßsystem und seine Erkrankungen. Handbuch Arzte Erfahr Weltkr 8:8-18
4. Aschoff L (1924) Atherosclerosis in lectures on pathology. Hoeber, New York, pp 131-153
5. Zinsesrling WD (1925) Untersuchungen über Atherosklerose. I. Uber die Aortaverfettung bei Kindern. Virchows Arch [Pathol Anat] 255:677-705
6. Zeek P (1930) Juvenile arteriosclerosis. Arch Pathol 10: 417-466
7. McGill HC Jr (ed) (1968) The geographic pathology of athero-sclerosis. Williams and Wilkins, Baltimore, or Lab Invest 18:463-467
8. Tejada C, Strong JP, Montenegro MR, Restrepo C, Solberg LA (1968) Distribution of coronary and aortic atherosclerosis by geographic location, race, and sex. Lab Invest 18:509-526
9. Duff GL, McMillan GC (1951) Pathology of atherosclerosis. Am J Med 11:92-108
10. Glagov S, Ozoa AK (1968) Significance of the relatively low incidence of atherosclerosis in the pulmonary, renal and mesenteric arteries, Ann NY Acad Sci 149(2):940-955
11. Schwartz CJ, Mitchell JRA (1962) Observations on the local-ization of arterial plaques. Circ Res 11:63-73
12. Holman R, McGill HC Jr, Strong JP, Geer JC (1958) The natural history of atherosclerosis: The early aortic lesions as seen in New Orleans in the middle of the 20th century. Am J Pathol 34:209-235
13. Mitchell JRA, Schwartz CJ (1965) Arterial disease. FA Davis Co, Philadelphia
14. Robertson WB, Geer JC, Strong JP, McGill HC Jr (1963) The fate of the fatty streak. Exp Mol Pathol 2 (Suppl. 1):28-39
15. Montenegro MR, Eggen DA (1968) Topography of atherosclerosis in the coronary arteries. Lab Invest 18:586-593
16. Solberg LA, Eggen DA (1971) Localization and sequence of development of atherosclerotic lesions in the carotid and vertebral arteries. Circulation 43:711-724
17. Strong JP, Eggen DA (1970) Risk factors and atherosclerotic lesions. In: Jones RJ (ed) Atherosclerosis. Springer-Verlag, New York, pp 355-364

18. Eggen DA, Solberg LA (1968)   Variations of atherosclerosis with age. Lab Invest 18:571-579
19. Strong JP (1972)   Atherosclerosis in human population. Atherosclerosis 16:193-201
20. Scrimshaw NS, Guzmán MA (1968)   Diet and atherosclerosis. Lab Invest 18:623-628
21. Robertson WB, Strong JP (1968)   Atherosclerosis in persons with hypertension and diabetes mellitus. Lab Invest 18:538-551
22. Strong JP, Richards ML, McGill HC Jr, Eggen DA, McMurry MT (1969) On the association of cigarette smoking with coronary and aortic atherosclerosis. J Atheroscler Res 10:303-317
23. Strong JP, Richards ML (1976) Cigarette smoking and atherosclerosis in autopsied men. Atherosclerosis 23:451-476
24. Auerbach O, Carter HW, Garfinkel L, Hammond EC (1976) Cigarette smoking and coronary artery disease. Chest 70:697-705
25. Auerbach O, Hammond EC, Garfinkel L (1965) Smoking in relation to atherosclerosis of the coronary arteries. N Engl J Med 273:775-779
26. Strong JP (1977) Unexplained variability in extent of atherosclerosis in homogenous subgroups of human populations. In: Schettler G, Goto Y, Hata Y, Klose G (eds) Atherosclerosis IV. Springer-Verlag, Berlin, pp 671-674
27. Garcia-Palmieri MR, Castillo MI, Oalmann MC, Sorlie PD, Costas R Jr (1977) The relation of antemortem factors to atherosclerosis. In: Schettler G, Goto Y, Hata Y, Klose G (eds) Atherosclerosis IV.   Springer-Verlag, Berlin, pp 108-113
28. Hatano S, Matsuzaki T (1977) Atherosclerosis in relation to personal attributes of a Japanese population in homes for the aged. In: Schettler G, Goto Y, Hata Y, Klose G (eds) Atherosclerosis IV.   Springer-Verlag, Berlin, pp 116-120
29. Solberg LA, Hjermann I, Helgeland A, Holme I, Leren PA, Strong JP (1977) Association between risk factors and atherosclerotic lesions based on autopsy findings in the Oslo study: A preliminary report. In: Schettler G, Goto Y, Hata Y, Klose G (eds) Atherosclerosis IV. Springer-Verlag, Berlin, pp 98-102
30. Stemmermann GN, Rhoads GG, Blackwelder WC (1977) Atherosclerosis and its risk factors in the Hawaiian Japanese. In: Schettler G, Goto Y, Hata Y, Klose G (eds) Atherosclerosis IV. Springer-Verlag, Berlin, pp 113-116
31. Sternby NH (1977) Atherosclerosis and risk factors. In: Schettler G, Goto Y, Hata Y, Klose G (eds) Atherosclerosis IV. Springer-Verlag, Berlin, pp 102-104
32. Strong JP (1977) An introduction to the epidemiology of atherosclerosis. In: Schettler G, Goto Y, Hata Y, Klose G (eds) Atherosclerosis IV. Springer-Verlag, Berlin, pp 92-98
33. Vartiainen I, Kanerva K (1947) Arteriosclerosis and war-time. Ann Med Intern Fenn 36:748-758
34. Wilens SL (1947) The resorption of arterial atheromatous deposits in wasting disease. Am J Pathol 23:793-804
35. Zelis R, Mason DT, Braunwald E, Levy RE (1970) Effects of hyperlipoproteinemias and their treatment on the peripheral circulation. J Clin Invest 49:1007-1015

36. Buchwald H, Moore RB, Varco RL (1974) The partial ileal bypass operation in treatment of the hyperlipidemias. Adv Exp Med Biol 63:221-230
37. Barndt R Jr, Blankenhorn DH, Crawford DW, Brooks SH (1977) Regression and progression of early femoral atherosclerosis in treated hyperlipoproteinemic patients. Ann Intern Med 86:139-146
38. Crawford DW, Sanmarco ME, Blankenhorn DH (1979) Spatial reconstruction of human femoral atheromas showing regression. Am J Med 66:784-789
39. DePalma RG, Hubay CA, Insull W Jr, Robinson AV, Hartman PH (1970) Progression and regression of experimental atherosclerosis. Surg Gynecol Obstet 131:633-647
40. Blankenhorn DH (1977) Studies of regression/progression of atherosclerosis in man. Adv Exp Med Biol. 82:453-458
41. Strong JP, Guzmán MA (1980) Decrease in coronary atherosclerosis in New Orleans. Lab Invest 43:297-301
42. McMahan CA (1960) Demographic aspects of the population of human autopsied cases. Hum Biol 31:185-196
43. McMahan CA (1962) Age-sex distributions of selected groups of human autopsied cases. Arch Pathol 73:40-47
44. McMahan CA (1968) Autopsied cases by age, sex, and "race". Lab Invest 18:468-478
45. Strong JP, Restrepo C (1978) Coronary and aortic atherosclerosis in New Orleans. I. Sampling bias due to source of autopsy specimens. Lab Invest 39:358-363

DISCUSSION: COLIN J. SCHWARTZ

This workshop addresses the very important subject of quantitative evaluation of atherosclerosis with an emphasis clearly on both lesion progression and regression. Before addressing some of the comments that have been made, I would like to draw your attention again to a view that was expressed by Dr. Michael DeBakey some years ago, which I think is important and tends to be forgotten. He has shown that within the spectrum of occlusive arterial disease one can identify at least two populations of people. One group is those that have rapidly progressive vascular disease, where in the course of weeks or months the outcome is arterial occlusion with resulting disability or death. The second is a subset of patients whose disease progresses slowly over many months or years. As we look at progression of disease we need to keep these two categories of patients in mind. Does the rapidly progressive type of disease reflect a thrombotic tendency in a subpopulation, or does it reflect accelerated atherogenesis? Are there noninvasive techniques by which one can identify the propensity of lesions to progress rapidly in some but not all patients?

The speakers this morning and yesterday have raised a number of important issues and I would like to address a few of these briefly. Dr. Newman has addressed the questions of whether fatty streaks progress, and whether these are the obligatory precursors of the fibrous plaque. This is still, we believe, an issue that is not fully resolved. Early fatty streaks in man, for example, occur in the aortic sinuses of Valsalva. This is a site that rarely becomes subsequently affected by advanced disease. And so while the issue is contentious it appears that not all fatty streaks necessarily progress to plaques, and that the factors responsible for their initiation and subsequent development may differ. Some important questions relating to the fatty streak issue need to be asked. Why do some but not all fatty streaks progress? Are there morphological characteristics of some fatty streaks that identify a propensity for progression? Why should coronary artery fatty streaks show a negative correlation with total plasma cholesterol levels, while fibrous plaques show a significant positive correlation? And, finally, can one on the basis of lesion composition identify biochemical characteristics of fatty streaks that predict their likelihood to progress?

Dr. Newman has commented on the International Atherosclerosis Project (IAP) experience comparing atherosclerosis severity during the period of 1960-64 and 1969-78. Notwithstanding the secular differences in disease during these periods when mortality from coronary heart disease has apparently declined, there is an urgent need to determine if the atherosclerotic substrate itself has really significantly diminished, or if we are dealing with a mortality change alone.

The mechanisms leading to progression or regression need considerable clarification and are best discussed in terms of plaque pathology. In this context I would like to summarize a few points of potential importance. There are many histologic changes present within the plaque itself, and the media, which exhibits prominent thinning in the presence of severe stenotic disease, and within the adventitia. In the latter we frequently see a triad of changes including fibrosis, increased vascularity, and in many instances a prominent lymphocyte infiltration. Progression or regression can clearly involve intimal, medial, or adventitial components.

While considerable emphasis is being placed on lesion regression, and correctly so, conceptually it is important to determine if intervention in man may slow the rate of lesion progression, or reduce the likelihood of plaque complications. Two features of the advanced atheromatous plaque are of particular importance in terms of regression, the large mass of collagen, and the extracellular lipid core on the other that presumably reflects a relatively inert metabolic pool. In particular what processes can facilitate the turnover of plaque collagen or extracellular lipid and thus enhance regression? Perhaps, as suggested by Dr. Daoud, the monocyte-derived macrophages play a role in both these areas, through the local release of proteolytic enzymes, and by phagocytosis of extracellular lipid.

In terms of lesion progression, with increasing disease severity adventitial lymphocytes emerge as an important feature of atherogenesis. In the later stages of progression these lymphocytes in all likelihood may reflect an immune or autoimmune process, perhaps due to changing composition and immunogenicity of one or more components of the plaque itself. Adventitial lymphocytosis occurs in some 80% of advanced human coronary, aortic, iliac, and carotid lesions, but is not a feature of fatty streaks, indicating yet another difference between these lesions and advanced disease.

The various cells involved in the atherosclerotic process have been discussed by Dr. St. Clair and by Dr. Daoud and fall into three categories. No attempt will be made to discuss further the endothelium at this time. The peripheral blood monocyte we believe to be an important progenitor of at least some of the arterial wall macrophages. Smooth muscle cells can also accumulate lipid and assume the features of foam cells. In various lesions one can identify a spectrum of foam cells, some of which are spherical and appear to have been derived from the blood monocyte, while others, somewhat more ellipsoid, appear to be the end result of lipid accumulation in smooth muscle cells.

The following comments merely emphasize the potentially important role of the peripheral blood monocyte in the atherogenic sequence. In the early stages of dietary-induced hyperlipidemia and atherosclerosis there are significant numbers of blood leukocytes attached to the overtly normal endothelium. In either scanning or transmission electron micrographs, they are readily seen in the process of migration, but at any time it is difficult to assess direction of movement ultrastructurally. Monocytes can be seen spread over the surface of the endothelium, a process which is quite impressive, and as activation of monocytes enhances cell spreading, one is encouraged to think that perhaps activation may play some part in this attachment and spreading process. Some leukocytes are deeply embedded in the endothelium, presumably in the process of migration. Intimal foam cells, with many of the morphologic features of the peripheral blood monocyte can be identified. These cells as described by Dr. Daoud are nonspecific esterase positive, providing some evidence of their monocyte origin, but definitive recognition of their monocyte derivation probably requires the demonstration of Fc and C3b receptors.

It has been suggested that the foam cells may leave the intima and contribute to the regression process by removing lipid. I suspect that we need to be cautious in assessing the direction of movement on the basis of the disposition of the endothelial margins around cells. Specifically we have seen migratory lymphocytes in which the location of the uropod and the disposition of the endothelial margins are not consistent.

What roles might the monocyte-derived macrophage play in progression or regression? This has been discussed in part by Dr. St. Clair and Dr. Daoud. It is difficult at this point, as was pointed out, to decide if the monocyte is a "good guy" or a "bad guy" in either the progression or regression phenomenon. In principle, however, the monocyte-derived macrophage may be important for a number of reasons and I would like to reemphasize these:

Because of its phagocyte potential as progenitor of at least some of the macrophages of the arterial wall and because of its secretory activity, with the secretion of hydrolytic and proteolytic enzymes, I believe that the enzymes may be important in regression and arterial remodeling. Lipoprotein uptake and metabolism is clearly an important role, and of course the monocyte-macrophage as a source of mitogen for smooth muscle cells has been discussed. One needs also to comment on the secretion of the enzyme, lipoprotein lipase, which is important in the catabolism of triglyceride-rich lipoproteins. Finally, activation of macrophages with their heightened secretory and phagocytic potential may prove to be an extremely important phenomenon in regression, a concept about which we need much more information.

21

Coronary Angiography Quality Control in the CASS Study

J. WARD KENNEDY, LLOYD D. FISHER, AND THOMAS KILLIP

The Coronary Artery Surgery Study (CASS) was organized in 1973 under the auspices of the National Heart, Lung, and Blood Institute. Enrollment of patients began in 1974 and continued through May 1979. CASS consists of a prospective, randomized study to compare the results of medical and surgical treatment in a subset of patients with anatomically proven coronary artery disease, and in a registry of consecutive patients undergoing coronary arteriography in 15 clinical sites in the United States and Canada. At the end of the enrollment period, 24,959 patients were entered into the registry, of which 780 patients were randomized to medical or surgical therapy. Extensive clinical and angiographic data are gathered on each subject at entry and during prolonged follow-up for both randomized and registry patients (1). Patients entered the CASS study when coronary arteriography and left ventriculography were carried out at a participating institution in a patient who was suspected of having coronary heart disease. Patients with other forms of heart disease were not entered, but patients who showed minimal or normal coronary arteries were retained in the registry. Therefore, at the end of enrollment in CASS, about 25,000 patients with carefully defined coronary artery anatomy are available for numerous types of investigations. This extensive data bank represents the largest collection of detailed anatomic information of heart disease in the world. For purposes of this

conference, we wish to describe the quality control processes
which were developed for entering arteriographic information into
the CASS data center and to describe some of the problems related
to the performance and interpretation of coronary arteriograms.

Coronary arteriography is the essential diagnostic technique
for defining the extent of coronary artery disease in man during
life. The performance and interpretation of coronary arteriograms
pose special problems when compared to arteriography of noncardiac
structures. The most important difference is cardiac motion.
Because of the motion of the heart, it became apparent early in
the development of coronary arteriography that it is necessary to
use cineangiographic techniques as opposed to static filming
techniques. This put the cardiac angiographer in the business of
making motion pictures, a technology far more complex than other
forms of angiography. It required the development of high-quality
image intensifiers, motion picture cameras, and television systems
that could operate with high resolution under limitations imposed
by x-ray generators, radiation dosages, and safe doses of contrast
material. This technology has evolved to the current high level
since its beginnings in the late 1950s at Dr. Wason Sones's
laboratory at the Cleveland Clinic. Although static filming
techniques were used in some laboratories in the early and
mid-1970s, by the time the CASS study had begun, it was clearly
recognized that cineangiographic filming techniques were by and
large superior for the visualization of the coronary arteries.
For this reason CASS relied on the cineangiographic filming
techniques. Because of the difficulties in standardization of
performance and interpretation of coronary arteriograms, an
angiographic quality control program was developed for the
CASS study. This consisted of the development of four quality
control laboratories at 4 of the 15 CASS sites. Each month, the
coordination center randomly selected from each clinical site
three films depicting at least minimal coronary lesions. These
films were then sent to a quality control site, where they were

reinterpreted. The interpretation from the quality control site was then compared with that of the original site and discrepancies were recorded. At regular meetings of participating angiographers, films over which there were substantial disagreement were reviewed in an effort to resolve the differences in interpretation. By the end of enrollment in CASS, 870 films had been read as a part of the quality control study. In addition to interpretation, films were judged for their diagnostic quality. Only 3% of these 870 films were considered poor or of unacceptable quality.

At the beginning of the CASS study, there was substantial variation in film quality among participating sites. In order to improve the technical quality, regular meetings were held for angiographers and laboratory technicians. These meetings, which were attended by technical experts from the film industry, concentrated on cineangiographic techniques and film processing. The 1meetings also dealt with difficulties in nomenclature of coronary artery anatomy, descriptive codes for the morphology of atherosclerotic lesions, and quality of distal segments. These numerous committee meetings and technical discussions resulted in an improved quality of cineangiograms during the course of the study.

This workshop is concerned with the measurement of change in atherosclerotic lesions and with evaluation of progression and regression of disease. At this time, the CASS study is not prepared to present data on progression or regression of coronary atherosclerotic lesions. The study is engaged in evaluation of change in the atherosclerotic process in the coronary arteries in randomized patients restudied five years after entry. In addition, numerous patients in CASS have undergone an additional study or studies following entry. Because of intense interest in the study of progression of disease following medical or surgical therapy, the angiography committee in the CASS has held several sessions dealing with the problems of the serial interpretation of coronary arteriograms. At one of these work sessions, held in St. Louis last year, numerous serial examinations were read by the committee.

In addition, many CASS angiographers have participated in group
readings of coronary arteriograms done as part of the National
Institutes of Health inhouse Type 2 study. From these experiences, the angiographic committee has established procedures
for the serial reading of coronary arteriograms in CASS. These
procedures require that both cine films be viewed simultaneously
on paired projectors by two angiographers and a technical assis-
tant to record the data. Each lesion is identified on both films;
than a judgment is made as to any change in the lesion. The
decision is scored as to the certainty of change, whether very
certain, probably accurate, or uncertain. A similar procedure
was used in the analysis of the Type 2 data, although in that
instance the coronary arteriograms for this purpose were recorded
on cut film. Fig. 1 presents the form for this purpose.

VARIATION IN THE INTERPRETATION OF CORONARY ARTERIOGRAMS

The quality control procedure in CASS as described above provided
a large amount of information with which to evaluate the variability in interpretation of coronary angiograms (2-5). This has
been the subject of prior evaluation by other investigators in
relatively small series of examinations (6-10). In the 870 arteriograms read independently by readers at different clinics, there
was an absolute difference in percent stenosis of between 5% and
10% depending on the arterial segment involved. Among proximal
segments, lesions of the left main coronary artery were the most
difficult to reproducibly interpret ($p < .02$) (2). In the left
main coronary artery where one reader may read a stenosis of 50%
or more, it is estimated that a second reader will find no stenosis 15.7% of the time. In 94.7% of the films the number of
significantly diseased vessels (>70% stenosis) was the same for
both readers (72.1%) or differed by one vessel (22.6%). When
comparing the reproducibility of numbers of diseased vessels
with film quality, it was clear that films of good or acceptable
quality yielded greater reproducibility of interpretation. It

is of interest that the mean absolute difference between the
readings of percent stenosis decreased over the time of the
patient enrollment between 1975 to 1978, a statistically significant drop. We believe this is due to the quality control program
for coronary angiography, which was active during this period.
One of the major difficulties in comparing the interpretation of
separate independent readers is the variability in the location of
the lesion. The CASS study identifies 26 separate segments of
the coronary vessels. Definition of those segments is complex
and open to variable interpretation. Therefore, when the reader
identifies a lesion in a particular segment, an independent reader
may identify the same lesion but place it in an adjacent segment.
For this reason, it was necessary to use a nearest neighbor rule
when making computer comparisons between readings. For example,
suppose a single high-grade stenosis is identified in the left
anterior descending coronary artery (LAD) by both readers. If
one places it in the middle segment, and the other places it in
the distal segment, but both read it as an 80% lesion, this would
be considered perfect agreement using the nearest neighbor rule.
This system works well when isolated lesions are present. However, when multiple lesions are present such as tight lesions in
both middle and distal segment of the LAD, the nearest neighbor
rule may fail to make the appropriate comparisons; in this case
the readers receive the benefit of the doubt.

There are many ways to present the variability in interpretation. In addition, because of the large number of segments of
the coronary arteries and various ways of interpreting variation
in reading, an immense amount of data is generated by this type
of analysis. For reasons of clarity and brevity we will limit
our presentation to a few examples as developed by the CASS study
(2,4). The first one is shown in Table 1. When one reader
records a lesion of a fixed amount, the table gives an estimate
of the percent of the time a second reader will record no lesion.
This interpretation uses the nearest neighbor rule. As you can

REPEAT ANGIOGRAPHY SUPPLEMENT

(TO BE USED WITH REPEAT ANGIOGRAPHY FORMS, 8B, 8C, 9A)

Instructions for comparison reading of initial and late (greater than 36 months) follow-up coronary and left ventricular angiograms:

1. Two CASS angiographers must be present for simultaneous interpretation.
2. Two projectors for simultaneous viewing of cine films must be used.
3. A CASS data technician must be present to record the data and to do a careful consistency check.
4. Readings must be accompanied by a judgment as to the certainty of the reading (confidence code).
5. Only films that are of technically adequate quality should be compared.
6. Both angiographers and the data technician must sign the completed form below. This form, after being completed and signed by both of the angiographers and the data technician, should then be mailed to the Coordinating Center. (Data on the corresponding Repeat Angiography form(s), 8B, 8C, and/or 9A, will be used for analysis only after this supplement form 19 has been received.)

Patient I.D. _____

Date of current angiography ___/___/___

Was the study initiated? By the site (routine)_____

By the clinical status of the patient _____

Was revascularization complete? Yes___ No___ No judgment___ Does not apply___

CASS Angiographer _____

CASS Angiographer _____

Data Technician _____

CASS 19 (10/27/81)
Page 1 of 1

---

affix computer I.D. here

REPEAT CHEST X-RAY AND
CORONARY ARTERIOGRAPHY

Name _____

Date of Angiography ___/___/___
No. Day Year

Angiography read comparatively with angiography of ___/___/___
No. Day Year

A. CHEST X-RAY

1. Heart

   Normal □   LV contour abnormal □
   Enlarged □   Other abnormality □
     1 slight □
     2 moderate □
     3 marked □

2. Cardiothoracic ratio _____
   Unable to determine □

3. Lungs and pleura

   Normal □   Increased upper lobe venous markings (P.V.C.) □
   Other abnormality □

B. ARTERIOGRAPHY

1. Was study complete   1 Yes □   2 No □
   If no, explain (20-keystroke limit)_____

2. Technique
   IV--Heparin: 1 Yes □   2 No □
   1 Cutdown □   2 Percutaneous □   3 Both □
   1 Brachial □   2 Femoral □   3 Both □   4 Other □

3. Complications   1 Yes □   2 No □
   If yes, complete "Complications" form

4. Congenital and other abnormalities   1 Yes □   2 No □
   If yes, explain (17-keystroke limit)_____

CASS 08B (4-1-79)
Page 1 of 3

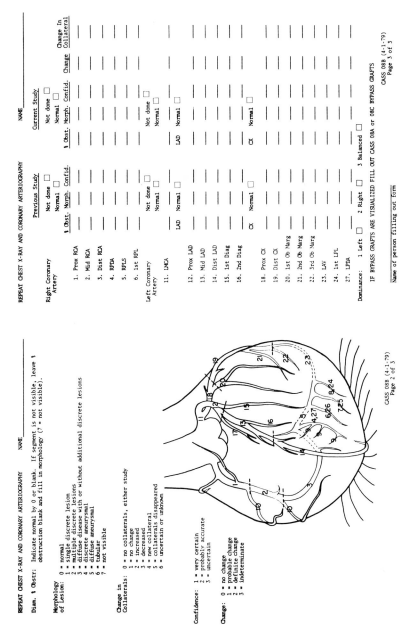

Fig. 1 Forms for evaluation of repeat coronary arteriography in the Coronary Artery Surgery Study, CASS.

Table 1. Likelihood of reader number 1 recording zero stenosis when reader number 2 reads a stenosis of >50% or more, >70% or more.

Segment	>50%	>70%
Proximal RCA[a]	2.2	2.1
Mid RCA	1.9	0.9
Distal RCA	10.5	8.6
PDA[b]	28.5	25.6
LMCA[c]	15.7	11.6
Proximal LAD[d]	2.9	1.5
Mid LAD	0.9	0.5
Distal LAD	10.2	6.4
Proximal Circumflex	3.0	2.4

[a] Right coronary artery.
[b] Posterior descending artery.
[c] Left main coronary artery.
[d] Left anterior descending coronary artery.

see, in the proximal right coronary artery (RCA) if one reader reads a lesion of greater than 50%, a lesion will be read by the other reader in all but 2.2% of the films. That is not to say that the lesion will be read as similar severity by both readers. If one reader reads it as greater than 70%, a lesion will be read by the other reader in all but 2.1% of the films. Stenosis of the mid-right coronary artery is read more reproducibly than the distal segment of that vessel. If one reader reads the distal right as greater than 50%, in 10.5% of films the other reader will not identify a lesion. For the left anterior descending artery, one reader will not identify a lesion in 28.5% of patients where the other reads a lesion of 50% or more. Of more importance clinically is the substantial variation in reading presence or absence of disease in the left main coronary artery (LMCA). When a single reader reads a lesion of greater than 50% in the left main coronary artery, 15.7% of the time the second reader will fail to identify a lesion. Likewise, the proximal and mid-left anterior descending arteries are read well, whereas the distal LAD is read relatively less consistently.

Another way to present this type of information is to look at the absolute value of the differences in the readings of the two readers. In Table 2 are listed the mean and standard deviations of the absolute value of the differences in angiographic readings between the two readers. In the proximal right coronary artery, the average difference was 9.4% stenosis and the standard deviation was 14.3%. The mid-right coronary artery has a difference of 6.8% and the distal right coronary artery has a difference of 8.9%. For the left main coronary artery, the mean difference was 5.8% with a standard deviation of 13.6%. The proximal LAD mean difference was 8.8%.

A second source of data on variability in angiographic readings resulted from a designed experiment within the CASS study. In this experiment, 30 films taken from the December 1975 CASS quality control films were used. The 30 films were read twice by each of three readers in a blinded fashion. The experiment was divided into three rounds. In the first round the films were randomly ordered, then separated into three groups of 10 films each. Three groups were circulated by mail in predetermined order among the three readers. When all readings were complete, the 30 films were reordered and grouped again for round two. The time between repeat readings of a film by a single reader was always greater than one month. It was found that the intrareader variability was

Table 2. Means and standard deviations of absolute value of differences in angiographic findings

Segment	Mean	Standard Deviation
Proximal RCA[a]	9.4	14.3
Mid RCA	6.8	12.2
Distal RCA	8.9	19.0
PDA[b]	8.7	21.4
LMCA[c]	5.8	13.6
Proximal LAD[d]	8.8	14.3
Mid LAD	7.1	11.6
Distal LAD	5.6	13.2
Proximal Circumflex	6.1	10.4

[a] Right coronary artery.
[b] Posterior descending artery.
[c] Left main coronary artery.
[d] left anterior descending coronary artery.

approximately one half of the interreader variability when
evaluating percent stenosis. This difference was statistically
significant (p < .00001) (4). The flavor of the data may be
obtained from Fig. 2. The left-hand panel shows the site, or
intrareader scatter diagram for percent stenosis in the proximal
left anterior descending coronary artery. The right-hand panel
shows the scatter comparing the readings between readers. As
one might predict, if you compare interpretations about other
aspects of the disease process, including the presence or absence
of collaterals, morphology of the lesion, morphology of the distal
vessel, size of the distal vessel, and presence or absence of
disease of the distal vessel, the variability between readers
increases.

We believe that this evaluation of the variability of interpretation of coronary arteriograms emphasizes the importance of
side-by-side double projection and interpretation of films by

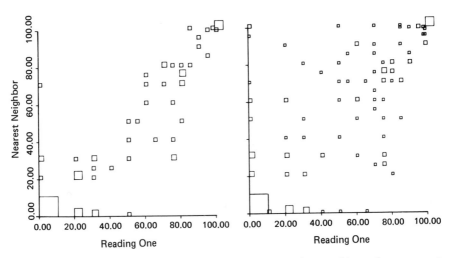

Fig. 2   Inter- and intrareader variability in reading the percent
stenosis in the proximal left anterior (PRXLAD) descending coronary artery.   The data came from the Coronary Artery Surgery Study
experiment.   Thirty films were read twice by each of three readers.

two angiographers when attempting to evaluate progression and regression of coronary atherosclerotic lesions. If studies like this are not done, the variability in the two readings will obscure any change or lack thereof. We have not yet mentioned the use of any calibration devices to aid the angiographer in interpreting the films. Numerous approaches to the quantification of coronary artery stenosis are either being developed or are currently in use. Among others, the work of Drs. Brown and Dodge at the University of Washington and the Wadsworth Veterans Administration Hospital deserves mention. These investigators have projected the coronary arteriograms onto digitizing tablets, traced the lesions in two views, 90° apart and perpendicular to the long axis of the lesion, and made measurements of diameter stenosis, cross-sectional area stenosis, and more importantly luminal diameter of the normal and stenotic portion of the vessel. These measurements, carried out over the length of the lesion, allow these investigators to estimate the mass of atherosclerotic material compromising the vessel lumen. By estimating the flow through the vessel, they can then estimate the theoretical drop in pressure across any given lesion. These investigators have also, with the use of this technique, measured the change in coronary artery diameter under the influence of various maneuvers and with different drugs. Another simpler approach is a digital caliper which allows an interpreter to measure the percent stenosis and percent cross-sectional area stenosis. The interpreter places the caliper on the area of maximum lumen stenosis and on the normal areas of the vessel above and below the stenosis. These data are entered into a minicomputer. This simple and relatively inexpensive device or other similar calibrating instruments may come into standard use in the future.

It seems likely that quantitative techniques such as these and others currently under development will be useful in future studies of progression and, hopefully, of regression of coronary atherosclerosis. The simpler of these calibration devices may come into standard clinical use and improve the physician's ability to communicate with his colleagues in a more uniform manner by reducing the variability in interpretation of coronary arteriograms. This would mean that interpretation of arteriograms in the future would contain relatively precise measurements of major coronary artery stenoses, present the reactivity of those lesions to vasodilating agents and give more precise information about the size and quality of the distal bed.

We would like to emphasize that in the near future better and more precise measurements of coronary artery lesions will depend upon the production of high-quality, high-resolution cineangiograms taken perpendicular to the long axis through the lesion in multiple views. Often, this will require special magnification techniques as well. At this time it does not appear that cut film techniques, despite their higher resolution, will be useful in this regard. Substantial improvement in the quality of cineangiograms is possible and undoubtedly will be forthcoming. In the design of future studies for the evaluation of progression and regression of disease in the coronary arteries obtaining the highest resolution, highest quality cineangiograms are essential.

We conclude with a few comments on designs to look at arteriographic changes over long time periods in a clinical setting. One may anticipate changes in equipment over an extensive time period. Even if the same equipment is used, over time there is always a question of the precision of standardization. Further, patient populations change with time. This leads us to conclude that in assessing a new therapy, control cases should be used because of the potential problems due to changing equipment, procedures, and population. This problem is particularly severe when the assessment of the amount of stenosis is made by human judgment, as in CASS, as opposed to an automated system. Even for an automated system, however, systematic changes in technique and equipment over time are always possible; the strongest inference will result with a parallel control group and blinded reading if human intervention is part of the evaluative process.

SUMMARY

The multi-institutional Coronary Artery Surgery Study (CASS) was developed to evaluate the efficacy of the surgical and medical management of patients with coronary artery disease. Selective coronary arteriography was performed on 24,959 patients who were entered into the CASS registry, including 780 patients who were randomized to medical or surgical therapy. During the development of the CASS, extensive efforts were made to control the quality and interpretation of coronary arteriograms. As part of this quality control program, 870 films were read at special quality control laboratories and at the participating site. In addition, a small angiographic interpretation experiment was carried out during the early period of CASS. This experiment involved the re-reading of 30 films at three different quality control laboratories. These data showed that readers have an average absolute difference of 5% to 10% in the interpretation of coronary artery narrowing. Because of this variability, CASS has developed special techniques and report forms for the reading of serial coronary arteriograms for the purpose of identifying progression and regression of atherosclerotic disease.

REFERENCES

1. CASS Principal Investigators and their associates (1981) National Heart, Lung, and Blood Institute Coronary Artery Surgery Study, Circulation 63 (Monograph #79)
2. Fisher LD, Judkins MP, Lesperance J, Cameron A, Swaye P, Ryan T, Maynard C, Bourassa M, Gosselin A, Kemp H, Faxon D, Wexler L, Davis K (to be published in Cathet Cardiovasc Diagn) Reproducibility of coronary arteriographic reading in the coronary artery surgery study (CASS)
3. Wexler LF, Lesperance J, Ryan TJ, Bourassa MG, Fisher LD, Maynard C, Kemp HG, Cameron A, Gosselin AJ, Judkins MP (to be published in Cathet Cardiovasc Diagn) Interobserver variability in interpreting contrast left ventriculograms (CASS)

4. Kemp HG, Davis KB, Judkins MP, Gosselin AJ, Kennedy JW, Cameron A, Swaye PS, Maynard C, Fisher LD (1981) Intrareader variability in the interpretation of coronary arteriograms from the Coronary Artery Surgery Study (CASS)
5. Cameron A, Kemp HG Jr, Fisher LD, Gosselin A, Judkins MP, Kennedy JW, Lesperance J, Mudd JG, Ryan TJ, Silverman JF, Tristani F, Vliestra RE, Wexler LF (to be published) Left main coronary artery stenosis: angiographic determination (CASS)
6. Zir LM, Miller SW, Dinsmore RE, Gilbert JP, Harthorne JW (1976) Interobserver variability in coronary angiography. Circulation 53:627-632
7. Detre KM, Wright E, Murphy ML, Takaro T (1975) Observer agreement in evaluating coronary angiograms. Circulation 53:979-986
8. DeRouen TA, Murray JA, Owen W (1977) Variability in the analysis of coronary arteriograms. Circulation 55:324-328
9. Sanmarco ME, Brooks SH, Blankenhorn DH (1978) Reproducibility of a consensus panel in the interpretation of coronary angiograms. Am Heart J 96:430-437
10. Galbraith JE, Murphy ML, DeSovza N (1978) Coronary angiogram interobserver variability. JAMA 240:2053-2056

APPENDIX

Cooperating Clinical Sites

University of Alabama in Birmingham William J. Rogers, M.D.*, Richard O. Russell, Jr., M.D., Albert Oberman, M.D., and Nicholas T. Kouchoukos, M.D.

Albany Medical College Julio A Sosa, M.D.*, Martin F. McKneally, M.D.*, Joseph MacIllduff, M.D., Thomas Older, M.D., and Eric K. Foster, M.D.

Boston University Thomas Ryan, M.D.*, David Faxon, M.D., Laura Wexler, M.D., Robert L. Berger, M.D., and Carolyn H. McCabe, B.S.

Loma Linda University Melvin P. Judkins, M.D.* and Joan Coggin, M.D.*

Marshfield Medical Foundation, Inc. and Marshfield Clinic William Myers, M.D.*, Richard D. Sautter, M.D.*, John N. Browell, M.D., Dieter M. Voss, M.D., and Robert D. Carlson, M.D.

---

*Principal Investigator

Massachusetts General Hospital   J. Warren Harthorne, M.D.*, W. Gerald Austen, M.D.*, Robert Dinsmore, M.D., Frederick Levine, M.D., and John McDermott, M.D.

Mayo Clinic and Mayo Foundation   Robert L. Frye, M.D.*, Hugh C. Smith, M.D., Ronald E. Vlietstra, M.D., Michael B. Mock, M.D., David R. Holmes, M.D., and Richard Fulton, M.D.

Miami Heart Institute   Arthur J. Gosselin, M.D.*, Parry B. Larsen, M.D., and Paul Swaye, M.D.

Montreal Heart Institute   Martial G. Bourassa, M.D.*, Bernard R. Chaitman, M.D., Claude Goulet, M.D., and Jacques Lesperance, M.D.

New York University   Ephraim Glassman, M.D.*, and Michael Schloss, M.D.

St. Louis University   George Kaiser, M.D.*, J. Gerard Mudd, M.D.*, Robert D. Wiens, M.D., Hendrick B. Barner, M.D., John E. Codd, M.D., Denis H. Tyras, M.D., and Vallee L. Willman, M.D.

St. Luke's Hospital Center   Harvey G. Kemp, Jr., M.D.* and Airlie Cameron, M.D.

Stanford University   Edwin Alderman, M.D.*, Francis H. Koch, M.D.*, Paul R. Cipriano, M.D.*, James F. Silverman, M.D.* and Edward B. Stinson, M.D.*

Medical College of Wisconsin   Felix Tristani, M.D.*, Harold L. Brooks, M.D.*, and Robert J. Flemma, M.D.

Yale University   Lawrence S. Cohen, M.D.*, Rene Langou, M.D., Alexander S. Geha, M.D., Graeme L. Hammond, M.D., and Richard K. Shaw, M.D.

Central Electrocardiographic Laboratory

University of Alabama   L. Thomas Sheffield, M.D.*, David Roitman, M.D., and Carol Troxell, B.S.

Coordinating Center

University of Washington   Lloyd Fisher, Ph.D.*, Mary Jo Gillespie, M.S., Kathryn Davis, Ph.D., J. Ward Kennedy, M.D., and Richard Kronmal, Ph.D.

Chairman of Steering Committee

Thomas Killip, M.D., Henry Ford Hospital

National Heart, Lung, and Blood Institute

Eugene R. Passamani, M.D., Peter L. Frommer, M.D., Suzanne M.
Mullin, R.N., M.P.H., Kent Bailey, Ph.D. and David DeMets, Ph.D.

DISCUSSION: LLOYD D. FISHER

Things are better than you think in terms of variability of angio-graphic complications. As I am a co-author on the paper and time is short, I will restrict my comments to two.

My comments only refer to the evaluation of the coronary arteries for reduction in luminal diameter. I have found it interesting within CASS, as a lay person (I am a biostatistician), to listen to the radiologists and cardiologists discuss interpre-tation of angiographic films. In particular, in listening to the discussion of serial angiography, I get an uneasy feeling; one person says we cannot talk about change because of overlap; another person will say this is obviously a slightly different view, and so on. The best hope is for quantitative techniques such as Dr. Brown's work and Dr. Blankenhorn's work. I am not sure this will be as useful in sequential angiography, taken say three to five years apart, as one might hope. I don't know how to quantify my insecurity; but because of changes in technique and changes in equipment that will occur it is extremely impor-tant that concurrent control groups be used in long-term studies at this time. Otherwise, it would be very difficult to decide whether the progression or regression was artifact.

You heard that the CASS films are viewed side by side. One thing I have given some thought to (but have not proceeded with because I am not involved in such a project) is how to quanti-tatively analyze *paired* films. We have seen two eloquent exam-ples of quantitative analysis. How might one actually evaluate the two sequential films quantitatively using their paired nature? The greatest promise in quantitative work, by having the most statistical power, will likely result not from methods that look at the films individually, but from methods that take into account the pairing of films on the same patient.

22

Vessel Injury, Thrombosis, and the Progression and Regression of Atherosclerotic Lesions

J. FRASER MUSTARD, RAELENE L. KINLOUGH-RATHBONE, AND MARIAN A. PACKHAM

The relationship of thrombosis to the development of early and advanced atherosclerotic lesions, and the clinical complications of atherosclerosis will be discussed in this presentation. Thrombosis is initiated by vessel injury and the platelets that adhere to an injury site cause smooth muscle cell proliferation. The duration of vessel wall reactivity after an injury also affects the extent of thrombosis and vessel wall changes. An important consideration in injury-mediated atherosclerosis is whether the extent of atherosclerosis can be reduced if the injurious factors are removed or inhibited. To investigate some of these relationships, several ways of monitoring vessel injury and thrombosis have been developed.

THROMBOSIS

Early Lesions

Endothelial injury that is associated with platelet accumulation on the damaged surface leads to a proliferative response of the smooth muscle cells in the wall and the formation of a thickened intima (1,2). This type of response appears to be largely mediated by a mitogen released from the platelets that adhere to the subendothelial structures (1,3). It seems unlikely, however, that this is the sole mechanism by which atherosclerosis occurs following

vessel injury, since other cells that can take part in the response to injury, such as monocytes, can also synthesize and
secrete a mitogen for smooth muscle cells (4). Other factors,
such as low-density lipoproteins (LDL) are also known to influence
smooth muscle cell proliferation (5). Vessel wall thickening can
be induced by mechanisms that do not appear to dislodge the
endothelium or cause platelet interaction with the vessel wall,
but do result in smooth muscle cell proliferation. The best
example of this is Marek's disease in chickens, in which the virus
stimulates the proliferation of smooth muscle cells and this
causes the development of atherosclerotic lesions (6).

The concept of the development of atherosclerosis in response
to vessel wall injury is compatible with the focal nature of
atherosclerotic lesions because effects of blood flow can cause
focal endothelial injury and can also localize the site of accumulation of injurious substances (2,7). The role of microthrombi
in the development of human atherosclerotic lesions was established by Geer and Haust (8).

Advanced Lesions

The role of thrombosis in the development of advanced atherosclerotic lesions is evident from human postmortem studies in which
mural thrombi have been observed to be organized into the wall to
produce intimal thickening (9-12). Experiments using animals have
shown that injury with mural thrombosis can lead to organization
of the thrombi, intimal thickening, and lesions that range from
those rich in smooth muscle cells to advanced atheroma (13,14).
The accumulation of lipids in lesions that are associated with
repeated vessel wall injury does not require elevation of serum
cholesterol, although the amount of lipid in the lesions and the
rate of its accumulation is increased if the serum cholesterol is
increased (15,16). The mechanism of lipid accumulation in lesions
in animals in which serum cholesterol is not elevated appears to
be mediated through the effects of endothelial cell regrowth over

the injury and on the formation of glycosaminoglycans, which can selectively trap LDL (17-19). It would appear from the human studies that the development of advanced atherosclerotic lesions may be largely dependent upon mural thrombi and their organization. In these lesions, the proliferative response associated with the organization of the thrombi can probably be further modified or enhanced by the monocytes that accumulate in such lesions; the monocytes can synthesize and release a factor that is mitogenic for smooth muscle cells (4).

Thromboembolic Complications

The evidence concerning thromboembolism and the development of the clinical complications of atherosclerosis is extensive but some aspects of this subject require further clarification. There is no doubt that thrombosis associated with atherosclerotic lesions in the major vessels to the head and neck is responsible for some attacks of cerebral ischemia and strokes (20-22). A similar relationship can be developed for myocardial ischemia and myocardial infarction. The problem, however, is that not all episodes of cerebral ischemia can be demonstrated to be associated with thromboembolic events, and sudden death associated with myocardial ischemia is usually not associated with occlusive thrombosis. There is debate about the relative importance of mural thrombi that embolize into the microcirculation, and coronary artery spasm as a cause of sudden death (23-26).

Some studies show that sudden death may be the result of small emboli from mural thrombi (26). When these emboli impact in the microcirculation they could cause ventricular fibrillation and sudden death. This mechanism is supported by early work in experimental animals (27), but it is not known how frequently it occurs in man. An interesting concept has emerged more recently about the possible role of vessel spasm in the initiation of ischemic events and sudden death, particularly in the coronary circulation (24,25,28-30). In studies of human coronary arteries

during angiography, spasm has been observed in association with
the development of ischemia, and, with release of the spasm, the
signs and symptoms of ischemic events disappear (24). The concept
of spasm is in keeping with the well-established observation that
when vessel walls are injured they do undergo a short period of
contraction (31,32). Injury to the surface of coronary arteries
with the adherence of formed elements that could form thromboxane
A_2 might be one of the mechanisms responsible for spasm (33),
although others have also been proposed (34). If focal spasm
lasted long enough and was in a vessel supplying a critical part
of the conduction system, it could precipitate ventricular fibrillation and sudden death. Alternatively, if spasm in a coronary
artery persisted, thrombosis might develop distal to the spasm and
the resultant infarction in the ischemic area would be clearly
associated with the thrombus in postmortem examination. In this
case, spasm would be the important initial response to vessel
injury, and thrombosis would be secondary to the spasm and not
the primary event initiating ischemia and myocardial infarction.

VESSEL INJURY

Endothelial injury and thrombosis are involved in the development
of both the early and advanced lesions of atherosclerosis and in
the thromboembolic complications of atherosclerosis. Endothelial
injury can be presumed to be mediated by blood-borne factors and
substances, the effects of blood flow, and possibly through the
effects of vessel wall changes that may affect the endothelium
(2). Among the blood-borne factors that may damage the endothelium are serum lipids, particularly LDL, high concentrations of
abnormal metabolites, such as homocystine, antigen-antibody
complexes, catecholamines, bacteria and bacterial products, and
viruses (35-42). Most of these blood-borne materials probably
exert their maximum effect in areas of altered blood flow. In
serum sickness it has been shown that the sites of maximum
interaction of antigen-antibody complexes with the vessel wall

tend to be around vessel orifices and branches, which are the sites where disturbed flow is likely to occur (35). The work of Goldsmith and Karino (7,43) provides considerable information about the way in which flow patterns could cause focal accumulation of plasma constituents. It is also possible that both the leucocytes and platelets could contribute to vessel injury through the release or formation of enzymes and other injurious materials when they interact with the vessel wall at sites of disturbed flow (44-49); the leucocyte may be more important in causing endothelial injury because it can adhere to the uninjured endothelium. It has recently been shown that activated neutrophils can adhere to endothelial cells in tissue culture and release proteases that can cause detachment of endothelial cells from the surface of the culture dish (47).

Blood flow may have a direct injurious effect on the endothelium itself. Experimentally, exposing the endothelium to a very high shear rate can result in the loss of endothelium from the vessel wall (50). Dislodgement of the endothelium from the proximal surface of stenotic lesions has been demonstrated by Gertz and his colleagues (33).

Smoking could contribute to vessel injury through causing the release of catecholamines, through the effects of nicotine, and through the formation of antigen-antibody complexes that may damage the vessel wall (51-59).

Vessel Wall Reactivity Following Injury

The contribution of the formed elements of the blood to the response of blood and vessel wall to injury is probably dependent in part upon the period during which the injury site remains reactive to the blood components. Experiments on thrombus formation in the microcirculation indicate that within an hour or so of an initial injury the site becomes relatively nonreactive to further platelet accumulation (31,60). The observations in larger arteries indicate that following a single injury the surface becomes nonreactive to further platelet or fibrin accumulation within hours (61-63). In rabbits, removal of the endothelium causes an immediate, extensive coating of platelets on the subendothelium. However, the ability of the surface to cause further platelet accumulation is rapidly lost and does not recur even though the platelets gradually leave the surface over a period of one to two days (62). When a diseased vessel wall or thickened intima is damaged, platelet-fibrin thrombi form on the surface and here again the surface rapidly becomes nonreactive to further thrombus formation (64). In cats, it has been demonstrated that injury to the carotid artery by endarterectomy leads to the formation of platelet-fibrin thrombi that can be inhibited by heparin administration (65). If thrombus formation is prevented by heparin therapy for a period of 6 h and then the heparin therapy is stopped, no thrombus forms on the damaged vessel wall. The factors that cause the surface to become nonreactive have not yet been identified. They obviously influence the time during which an injury site could be reactive and could contribute to the development of atherosclerotic lesions or thromboembolic complications. These observations strongly indicate that the thromboembolic events associated with the development of atherosclerotic lesions and clinical complications are episodic. This concept has important implications for the attempts to establish methods to determine whether thromboembolic events resulting from vessel injury are actually occurring.

A practical illustration of this comes from studies of platelet survival. A single injury such as the removal of the endothelium or damage to the neointima does not shorten platelet survival (62). This is not unexpected since the amount of platelet material that interacts with the damaged vessel wall is less than 1 to 2% of the circulating platelet mass. Repeated injury to the vessel wall during the period of measurement of platelet survival is associated with shortened platelet survival (66-68). This is probably due to repeated interaction of platelets with the vessel wall, and platelet changes resulting from this interaction that lead to their loss from the wall and subsequent removal from the circulation. Thus, the observations that cigarette smokers have a shorter platelet survival when they are smoking than when they are not smoking (69), and nonsmokers have longer platelet survival times than smokers (70) could be related to repeated injury to the vessel wall by materials in cigarette smoke.

REGRESSION OF ATHEROSCLEROTIC LESIONS

In almost all experimental studies, removal of the stimulus causing the development of atherosclerosis leads to regression of the lesions (71,72). Experimental atherosclerosis produced by feeding hypercholesterolemic diets regresses when cholesterol is removed from the diet, probably because the injurious effects of LDL on the vessel wall no longer occur (73). Armstrong (74) demonstrated in pigs, that when a hypercholesterolemic diet is discontinued, the lesions regress. More direct experiments have been carried out in animals with immunologically-induced athero-sclerosis of the carotid arteries. In these studies, Friedman and his associates (75) showed that removal of the injurious material led to the resolution of advanced atheromatous lesions, fatty streaks, and fibrous plaques.

It may be difficult, however, to prevent further injury at sites of advanced atherosclerotic lesions where hemodynamic factors may be responsible for injury (33,76,77). Under these circumstances the hemodynamic forces may cause repeated injury that leads to the progression of the atherosclerotic lesions and the development of thromboembolic complications.

Studies in man are more difficult to interpret than studies with experimental animals because it is not possible to establish as clear a relationship among exposure to an injury stimulus, the development of atherosclerosis, withdrawal of the stimulus, and regression of the lesions. It does seem, however, that the decrease in ischemic heart disease that has been observed among

North Americans in the last decade is associated with a decrease in the amount of coronary atherosclerosis (78,79). If this decrease in the incidence of ischemic heart disease is related to changes in smoking habits and in the lipid content of the diet, the observations would be compatible with a reduction in the amount of injury to which vessel walls are subjected (80,81). The available data indicate that when individuals stop smoking they have a reduced risk of developing the complications of coronary artery disease (82,83). It has recently been reported that reduction of serum cholesterol and decreased smoking in normotensive men at high risk of coronary heart disease significantly reduced the incidence of sudden death and death from myocardial infarction (84). As mentioned earlier, cessation of smoking is associated with lengthening of shortened platelet survival in subjects who are chronic smokers. This observation is compatible with the concept of a reduction in the risk of the clinical manifestations of atherosclerosis when injurious agents are withdrawn. In the case of cigarette smoking, however, this could be caused by a reduction in the risk of thromboembolic complications as well as by a reduction in the extent of atherosclerosis.

Further evidence supporting the concept of regression of atherosclerosis comes from postmortem studies and studies in which coronary artery imaging has been used. Strong and Guzmán (85) reported that the extent of coronary atherosclerosis in black and white males in New Orleans decreased in the years between 1960 and 1972. Preliminary studies indicate that modern imaging techniques may make it possible to demonstrate regression of atherosclerotic lesions (86-88). There has been concern, however, that atherosclerotic lesions rich in collagen are more advanced than lipid-rich lesions and that the former may not regress (71,89).

MONITORING VESSEL INJURY AND THROMBOSIS

No simple methods have been established to estimate the extent of vessel injury. Attempts have been made to determine the number of endothelial cells in the plasma in circumstances in which endothelial injury is suspected, but this is a tedious process that is difficult to quantitate (90,91). Another approach has been to examine the concentration in plasma of products formed or secreted by the endothelial cells as a result of stimulation or injury. One such product is the factor VIII related antigen (von Willebrand factor) that is synthesized by the endothelial cells (92-94). Increased fibrinolytic activity in plasma could be another measure of endothelial injury or stimulation since endothelial cells are known to be able to form plasminogen activator (95,96).

A different approach to assessing the extent of vessel wall injury is to monitor changes in platelets, or the plasma concentration of materials released from or formed by platelets when they interact at injury sites. Shortened platelet survival probably reflects platelet interaction with a damaged vessel wall and the subsequent platelet changes that result in their removal from the circulation (97,98). Platelets can interact with the vessel wall but not take part in thrombus formation, and under these circumstances the only monitor of changes in platelets would be the changes in platelet survival that occur with repeated vessel wall injury (67). The extent of release of platelet granule contents that occurs when a single layer of platelets adheres to injury sites on the vessel wall is probably too small for the products to be detected in the plasma. Adelman and his colleagues (99) have shown that the interaction of platelets with an injured vessel wall is not sufficient to lead to an increase in platelet factor 4 (PF4) in plasma. No evidence is available about the effect on the plasma concentration of PF4 of repeated endothelial injury that is associated with shortened platelet survival. A large part of the released material may penetrate the vessel wall, as demonstrated by Goldberg and his associates (100), and therefore not be demonstrable in the plasma.

On the other hand, when the platelets are involved in thrombosis associated with endothelial injury, it may be possible to

detect increased amounts of constituents released or formed by the
platelets in the plasma (101,102). Increases in PF4, β-thromboglobulin, and thromboxane B_2 have been detected in the plasma
during extracorporeal circulation (103-105) and these increases
are compatible with the extensive platelet thromboembolism that
occurs with such devices. In patients with the clinical manifestations of myocardial ischemia, a number of studies indicate that
there may be increased concentrations of these products in the
plasma, particularly in the blood from the coronary sinus (106-110).
In a study of the value of the measurement of these platelet
products in patients with myocardial ischemia, de Boer and his
associates concluded that measurement of β-thromboglobulin and
thromboxane B_2 was of limited clinical value (111,112). They did
conclude, however, that their results were compatible with the
concept that platelets were frequently, but not invariably,
activated in patients with myocardial ischemia or infarction. In
patients with prosthetic heart valves, however, they were able
to show increased levels of PF4 and β-thromboglobulin in the
circulation; these data are in agreement with those reported by
other investigators (113,114). Thus, it seems reasonable to
conclude that these materials are only likely to be detectable in
the circulation if there is repeated platelet stimulation.

Another change in platelets resulting from their participation
in thrombosis is a decrease in their density (115). Although it
may eventually be possible to monitor thromboembolic events by
measuring platelet density changes, the wide differences among
individuals may preclude such an approach. However, further
studies are needed to determine whether it is possible to use
this technique to identify the presence of altered platelets in
the circulation. Decreased amounts of serotonin and ADP in
platelets have been demonstrated in association with thromboembolic events that would be expected to cause the release of
platelet granule contents (116,117).

Since thrombosis involves coagulation and thrombin formation,
the action of thrombin on fibrinogen can also be used to determine

whether or not thrombosis is occurring. Measurement of fibrinopeptides A and B in plasma has been developed to assess the amount
of fibrinogen cleaved by thrombin (101,118-120). This technique
may be limited by the episodic nature of thrombosis and the removal of the fibrinopeptides from plasma between episodes. This
limitation also applies to measurements of PF4, β-thromboglobulin
and thromboxane B_2 (101). With cardiopulmonary bypass, the
concentration of FPA in plasma is increased (104). The elevated
FPA levels associated with thromboembolism return to normal upon
the administration of heparin (120).

Attempts to measure the extent of thrombosis have been made
using radioactively labeled fibrinogen, platelets, or white cells
(121-123). In thrombi that have a large platelet and/or white
cell component, the use of [111]Indium-labeled platelets or white
cells does appear to give some indication of the extent of thrombosis and the turnover of the thrombus material (122,123). Modern
imaging techniques in which subtraction is used enhance the
definition in such studies and it is possible that this technology
and other noninvasive techniques may prove valuable in monitoring
thromboembolic events in vivo.

SUMMARY

Vessel injury and thrombosis can contribute to the development of
all stages of atherosclerosis and its clinical complications. In
the early lesions, platelet interaction with the subendothelium
leads to the release of substances that cause migration and
proliferation of smooth muscle cells in the intima. With more
advanced atherosclerosis, vessel injury is associated with the
formation of thrombi that may persist and become organized,
contributing to vessel wall thickening. Thrombi forming on
advanced lesions may cause clinical complications by showering the
microcirculation with emboli or by occluding a main vessel,
causing infarction. Vessel injury may also cause spasm, leading
to ischemia and the formation of thrombi as a secondary event.

Experimentally it can be shown that repeated injury to the endothelium can cause the full spectrum of atherosclerotic lesions and that withdrawal of the injury stimulus leads to regression of the lesions. The key to the control of vessel injury, thrombosis, and atherosclerosis is control of the factors that injure the endothelium. At present we have only limited knowledge about endothelial injury and no simple, accurate ways of quantitating the frequency and extent of endothelial injury in man. Techniques are being developed to measure products formed or released by injured endothelial cells, products formed or released by platelets, or products formed as a result of blood coagulation. These new techniques, as well as others for imaging of thrombi with isotopically labeled white cells, platelets, or fibrinogen, and imaging of diseased vessels, may provide new approaches for studying vessel injury, thrombosis, and the development of atherosclerosis.

REFERENCES

1. Ross R (1981) Atherosclerosis: A problem of the biology of arterial wall cells and their interactions with blood components. Arteriosclerosis 1:293-311
2. Mustard JF, Packham MA, Kinlough-Rathbone RL (1981) Platelets, atherosclerosis and clinical complications. In: Moore S (ed) Vascular injury and atherosclerosis. Marcel Dekker Inc, New York, pp 79-110
3. Ross R, Vogel A (1978) The platelet-derived growth factor. Cell 14:203-210
4. Glenn K, Ross R (1981) Human monocyte-derived growth factor(s) for mesenchymal cells: activation of secretion by endotoxin and concanavalin A [Con A]. Cell 25:603-615
5. Dzoga K, Vesselinovitch D, Fraser R, Wissler RW (1971) The effect of lipoproteins on the growth of aortic smooth muscle cells in vitro. Am J Pathol 62:32a
6. Minick CR, Fabricant CG, Fabricant J, Litrenta MM (1979) Atheroarteriosclerosis induced by infection with a herpesvirus. Am J Pathol 96:673-706
7. Goldsmith HL (1972) The flow of model particles and blood cells and its relation to thrombogenesis. In: Spaet TH (ed) Progress in hemostasis and thrombosis, vol 1. Grune and Stratton, New York, pp 97-139
8. Geer JC, Haust MD (1972) Smooth muscle cells in atherosclerosis. In: Pollak OJ, Simms HS, Kirk JE (eds) Monographs on atherosclerosis vol 2. S Karger, Basel, pp 1-140

9. Duguid JB (1946) Thrombosis as a factor in the pathogenesis of coronary atherosclerosis. J Pathol Bacteriol 58:207-212

10. Morgan AD (1956) The pathogenesis of coronary occlusion. Blackwell Scientific Publications, Oxford

11. Crawford T (1977) Pathology of ischaemic heart disease. Butterworths, London, pp 1-170

12. Woolf N, Bradley JWP, Crawford T, Carstairs KC (1968) Experimental mural thrombi in the pig aorta. The early natural history. Br J Exp Pathol 49:257-264

13. Jørgensen L, Rowsell HC, Hovig T, Mustard JF (1967) Resolution and organization of platelet-rich mural thrombi in carotid arteries of swine. Am J Pathol 51:681-719

14. Moore S (1973) Thromboatherosclerosis in normolipemic rabbits: a result of continued endothelial damage. Lab Invest 29:478-487

15. Björkerud S, Bondjers G (1976) Repair responses and tissue lipid after experimental injury to the artery. Ann NY Acad Sci 275:180-198

16. Bondjers G, Brattsand R, Hansson GK, Björkerud S (1976) Cholesterol transfer and content in aortic regions with defined endothelial integrity from rabbits with moderate hypercholesterolemia. Nutr Metab 20:452-460

17. Richardson M, Ihnatowycz I, Moore S (1980) Glycosaminogly-can distribution in rabbit aortic wall following balloon catheter deendothelialization. An ultrastructural study. Lab Invest 43:509-516

18. Minick CR (1981) Synergy of arterial injury and hypercho-lesterolemia in atherosclerosis. In: Moore S (ed) Vascular injury and atherosclerosis. Marcel Dekker Inc, New York, pp 149-173

19. Moore S (1981) Injury mechanisms in atherogenesis. In: Moore S (ed) Vascular injury and atherosclerosis. Marcel Dekker Inc, New York, pp 131-148

20. Barnett HJM (1976) Pathogenesis of transient ischemic attacks. In: Scheinberg P (ed) Cerebrovascular diseases. Raven Press, New York, pp 1-21

21. Gunning AJ, Pickering GW, Robb-Smith AHT, Russell RR (1964) Mural thrombosis of the internal carotid artery and subsequent embolism. Q J Med 33:155-195

22. Russell RWR (1961) Observations on the retinal blood vessels in monocular blindness. Lancet 2:1422-1428

23. Chandler AB, Chapman I, Erhardt LR, Roberts WC, Schwartz CJ, Sinapius D, Spain DM, Sherry S, Ness PM, Simon TL (1974) Coronary thrombosis in myocardial infarction. Report of a workshop on the role of coronary thrombosis in the patho-genesis of acute myocardial infarction. Am J Cardiol 34:823-833

24. Maseri A, L'Abbate A, Baroldi G, Chierchia S, Marzilli M, Ballestra AM, Severi S, Parodi O, Biagini A, Distante A, Pesola A (1978) Coronary vasospasm as a possible cause of myocardial infarction. A conclusion derived from the study of "preinfarction" angina. N Engl J Med 299:1271-1277

25. Braunwald E (1978) Coronary spasm and acute myocardial infarction--new possibility for treatment and prevention. N Engl J Med 299:1301-1302
26. Haerem JW (1978) Sudden, unexpected coronary death. The occurrence of platelet aggregates in the epicardial and myocardial vessels of man. Acta Pathol Microbiol Scand [A] 265:7-47
27. Jørgensen L, Rowsell HC, Hovig T, Glynn MF, Mustard JF (1967) Adenosine diphosphate-induced platelet aggregation and myocardial infarction in swine. Lab Invest 17:616-644
28. Conti CR (1980) Coronary artery spasm. Circulation 61:862-864
29. Oliva PB, Breckenridge JC (1977) Arteriographic evidence of coronary artery spasm in acute myocardial infarction. Circulation 56:366-374
30. Ganz W (1981) Editorial. Coronary spasm in myocardial infarction: fact or fiction? Circulation 63:487-488
31. Fulton GP, Akers RP, Lutz BR (1953) White thromboemboli and vascular fragility in hamster cheek pouch after anticoagulants. Blood 8:140-152
32. McFarlane RG (1972) Haemostasis. In: Biggs R (ed) Human blood coagulation, haemostasis and thrombosis. Blackwell Scientific Publications, Oxford, pp 543-585
33. Gertz SD, Uretsky G, Wajnberg R, Navot N, Gotsman MS (1981) Endothelial cell damage and thrombus formation after partial arterial constriction: relevance to the role of coronary artery spasm in the pathogenesis of myocardial infarction. Circulation 63:476-486
34. Maseri A, Chierchia S, L'Abbate A (1980) Pathogenetic mechanisms underlying the clinical events associated with atherosclerotic heart disease. Circulation 62 (Suppl V): 3-13
35. Kniker WT, Cochrane CG (1968) The localization of circulating immune complexes in experimental serum sickness. The role of vasoactive amines and hydrodynamic forces. J Exp Med 127:119-135
36. Harker LA, Ross R, Slichter SJ, Scott CR (1976) Homocystine-induced arteriosclerosis. The role of endothelial cell injury and platelet response in its genesis. J Clin Invest 58:731-741
37. Mason RG, Sharp D, Chuang HYK, Mohammad F (1977) The endo-thelium. Roles in thrombosis and hemostasis. Arch Pathol Lab Med 101:61-64
38. Mustard JF, Packham MA, Kinlough-Rathbone RL (1981) Mechanisms in thrombosis. In: Bloom AL, Thomas DP (eds) Haemostasis and thrombosis. Churchill Livingstone, London, pp 503-526
39. Hendriksen T, Evensen SA, Carlander B (1979) Injury to human endothelial cells induced by low-density lipoproteins. Scand J Clin Lab Invest 39:361-368
40. Hessler JR, Robertson AL Jr, Chisholm GM (1979) LDL-induced cytotoxicity and its inhibition in human vascular smooth

muscle and endothelial cells in culture. Atherosclerosis
32:213-229

41. Gerrity RG, Caplan BA, Richardson M, Cade JF, Hirsh J,
    Schwartz CJ (1975) Endotoxin-induced endothelial injury
    and repair. 1. Endothelial cell turnover in the aorta of
    the rabbit. Exp Mol Pathol 23:379-385

42. Curwen KD, Gimbrone MA Jr, Handin RI (1980) In vitro
    studies of thromboresistance. The role of prostacyclin
    (PGI$_2$) in platelet adhesion to cultured normal and virally
    transformed human vascular endothelial cells. Lab Invest
    42:366-374

43. Goldsmith HL, Karino T (1979) Mechanically induced thrombo-
    emboli. In: Hwang NHC, Gross DR, Patel DJ (eds) Quanti-
    tative cardiovascular studies. Clinical and research
    applications of engineering principles. University Park
    Press, Baltimore, pp 289-351

44. Chesney CM, Harper E, Colman RW (1974) Human platelet
    collagenase. J Clin Invest 53:1647-1654

45. Legrand Y, Pignaud G, Caen JP (1977) Human blood platelet
    elastase and proelastase. Activation of proelastase and
    release of elastase after adhesion of platelets to collagen.
    Haemostasis 6:180-189

46. Sacks T, Moldow CF, Craddock PR, Bowers TK, Jacob HS (1978)
    Oxygen radicals mediate endothelial cell damage by
    complement-stimulated granulocytes. An in vitro model of
    immune vascular damage. J Clin Invest 61:1161-1167

47. Harlan JM, Killen PD, Harker LA, Striker GE, Wright DG
    (1981) Neutrophil-mediated endothelial injury in vitro.
    Mechanisms of cell detachment. J Clin Invest 68:1394-1403

48. Mustard JF, Movat HZ, MacMorine DRL, Senyi A (1965)
    Release of permeability factors from the blood platelet.
    Proc Soc Exp Biol Med 119:988-991

49. Mustard JF, Packham MA (1978) The reaction of the blood
    to injury. In: Movat HZ (ed) Inflammation, immunity and
    hypersensitivity. Harper & Row, New York, pp 557-664

50. Fry DL (1976) Hemodynamic forces in atherogenesis. In:
    Scheinberg P (ed) Cerebrovascular diseases. Raven Press,
    New York, pp 77-95

51. Shimamoto T (1974) Contraction of endothelial cells as a
    key mechanism in atherogenesis and treatment of atheroscle-
    rosis with endothelial cell relaxants. In: Schettler G,
    Weizel A (eds) Atherosclerosis III. Springer-Verlag,
    New York, pp 64-82

52. Constantinides P, Robinson M (1969) Ultrastructural injury
    of arterial endothelium. II. Effects of vasoactive amines.
    Arch Pathol 88:106-112

53. Robertson AL Jr, Khairallah PA (1973) Arterial endothelial
    permeability and vascular disease: the "trap door" effect.
    Exp Mol Pathol 18:241-260

54. Joris I, Majno G (1981) Medial changes in arterial spasm
    induced by L-norepinephrine. Am J Pathol 105:212-222

55. Booyse FM, Osikowicz G, Quarfoot AJ (1981) Effects of chronic oral consumption of nicotine on the rabbit aortic endothelium. Am J Pathol 102:93-102

56. Becker CG, Dubin T, Wiedemann HP (1976) Hypersensitivity to tobacco antigen. Proc Natl Acad Sci USA 73:1712-1716

57. Becker CG, Levi R, Zavecz J (1979) Induction of IgE antibodies to antigen isolated from tobacco leaves and from cigarette smoke condensate. Am J Pathol 96:249-256

58. Asmussen I, Kjeldsen K (1975) Intimal ultrastructure of human umbilical arteries. Observations on arteries from newborn children of smoking and nonsmoking mothers. Circ Res 36:579-589

59. Editorial (1980) How does smoking harm the heart? Br Med J 3:573-574

60. Honour AJ, Russell RWR (1962) Experimental platelet embolism. Br J Exp Pathol 43:350-362

61. Baumgartner HR (1973) The role of blood flow in platelet adhesion, fibrin deposition and formation of mural thrombi. Microvasc Res 5:167-179

62. Groves HM, Kinlough-Rathbone RL, Richardson M, Moore S, Mustard JF (1979) Platelet interaction with damaged rabbit aorta. Lab Invest 40:194-200

63. Clowes AW, Collazzo RE, Karnovsky MJ (1978) A morphologic and permeability study of luminal smooth muscle cells after arterial injury in the rat. Lab Invest 39:141-150

64. Groves HM, Kinlough-Rathbone RL, Richardson M, Jørgensen L, Moore S, Mustard JF (1982) Thrombin generation and fibrin formation following injury to rabbit neointima: studies of vessel wall reactivity and platelet survival. Lab Invest 46:605-612

65. Piepgras DG, Sundt TM Jr, Didisheim P (1976) Effect of anticoagulants and inhibitors of platelet aggregation on thrombotic occlusion of endarterectomized cat carotid arteries. Stroke 7:248-254

66. Meuleman DG, Vogel GMT, van Delft AML (1980) Effects of intra-arterial cannulation on blood platelet consumption in rats. Thromb Res 20:45-55

67. Winocour PD, Cattaneo M, Kinlough-Rathbone RL, Mustard JF (1981) Vessel injury, thrombosis and platelet survival. Thromb Haemost 46:290

68. Kinlough-Rathbone RL, Packham MA, Mustard JF (1981) Platelet survival in relation to vessel wall injury. Thromb Haemost 46:248

69. Mustard JF, Murphy EA (1963) Effect of smoking on blood coagulation and platelet survival in man. Br Med J 1: 846-849

70. Fuster V, Cheseboro JH, Frye RL, Elveback LR (1981) Platelet survival and the development of coronary artery disease in the young adult: effects of cigarette smoking, strong family history and medical therapy. Circulation 63:546-551

71. Constantinides P (1981) Overview of studies on regression of atherosclerosis. Artery 9:30-43

72. Malinow MR (1980) Brief reviews. Atherosclerosis: regression in nonhuman primates. Circ Res 46:311-320

73. Berenson GS, Radhakrishnamurthy B, Srinivasan SR, Dalferes ER Jr, Malinow MR (1981) Chemical changes in the arterial wall during regression of atherosclerosis in monkeys. Artery 9:44-58

74. Armstrong ML (1976) Regression of atherosclerosis. Atheroscler Rev 1:137-182

75. Friedman RJ, Moore S, Singal DP, Gent M (1976) Regression of injury-induced atheromatous lesions in rabbits. Arch Pathol Lab Med 100:189-195

76. Fry DL (1976) Hemodynamic forces in atherogenesis. In: Scheinberg P (ed) Cerebrovascular diseases. Raven Press, New York, pp 77-95

77. Caro CG (1977) Mechanical factors in atherogenesis. In: Hwang NHC, Normann NA (eds) Cardiovascular flow dynamics and measurements. University Park Press, Baltimore, pp 473-487

78. Cooper R, Stamler J, Dyer A, Garside D (1978) The decline in mortality from coronary heart disease, USA 1968-1975. J Chronic Dis 31:709-720

79. Levy RI (1981) Declining mortality in coronary heart disease. Arteriosclerosis 1:312-325

80. Walker WJ (1977) Changing United States life-style and declining vascular mortality: cause or coincidence? N Engl J Med 297:163-165

81. Stamler J (1979) Research related to risk factors. Circulation 60:1575-1587

82. Gordon T, Kannel WB, McGee D, Dawber TR (1979) Death and coronary attacks in men after giving up cigarette smoking. Lancet 2:1345-1348

83. Wilhelmsson C, Vedin JA, Elmfeldt D, Tibblin G, Wilhelmsen L (1975) Smoking and myocardial infarction. Lancet 1:415-420

84. Hjermann I, Byre KV, Holme I, Leren P (1981) Effect of diet and smoking intervention on the incidence of coronary heart disease. Report from the Oslo Study Group of a randomised trial in healthy men. Lancet 2:1303-1316

85. Strong JP, Guzmán MA (1980) Decrease in coronary atherosclerosis in New Orleans. Lab Invest 43:297-301

86. Roth D, Kostuk WJ (1980) Noninvasive and invasive demonstration of spontaneous regression of coronary artery disease. Circulation 62:889-896

87. Blankenhorn DH, Sanmarco ME (1979) Editorial. Angiography for study of lipid-lowering therapy. Circulation 59:212-214

88. Rafflenbeul W, Smith LR, Rogers WJ, Mantle JA, Rackley CE, Russell RO Jr (1979) Quantitative coronary arteriography. Coronary anatomy of patients with unstable angina pectoris re-examined one year after optimal medical therapy. Am J Cardiol 43:699-707

89. Hollander W, Kirkpatrick B, Paddock J, Colombo M (1979)

Studies on the progression and regression of coronary and peripheral atherosclerosis in the cynomolgus monkey. 1. Effects of dipyridamole and aspirin. Exp Mol Pathol 30:55-73

90. Gaynor E, Bouvier CA, Spaet TH (1968) Circulating endothelial cells in endotoxin treated rabbits. Clin Res 16:535

91. Hladovec J, Rossmann P (1973) Circulating endothelial cells isolated together with platelets and the experimental modification of their counts in rats. Thromb Res 3:665-674

92. Bensoussan D, Levy-Toledano S, Passa P, Caen J, Canivet J (1975) Platelet hyperaggregation and increased level of von Willebrand factor in diabetics with retinopathy. Diabetologia 11:307-312

93. Brinkhous KM, Sultzer DL, Reddick RL, Griggs TR (1980) Elevated plasma von Willebrand factor (vWF) levels as an index of acute endothelial injury: use of a hypotonic injury model in rats. Fed Proc 39:630

94. Cucuianu MP, Missits I, Olinic N, Roman S (1980) Increased ristocetin-cofactor in acute myocardial infarction: a component of the acute phase reaction. Thromb Haemost 43:41-44

95. Loskutoff DJ, Edgington TS (1977) Synthesis of a fibrinolytic activator and inhibitor by endothelial cells. Proc Natl Acad Sci USA 74:3903-3907

96. Shepro D, Schleef R, Hechtman HB (1980) Plasminogen activator activity by cultured bovine aortic endothelial cells. Life Sci 26:415-422

97. Mustard JF (1978) Platelet survival. Thromb Haemost 40:154-162

98. Mustard JF, Packham MA, Kinlough-Rathbone RL (1978) Platelet survival. In: Day HJ, Holmsen H, Zucker MB (eds) Platelet function testing. DHEW Publication no. (NIH) 78-1087, US. Govt Printing Office, Washington, DC, pp 545-560

99. Adelman B, Stemerman MB, Mennell D, Handin RI (1981) The interaction of platelets with aortic subendothelium: Inhibition of adhesion and secretion by prostaglandin I_2. Blood 58:198-205

100. Goldberg ID, Stemerman MB, Handin RI (1980) Vascular permeation of platelet factor 4 after endothelial injury. Science 209:611-612

101. Kaplan KL, Owen J (1981) Plasma levels of β-thromboglobulin and platelet factor 4 as indices of platelet activation in vivo. Blood 57:199-202

102. Zahavi J, Kakkar VV (1980) β-thromboglobulin - a specific marker of in vivo platelet release reaction. Thromb Haemost 44:23-29

103. Addonizio VP Jr, Smith JB, Guiod LR, Strauss JF III, Colman RW, Edmunds LH Jr (1979) Thromboxane synthesis and platelet protein release during simulated extracorporeal circulation. Blood 54:371-376

104. Davies GC, Sobel M, Salzman EW (1980) Elevated plasma fibrinopeptide A and thromboxane B_2 levels during cardio-pulmonary bypass. Circulation 61:808-814

105. Files JC, Malpass TW, Yee EK, Ritchie JL, Harker LA (1981) Studies of human platelet α-granule release in vivo. Blood 58:607-618

106. Sobel M, Salzman EW, Davies GC, Handin RI, Sweeney J, Ploetz J, Kurland G (1981) Circulating platelet products in unstable angina pectoris. Circulation 63:300-306

107. Smitherman TC, Milam M, Woo J, Willerson JT, Frenkel EP (1981) Elevated beta-thromboglobulin in peripheral venous blood of patients with acute myocardial ischemia: direct evidence for enhanced platelet reactivity in vivo. Am J Cardiol 48:395-402

108. Lewy RI, Wiener L, Walinsky P, Lefer AM, Silver MJ, Smith JB (1980) Thromboxane release during pacing-induced angina pectoris: possible vasoconstrictor influence in the coronary vasculature. Circulation 61:1165-1171

109. Hirsh PD, Hillis LD, Campbell WB, Firth BG, Willerson JT (1981) Release of prostaglandins and thromboxane into the coronary circulation in patients with ischemic heart disease. N Engl J Med 304:685-691

110. Robertson RM, Robertson D, Roberts LJ, Maas RL, Garret AF, Friesinger GC, Oates JA (1981) Thromboxane A_2 in vasotonic angina pectoris. Evidence from direct measurements and inhibitor trials. N Engl J Med 304:998-1003

111. de Boer AC, Turpie AGG, Butt RW, Johnston RV, Genton E (1982) Platelet release and thromboxane synthesis in symptomatic coronary artery disease. Circulation 66:327-333

112. de Boer AC, Turpie AGG, Genton E (1982) Chemistry, measure-ment and clinical significance of platelet specific proteins. In: Clinical reviews in clinical and laboratory sciences. Vol 18. CRC Press Inc, Boca Raton, Florida, pp 183-211

113. Pumphrey CW, Dawes J (1981) Elevation of plasma β-thrombo-globulin in patients with prosthetic cardiac valves. Thromb Res 22:147-155

114. Dudczak R, Niessner H, Thaler E, Lechner K, Kletter K, Frischauf H, Domanig E, Aicher H (1981) Plasma concentra-tion of platelet-specific proteins and fibrinopeptide A in patients with artificial heart valves. Haemostasis 10: 186-194

115. Packham MA, Mustard JF, Guccione MA, Winocour PD, Groves HM, Rand ML, Kinlough-Rathbone RL (1979) Investigation of in vivo factors that may influence platelet survival and density. Thromb Haemost 42:328 (abstr)

116. Clagett GP, Russo M, Hufnagel H, Collins GJ Jr, Rich NM (1980) Platelet serotonin changes in dogs with prosthetic aortic grafts. J Surg Res 28:223-229

117. Beurling-Harbury C, Galvan CA (1978) Acquired decrease in platelet secretory ADP associated with increased postoper-ative bleeding in post-cardiopulmonary bypass patients and

in patients with severe valvular heart disease.   Blood
52:13-23

118. Kaplan KL, Nossel HL, Drillings M, Lesznik G (1978)
Radioimmunoassay of platelet factor 4 and β-thromboglobulin:
development and application to studies of platelet release
in relation to fibrinopeptide A generation.   Br J Haematol
39:129-146

119. Nossel HL, Butler VP Jr, Canfield RE, Yudelman I, Ti M,
Spanondis K, Soland T (1975) Potential use of fibrinopeptide A measurements in the diagnosis and management of
thrombosis.   Thromb Haemost 33:426-434

120. Bilezikian SB, Nossel HL, Butler VP Jr, Canfield RE (1975)
Radioimmunoassay of fibrinopeptide B and kinetics of fibrinopeptide cleavage by different enzymes.   J Clin Invest
56:438-445

121. Salimi A, Oliver GC Jr, Lee J, Sherman LA (1977) Continued
incorporation of circulating radiolabeled fibrinogen into
preformed coronary artery thrombi.   Circulation 56:213-217

122. Ritchie JL, Stratton JR, Thiele B, Hamilton GW, Warrick LN,
Huang TW, Harker LA (1981) Indium-111 platelet imaging
for detection of platelet deposition in abdominal aneurysms
and prosthetic arterial grafts.   Am J Cardiol 47:882-889

123. Davies RA, Thakur ML, Berger HJ, Wackers FJT, Gottschalk A,
Zaret BL (1981) Imaging the inflammatory response to acute
myocardial infarction in man using indium-111-labeled
autologous platelets.   Circulation 63:826-832

A DISCUSSION OF PLATELET THROMBI IN ATHEROGENESIS: M. DARIA HAUST

Dr. Mustard's address on the subject matter under consideration not only was thorough and complete, but the contents of his presentation are in agreement with my own views. Therefore, instead of discussing his address it may be more useful to draw the attention to some still-existing controversy on the topic of microthrombi and add in brief a few data from our work regarding the mode of their organization.

The controversy regarding the arterial microthrombi relates largely to two areas: whether they occur at all, and if so, do they play any role in atherogenesis? The latter controversy is perhaps best illustrated by Dr. Small's presentation in which microthrombi were not even mentioned as precursor lesions of atherosclerotic plaques. Some investigators, however, firmly believe that arterial microthrombi represent one form of the early lesions of atherosclerosis, and have no problem in finding the tiny thrombi in the arteries of man (1-14) and experimental animal (15). In support of the contention that these deposits represent lesions of inception of atherosclerosis are the observations that they occur on the intima of normal porcine aorta at the orifices of the intercostal arteries and at bifurcations (15), i.e., in a distribution resembling that of atherosclerotic lesions developing in the pig. Moreover, the sites of deposition of microthrombi in extracorporeal circulation of swine are similar to those of early atherosclerotic lesions in vivo of the same species (16).

The difficulty in establishing the true incidence of occurrence of microthrombi on arterial intimal surface may be attributed to our inability to detect the minute thrombotic deposits on gross examination. Thus, microthrombi are observed incidentally on microscopic examination only. They were found in several arteries (aorta and coronary, renal, and testicular arteries) and

This work was supported by a grant-in-aid of research T.3-11 from the Ontario Heart Foundation, Toronto, Canada.

at all ages, even in young children (3,7,8). As documented by
the examples shown at this Workshop, the microthrombi may be of
different shapes, size, and composition. They may consist
largely of fibrin or of platelets, but most commonly are of a
"mixed" variety. Endothelium may cover these deposits entirely
or in part, but not all microthrombi are endothelialized and thus
may be resolved or dislodged (1).

Microthrombi have been observed on an unaltered intima
displaying only the presence of diffuse intimal thickening
(1,3,5,8,9), but at times a slight edema (See Fig. 10 in Ref. 4)
or a tiny yellow dot are evident in the immediately adjacent
intima (7). In the latter two instances it is difficult to
assess whether the microthrombus preceded or followed the changes
in the intima.

The size and shapes of these small mural deposits also vary
(1). Some microthrombi are flat or molded into the intimal
substance, and may extend over a considerable surface (1,9).
Other microthrombi protrude slightly or considerably into the
arterial lumen (1,3).

The largest problem with respect to the arterial microthrombi
relates to their incidence. In one study undertaken in systematic search of microthrombi at a specific site in aortae of
young children, no such deposits were found (17). In another
study, microthrombi were present in seven serially sectioned
segments of left coronary arteries obtained at autopsy from nine
patients ranging in age from 12 to 30 years (12-14). In three of
these instances the microthrombi were found on normal intima and
in six they were superimposed on an underlying intimal lesion.

Microthrombi that are endothelialized are ultimately organized to connective tissues similar to those of the surrounding
intima, but their connective tissue components are "young" and
may be the hallmark of their thrombotic derivation for some time
(See Fig. 21 in Ref. 3). A microthrombus when organized may
become a nidus for repeated deposition of small or larger

thrombi. Moreover, secondary changes within its substance and/or the underlying intima all may contribute to the progression of the "compounded" alterations culminating in the formation of an advanced atherosclerotic lesion.

The process of organization of a microthrombus is in itself an interesting phenomenon and was studied in our laboratories in man and in experimental animals (rabbits). Endothelium overgrows the tiny deposit in approximately 24 h although all components of the mural deposit may be still well preserved with the platelets within it retaining their granules (See Fig. 6.35 in Ref. 7). Soon thereafter, smooth muscle cells from the underlying intima migrate into the substance of the microthrombus, multiply here and "organize" the now altered blood components into connective tissues (See Fig. 5 in Ref. 18). Ultimately, the entire small thrombus is converted to connective tissues, and smooth muscle cells--best identified on electron microscopic examination (See Fig. 8 in Ref. 2)--are the only cellular elements present. They are usually arranged in rows parallel to each other and to the intimal surface.

In conclusion, it may be stated that arterial microthrombi do occur and when organized, should be viewed as precursor-lesions of the advanced atherosclerotic plaques. Intimal smooth muscle cells migrate into the substance of these deposits and are instrumental in the process of their organization.

REFERENCES

1. Haust MD (1971) The morphogenesis and fate of potential and early atherosclerotic lesions in man. Hum Pathol 2:1-29
2. Haust MD (1977) Thrombosis in the inception and progression of coronary atherosclerotic lesions. In: Schettler G, Horsch A, Morl H, Orth H, Weizel A (eds) Der Herzinfarkt. FK Schattauer Verlag, Stuttgart-New York, pp 120-135
3. Haust MD (1978) Atherosclerosis in childhood. In: Rosenberg HS, Bolande RP (eds) Perspectives in pediatric pathology, Vol 4. Year Book Medical Publishers Inc, Chicago, pp 155-216

4. Haust MD (1978) Light and electron microscopy of human atherosclerotic lesions. Adv Exp Med Biol 104:33-59

5. Haust MD (1978) Zur Morphologie der Arteriosklerose. Internist (Berlin) 19:621-626

6. Haust MD (1981) The natural history of atherosclerotic lesions. In: Moore S (ed) Vascular injury and atherosclerosis, Marcel Dekker Inc, New York, pp 1-23

7. Haust MD (1982) Atherosclerosis; - lesions and sequelae. In: Silver MD (ed) Cardiovascular pathology. Churchill-Livingston, New York

8. Haust MD, More RH (1960) The thrombotic basis of arteriosclerosis. Heart Bull 9:90-92

9. Movat HZ, Haust MD, More RH (1959) The morphologic elements in the early lesions of arteriosclerosis. Am J Pathol 35: 93-101

10. Mustard JF (1967) Recent advances in molecular pathology: a review. Platelet aggregation, vascular injury and atherosclerosis. Exp Mol Pathol 7:366-377

11. Mustard JF (1975) Function of blood platelets and their role in thrombosis. Trans Am Clin Climatol Assoc 87:104-127

12. Chandler AB (1972) Thrombosis in the development of coronary atherosclerosis. In: Likoff W, Segal BL, Insull W Jr, Moyer JH (eds) Atherosclerosis and coronary heart disease. Grune and Stratton Inc, New York, p 28

13. Chandler AB (1974) Mechanisms and frequency of thrombosis in the coronary circulation. Thromb. Res. 4(Suppl):3-23

14. Chandler AB, Pope JT (1975) Arterial thrombosis in atherogenesis. A survey of the frequency of incorporation of thrombi into atherosclerotic plaques. In: Hautvast JGAJ, Hermus RJJ, Van Der Haar F (eds) Blood and arterial wall in atherogenesis and arterial thrombosis. EJ Brill, Leiden, The Netherlands, pp 111-118

15. Geissinger HD, Mustard JF, Rowsell HC (1962) The occurrence of microthrombi on the aortic endothelium of swine. Can Med Assoc J 87:405-408

16. Murphy EA, Rowsell HC, Downie HG, Robinson GA, Mustard JF (1962) Encrustation and atherosclerosis: the analogy between early in vivo lesions and deposits which occur in extracorporeal circulations. Can Med Assoc J 87:259-274

17. Hudson J, McCaughey WTE (1974) Mural thrombosis and atherogenesis in coronary arteries and aorta. An investigation using antifibrin and antiplatelet sera. Atherosclerosis 19: 543-553

18. Haust MD (to be published) Atherosclerosis and smooth muscle cells. In: Stephens NL (ed) Biochemistry of smooth muscle. CRC Press Inc, Boca Raton

23

Review of Clinical Studies on the Quantification and Progression of Atherosclerosis

MICHAEL B. MOCK

EPIDEMIOLOGIC POPULATION STUDIES

Beginning in the early 1950s, a number of epidemiologic population studies were carried out to identify those persons who were at high risk for the development of atherosclerotic disease and death. The most notable of these population studies is the Framingham Study, supported by the National Heart, Lung, and Blood Institute (NHLBI) (1). This large community study of an asymptomatic population with subsequent long-term follow-up has firmly established a relationship between certain clinical risk factors and the development of clinical manifestations of atherosclerotic disease. The most important risk factors that have been identified are age, sex, cigarette smoking, serum cholesterol levels, hypertension, family history, and diabetes. A shortcoming of the epidemiologic community studies is that they are most useful in identifying high risk that is concentrated on the high end of the frequency distribution for each of these particular risk factors. Rose (2) has pointed out that a strategy of atherosclerotic disease control based on a few persons with high values for these individual risk factors is not likely to contribute much to the control of the disease as a whole. This can be illustrated by using the cholesterol data from men, aged 55 to 64, in the Framingham Study. When the relationship between the serum cholesterol

levels and attributable coronary heart disease mortality was
correlated in 1000 men of ages 55 to 64 who were enrolled in the
Framingham Study and followed for a 10-year period, only one death
occurred, in a man whose cholesterol level was more than 310 mg/dl.
Seven deaths occurred in men with cholesterol levels of 250 mg/dl
or less (Fig. 1). Another major shortcoming of community epidemiologic studies is the rather low sensitivity and lack of specificity of the clinical endpoints that are used in these studies.
Many asymptomatic patients who have been identified as having one
or more of the major risk factors have, with long-term follow-up,
remained free of clinical manifestations of coronary artery
disease.

CONTROLLED INTERVENTION STUDIES WITH CLINICAL ENDPOINTS

The epidemiologic population studies provided the first substantial
data suggesting that medical intervention might affect the progression of coronary artery disease. There were many in the health
care community who were ready to accept the total validity of the
available data regarding the major risk factors and to apply them

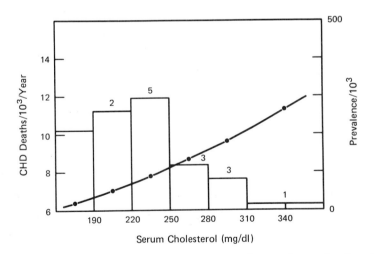

Fig. 1   Epidemiological population study: the relationship
between serum cholesterol and 1-year (CHD) mortality in 1000 men
in the Framingham Study.   (From Ref. 2 with permission from
Blackwell Scientific Publications, Ltd.)

to the population as a whole. There were others, stressing the
need for more information concerning the effectiveness of inter-
vening to counter these presumed risk factors, who asked for more
information on the possible hazards or undesirable consequences
of such intervention. This led to the development of the large
controlled intervention studies with clinical endpoints. One of
these studies, the Oslo Randomized Trial on the Effect of Diet and
Smoking Intervention on the Incidence of Coronary Heart Disease,
has recently reported on the outcome of its trial (3). In the
Oslo trial, 1232 asymptomatic, normotensive men were identified
as being at possible high risk for coronary heart disease on the
basis of cholesterol levels and smoking habits. The men in the
intervention group were advised to lower their lipids by a change
in diet and to stop smoking. Over the 5 years of the study, the
mean fasting serum cholesterol concentrations were 13% lower in
the intervention group than in the control group. The mean
tobacco consumption decreased by 45% more in the intervention
group than in the control group. It is of interest to note,
however, that only 25% of the smokers in the intervention group
stopped smoking completely compared with 17% in the control group.
Over the course of the 5-year follow-up, the incidence of fatal
and nonfatal myocardial infarction and sudden death considered
together as clinical events was significantly lower in the intervention group as compared with the control (Fig. 2). On the basis
of the 47% lower event rate in the intervention group, these
investigators concluded that a change in eating habits and cessation of smoking significantly reduces the incidence of the first
event of myocardial infarction and of sudden death.

In the United States a national study of primary prevention
of coronary heart disease, called the Multiple Risk Factor Intervention Trial (MRFIT) is scheduled to release the results of its
study later this year. The MRFIT study is a much larger, more
rigorously controlled study, with 20 geographically separate
clinical centers and with laboratories and a data center that are

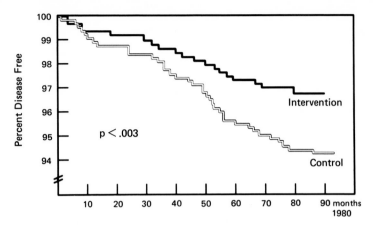

Fig. 2 Controlled intervention study with clinical endpoints:
Oslo randomized trial on the effect of diet and smoking inter-
vention on the incidence of coronary heart disease. (From
Ref. 3 with permission from The Lancet Ltd.)

independent of the clinical centers (4). Twelve thousand men aged
35-57 were enrolled and randomized to either "active" intervention
of dietary instruction, drug treatment of hypertension and advice
on stopping smoking or to "usual care." The endpoint was defined
as death by coronary heart disease (CHD).

Another major randomized intervention study with clinical endpoints is the NHLBI Coronary Primary Prevention Trial, which is a
national multicenter study being carried out at 12 lipid research
clinics (5). In this study, men 40-49 years of age with no history
of hypertension, angina, or myocardial infarction but with plasma
cholesterol levels above 265 mg/dl were randomized to treatment
with the cholesterol-lowering drug cholestyramine or a placebo.
The 12 collaborating lipid research clinics had recruited 3810 men
by 1976, and the plan is for a minimum follow-up of 7 years. The
primary endpoints are CHD death and nonfatal myocardial infarction.
Secondary endpoints for this study will be atherothrombotic brain
infarction, arterial peripheral vascular disease, angina pectoris,
intermittent claudication, transient cerebral ischemic attacks,
abnormal exercise electrocardiographic study, and other mortality
attributed by death certificate to atherosclerotic vascular

disease. This trial is, in a manner of speaking, the flagship of
the "lipid theory" for coronary atherosclerotic disease. It is
an impeccably designed randomized, double-blind trial that has
recruited a sufficient number of participants who are receiving
a cholesterol-lowering drug that should achieve a sufficient
cholesterol differential between the treatment group and the
control group. It would also seem that they have selected participants who have potentially reversible lesions. This study
certainly has satisfactory laboratory and data-handling support
and sound statistical methods for data analysis. We await with
great interest the results of this controlled study, which are
scheduled to be reported in 1983.

The epidemiologic studies of large populations have clearly
demonstrated that atherosclerosis is a degenerative arterial
disease that progresses over time and that persons with certain
identified risk factors experience higher incidence of myocardial
damage or death. However, since these studies only evaluate
clinical endpoints, we cannot be certain that the myocardial
infarction or death is always related to the extent of obstructive
disease in the coronary arteries. We must also consider the
possibility that these risk factors could also act directly on the
myocardium and its conduction system, causing disorders that could
lead to the development of clinical cardiovascular endpoints.

CLINICAL ANGIOGRAPHIC STUDIES

The advent of coronary arteriography in the late 1950s provided a
graphic anatomic delineation of the presence and extent of obstructive coronary artery disease in life. A number of clinical studies
have demonstrated the correlation between the anatomic extent of
disease and cumulative survival. One of the most recent studies
reporting a direct correlation between anatomic extent of disease
and cumulative survival is the Coronary Artery Surgery Study,
CASS, sponsored by the National Institutes of Health (6). This
study reports on 20,088 patients enrolled in the CASS registry

without previous coronary artery bypass surgery who are receiving
medical therapy. The 4-year survival of medically treated patients with no significant obstructive disease is 97%, in contrast
to 92%, 84%, and 68% in patients with one-, two-, and three-vessel
disease, respectively on the basis of 70% obstruction.

Coronary angiographic studies in large populations of patients
also offered an opportunity to examine the correlation between
occurrence of clinical risk factors and significant obstruction in
the coronary arteries. Vlietstra and coworkers (7) utilized the
CASS registry to demonstrate that certain risk factors (sex, cigarette smoking, and serum cholesterol level) were significantly
correlated with the finding of obstructive coronary artery disease.

These studies have demonstrated that there is substantial
independence among the major risk factors. Therefore, the absolute
risk of a particular factor is interdependent on the presence or
absence of the other major risk factors. Thus, the absolute risk
for a person who smokes cigarettes is significantly higher for one
who also has an elevated cholesterol level and hypertension than for
one who is normotensive and is not hypercholesterolemic (Fig. 3).

Coronary angiography has also provided a tool for the quantitative estimate of the progression of the arterial stenotic lesion
in living persons. Shub and his associates (8) at the Mayo Clinic
analyzed serial coronary angiograms in 65 symptomatic patients to
study the relationships among risk factors and coronary angiographic data, seeking to determine what factors might lead to the
progression of arterial stenosis in coronary artery disease. They
studied the relationships among the various clinical and laboratory risk factors and the angiographic data on the progression of
stenotic lesions in the coronary artery, using stepwise linear
discriminant analysis. They could not find any clinical risk
factor or laboratory data that significantly correlated with
progression (Fig. 4). They did find that the probability of
having progression to complete occlusion was related to the
severity of the stenosis at the time of the initial angiography.

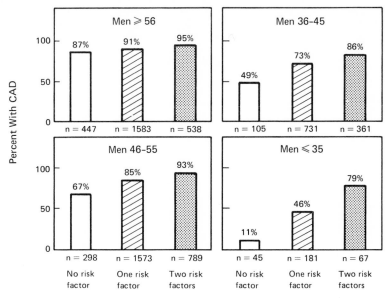

Fig. 3   Clinical angiographic study: the relationship between coronary artery disease (CAD) risk factors and coronary artery disease: the Coronary Artery Surgery Study.   (From Ref. 7 with permission from the American Heart Association, Inc.)

When an initial lesion was 98% to 99% occluded, the progression to complete occlusion on repeat angiography was 90% (Fig. 5).   In a similar serial clinical angiographic study, Rösch and Rahimtoola (9) evaluated 77 patients with coronary artery disease and correlated the progression of coronary arterial stenosis with the type of the initial stenosis demonstrated on angiography.   They discovered that the highest tendency to progression was found in patients with tubular stenosis with ulcerating plaques. Tubular, irregular and short eccentric stenoses also showed a high tendency to progress (Fig. 6).   They further reported an increased rate of progression of coronary artery disease in lesions that were located in the proximal segments of the coronary artery, particularly in the right coronary artery.

Campeau and his associates (10) at the Montreal Heart Institute performed coronary angiograms on 75 unselected patients after coronary artery bypass graft surgery.   They demonstrated that the loss

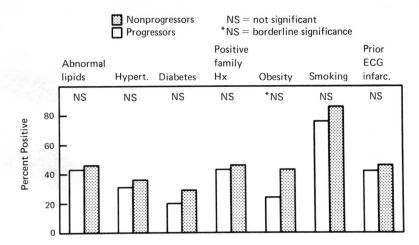

Fig. 4 Clinical angiographic study: the effect of risk factors
on the progression of coronary artery disease. (From Ref. 8
with permission.)

of symptomatic benefit and the return of angina pectoris in these
patients were related to the progression of the atherosclerotic
process, both in the graft and, more significantly, in the ungrafted
coronary arteries. They reported that progressive changes in these
grafts were observed in 5.1% of the patients who had continued
improvement versus 27.3% of patients in whom angina pectoris
redeveloped. Even more striking was the finding that 12.8% of the
patients who continued to improve showed significant changes in
the arteries, compared with 50% of those whose improvement had not
persisted (Fig. 7).

Although these serial angiographic studies have provided
valuable information, they are fraught with severe logistic
problems. They represent very selective populations of symptomatic patients and may not be representative of the natural history
of the disease in asymptomatic patients. The patients selected
for repeat studies generally are those with persistent or progressive clinical symptoms. Thus, these study populations represent a smaller number of patients with stable disease and, of
course, exclude all patients whose disease was fatal.

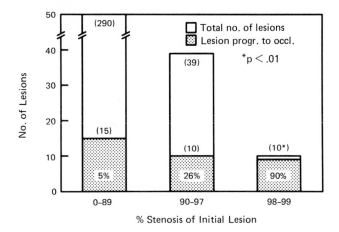

Fig. 5   Clinical angiographic study: the effect of initial percent stenosis on the progression to complete occlusion.   (From
Ref. 8 with permission.)

CONTROLLED INTERVENTION STUDIES WITH ANGIOGRAPHIC ENDPOINTS

Controlled randomized studies in which all enrolled patients
undergo angiography at baseline and at a predetermined future date
in spite of the progression of symptoms overcome some of the
problems of retrospective clinical angiographic studies.   The
first major study with this experimental design is the NHLBI Type
II Coronary Intervention Study (11).   In this study, 143 patients
with type II hyperlipoproteinemia and coronary artery disease were
enrolled between 1972 and 1976.   Patients were randomly assigned
to a daily dosage of 24 g cholestyramine and a diet, or placebo
and a diet.   The type II Coronary Intervention Study is the first
multicenter secondary prevention trial of a cholesterol-lowering
agent employing as its endpoint the arteriographic changes in the
coronary arteries.   By their use of angiographic changes in the
coronary artery, more "positive endpoints" should potentially be
determined so that a smaller number of patients is required than
in the larger epidemiologic-type trials discussed earlier, which
have clinical endpoints of mortality or morbidity.   However,
because the lesion change in the coronary arteries is a unique
and more "fragile" endpoint, it is essential that it be measured

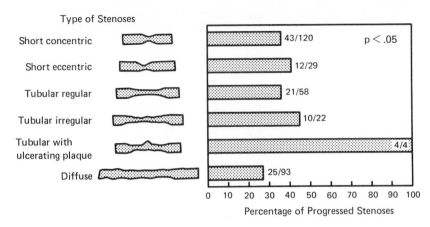

Fig. 6 Clinical angiographic study: the effect of initial type
of stenosis on the progression of coronary artery disease.
(From Ref. 9 with permission from the F. A. Davis Company.)

accurately.   In the type II study, an elaborate methodological
process for reading sequential angiograms has been developed.
For each participant in the type II study, the baseline and
5-year follow-up angiograms were evaluated with side-by-side
comparison by three separate panels. These panels consist of
three expert angiographers, who reached a consensus evaluation.
The quality control procedures were rigid and demanded that 20%
of the pairs be read by each of the three panels a second time
6 months after the first reading. The task for the panels was
to measure the reduction in luminal diameter for each lesion on
the two films and to indicate whether a change was noted.   When
the films were evaluated side by side, the temporal sequence of
the set of films was not known to the panel. Thus, they did not
know whether they were reading an improvement or a deterioration.
Readings were made by the use of cut films, and the readers
located the site of lesions of 50% or greater on copies of cut
films. We await with great interest the report of the data
analysis from the NHLBI Type II Coronary Intervention Study
later this year.

Another intervention trial using angiographic endpoints is the
clinical trial of the partial ileal bypass operation used in the

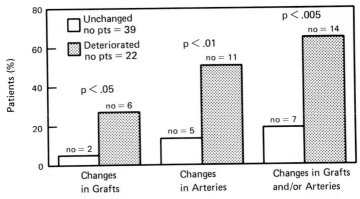

Fig. 7 Clinical angiographic study: the progression of coronary atherosclerotic disease 6 years or less after aortocoronary by-pass surgery correlated with angina pectoris. (From Ref. 10 with permission from the American Heart Association, Inc.)

treatment of patients with hyperlipidemia being conducted by Dr. Buchwald and associates (12,13) at the University of Minnesota Medical School. Dr. Buchwald's group performed the first human partial ileal bypass operation specifically for cholesterol reduction in 1963. In their series of more than 100 patients, they reported that the cholesterol level was reduced an average of 41% from the preoperative level. However, they do report great variability from patient to patient, with the cholesterol response varying from a 5% to a 79% reduction. They reported that 66% experienced improvement in angina, and 55% exhibited apparent nonprogression on serial coronary angiogram (mean 3.6 years). Twenty-two patients had comparable serial angiograms, 9 patients had comparable pelvic arteriograms with no apparent progression (mean 4.3 years), and 3 patients (13.6%) exhibited apparent coronary artery "true plaque" regression. An on-going randomized study is in progress.

In preliminary reports from the serial arteriography of the coronary arteries, Buchwald and associates (12) report an apparent nonprogression rate of coronary artery disease in 55% of the patients who were followed for up to 3 years after ileal bypass. They reported coronary arteriographic evidence of true plaque

regression in three of their partial ileal bypass patients. This
group of investigators has an ongoing randomized clinical trial
evaluating the effect of ileal bypass surgical treatment of hyperlipidemic patients; the endpoint is serial coronary arteriograms.

Barndt and his associates (14) have reported a serial angiographic study in which they evaluated the femoral arteries in 25
patients with hyperlipoproteinemia who were subsequently treated
with diet and, when indicated, drug therapy. They found 13
patients who showed progression, 9 who had regression, and 3 who
had no change. Within the group of 25 patients as a whole, the
magnitude and rate of change were almost a continuum. Evaluation
of the rate of change showed that progression occurred at a faster
rate (Fig. 8). During the 13-month interval between the baseline
and the follow-up angiograms, the average cholesterol level of the
group showing regression was significantly lower than that of the
group showing progression. The average reduction of the cholesterol level in the group showing regression was 65.2 mg/dl,
compared with an average reduction of 19.3 mg/dl in the group of
patients showing progression. In addition to the standard visual
evaluation of the angiograms, the investigators also evaluated the
femoral angiograms by a computer-controlled image-sectoring method
developed by Dr. Blankenhorn's laboratory (15). They found the
correlation between the visual readings and the computer-controlled
image readings was good ($r = 0.68$). Although they were encouraged
by their findings of regression of femoral atherosclerotic lesions,
they realized that their sample size was small and they emphasized
that they had studied patients with early disease. Their patients'
average age was 48 years, and only one of their patients had the
symptoms of claudication. Dr. Blankenhorn's laboratory has now
undertaken a randomized intervention trial and is utilizing
angiographic endpoints. To date, 80 patients have been randomized
to treatment with cholestyramine in order to lower the cholesterol
level, and 80 patients have received a placebo.

Although the angiographic technique has provided an excellent
tool for quantifying the extent of atherosclerotic vascular disease

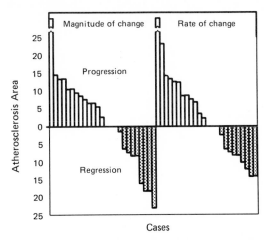

Fig. 8 A clinical intervention study with angiographic endpoints: the progression and regression of femoral atherosclerosis in treated hyperlipoproteinemic patients. (From Ref. 14 with permission from the American College of Physicians.)

there are certain drawbacks to this method. We must remember that, when we use the angiographic technique to define stenotic lesions, what is measured is the lumen that is filled with contrast dye. The actual nature of the obstructing plaque and altered vessel wall is not demonstrated by this method.

Some of the problems that complicate the use of serial angiograms for evaluating the extent of vascular disease are the invasive nature of the technique, the high cost of each study, the rather high level of radiation exposure, the interobserver variability in interpreting serial studies, the possibility that vascular spasm is being interpreted as a fixed lesion and technical variability in serial studies.

Ultrasound B-mode and intravenous subtraction angiography are two techniques for visualizing atherosclerotic obstructions in the arteries of living patients in a less invasive way than intraarterial angiography. Although both of these techniques have gone beyond the investigational stage and are receiving broad clinical use in a number of institutions, their efficacy for quantifying baseline atherosclerotic disease and then measuring progression

and regression in the clinical setting has not yet been fully
demonstrated. The NHLBI Ultrasound B-mode Assessment Program for
Iliofemoral and Carotid Atherosclerotic Disease being carried
out by the Devices and Technology Branch of the NHLBI, is now
beginning pilot studies at seven cooperating institutions. This
important program for validating the ultrasound B-mode method will
provide quantitative information on the reliability of this technique used in a clinical setting. The B-mode results will be
compared with the angiographic, functional, surgical, and pathologic findings. The common protocols, which will be carried out
at a number of geographically separate institutions, with the data
being analyzed at a distant data coordinating center, will answer
important questions regarding operator and interpreter variability. The design of this validation study of a noninvasive imaging
technique for atherosclerotic vascular disease can serve as a
model that could be applied to other noninvasive techniques for
evaluating the extent of atherosclerotic vascular disease. The
interdisciplinary effort being used in this project, including
bioengineers, radiologists, pathologists, neurologists, vascular
surgeons, and cardiologists, is laudable. Similar efforts with
other techniques are needed if we are to develop a suitable,
noninvasive technique for evaluating the entire vascular system
of patients of both sexes and of all ages over a number of years.
These techniques offer the promise that in the future we will be
able to design clinical studies in which we can accurately and
safely locate and quantify this insidious process in each individual patient and determine the most appropriate medical inter-
vention--be it diet control or pharmacologic--or surgical intervention at an early stage of the process. Such methods will also
allow follow-up of the individual patient's response and accurately
and affordably identify those patients requiring treatment before
the occurrence of the clinical events of atherosclerotic vascular
disease, that currently often precipitate unheralded death and
disability.

REFERENCES

1. Kannel WB, Gordon T, Sorlie P (eds) (1971) The Framingham study: an epidemiological investigation of cardiovascular disease. Section 27: coronary heart disease, atherothrombotic brain infarction, intermittent claudication--a multivariate analysis of some factors related to their incidence: Framingham study, 16-year followup. Government Printing Office, Washington, DC

2. Rose G (1976) Detection of high coronary risk. Postgrad Med J 52:452-455

3. Hjermann I, Velve Byre K, Holme I, Leren P (1981) Effect of diet and smoking intervention on the incidence of coronary heart disease: report from the Oslo Study Group of a randomised trial in healthy men. Lancet 2:1303-1310

4. The multiple risk factor intervention trial (MRFIT) (1976) A national study of primary prevention of coronary heart disease. JAMA 235:825-827

5. The Lipid Research Clinics Program (1979) The coronary primary prevention trial: design and implementation. J Chronic Dis 32:609-631

6. Mock MB, Ringqvist I, Fisher LD, Davis KB, Chaitman BR, Kouchoukos NT, Kaiser GC, Alderman E, Ryan TJ, Russell RO Jr, Mullin S, Fray D, Killip T III, and participants in the Coronary Surgery Study (1982) Survival of medically treated patients in the Coronary Artery Surgery Study (CASS) registry. Circulation 66:562-574

7. Vlietstra RE, Frye RL, Kronmal RA, Sim DA, Tristani FE, Killip T III, and participants in the Coronary Artery Surgery Study (1980) Risk factors and angiographic coronary artery disease: A report from the Coronary Artery Surgery Study (CASS). Circulation 62:254-261

8. Shub C, Vlietstra RE, Smith HC, Fulton RE, Elveback LR (1981) The unpredictable progression of symptomatic coronary artery disease: A serial clinical-angiographic analysis. Mayo Clin Proc 56:155-160

9. Rösch J, Rahimtoola SH (1977) Progression of angiographically determined coronary stenosis. Cardiovasc Clin 8:55-70

10. Campeau L, Lespérance J, Hermann J, Corbara F, Grondin CM, Bourassa MG (1979) Loss of the improvement of angina between 1 and 7 years after aortocoronary bypass surgery: Correlations with changes in vein grafts and in coronary arteries. Circulation 60:1-5

11. Brensike JF, Kelsey SF, Passamini ER, Fisher MR, Richardson JM, Loh IK, Stone NJ, Aldrich RF, Battaglini JW, Moriarty DJ, Myrianthopoulos MB, Detre KM, Epstein SE, Levy RI (1982) National Heart, Lung, and Blood Institute Type II Coronary Intervention Study: Design, methods, and baseline characteristics. Controlled Clin Trials 3:91-111

12. Buchwald H, Moore RB, Varco RL (1974) The partial ileal

bypass operation in treatment of the hyperlipidemias. Adv Exp Med Biol 63:221-230

13. Knight L, Scheibel R, Amplatz K, Varco RL, Buchwald H (1972) Radiographic appraisal of the Minnesota partial ileal bypass study. Surg Forum 23:141-142

14. Barndt R Jr, Blankenhorn DH, Crawford DW, Brooks SH (1977) Regression and progression of early femoral atherosclerosis in treated hyperlipoproteinemic patients. Ann Intern Med 86: 139-146

15. Crawford DW, Sanmarco ME, Blankenhorn DH (1979) Spatial reconstruction of human femoral atheromas showing regression. Am J Med 66:784-789

DISCUSSION: DAVID H. BLANKENHORN

A number of trials are now in progress where the primary endpoint
is a measured change in atherosclerosis. One of these, an intramural trial at the National Heart, Lung, and Blood Institute, is
reported to be in final stages of film reading and data analysis.
Seven other trials are at an earlier stage; Table A.1 presents an
overview of these seven trials drawn from personal communication
with the principal investigators.

Five of the seven studies are in the United States, two are
in Europe. Four of the seven studies are randomized. The age
of subjects ranges from 20 years to 69 years; two of the trials
include only men. The major criterion for entry is either an
elevation of blood lipid level or manifest atherosclerosis. The
trial in Northern California conducted by Havel is limited to
patients with familial Type II hyperlipoproteinemia. The other
trials for which the major entry criterion is blood lipid level
accept other hyperlipoproteinemic types.

By far the largest trial is the Minnesota/Multicenter trial,
for which the principal endpoint is ischemic heart disease (IHD),
mortality, or morbidity; angiographic endpoints are a secondary
feature. The 800 subjects in this study provide a relatively
small sample size to test an IHD mortality endpoint, but constitute a very large angiographic trial. The principal reason why
angiographic trials are smaller than mortality-based trials is
that a measurement of atherosclerosis change is obtained in every
subject for whom angiograms are obtained; and so all subjects
provide endpoint data. In a mortality trial only the subjects
who die provide endpoint data.

Most trials are attempting to produce a major change in blood
lipid levels through use of vigorous drug therapy or partial ileal
bypass. One trial is testing the effect of diet.

Four of the seven trials will employ computerized angiographic
measurement of lesions. The location of the laboratory where
computer analysis will be performed is indicated. Three trials

M. B. Mock

Table A.1. Clinical trials in progress.

Principal Investigator	Location	Randomized	Age	Sex	Major Entry Criterion
Arntzenius	The Netherlands	No	Under 60	M/F	Angina
Blankenhorn	South. Calif.	Yes	40-59	M	Coronary artery bypass graft
Buchwald	Minnesota/ Multicenter	Yes	30-64	M/F	Myocardial infarct
Havel	North. Calif.	Yes	21-55	M/F	Type II
Kuo	New Jersey	No	20-65	M/F	Type II, IV, and Mixed
Nash	New York	No	30-69	M/F	Coronary angiogram positive
Olsson	Sweden	Yes	40-69	M	Type II, III, and IV

[a]Jet Propulsion Laboratory of the California Institute of Technology and the University of Southern California School of Medicine.

plan to interpret films with a panel of human readers. A variety of additional endpoint measures are planned, but only major auxiliary endpoint measures are listed in Table A.1.

Number Now in Trial	Total Number to be Enrolled	Angiogram Vessel Sites	Angiographic Interval (years)	Principal Therapy Agent Under Test	Endpoint Measurement
52	52	Coronary	2	Diet with increased linoleic acid	Computerized angiograms (Ultrecht)
58	160	Femoral, Coronary, Carotid	2	Colestid-Niacin	Computerized angiograms and Ultrasound (JPL/USC)[a]
540	800	Coronary, Pelvic	3 & 5	Ileal bypass	Panel Reading of angiograms Mortality/morbidity
2	70	Coronary, Femoral	4	Colestid-Niacin	Computerized angiograms (UCSF and JPL/USC)
75	100	Coronary	3-5	Colestid-Niacin Colestid-Probucol	Panel Reading of angiograms
57	57	Coronary	2	Colestid Clofibrate	Panel Reading of angiograms
40	40	Right Femoral	0.5	Niacin-Phenofibrate	Computerized angiograms (Uppsala)

24

Experimental Design Problems
Interpretation of Statistical Arithmetic

ELMER C. HALL

When first asked to speak on experimental design problems in the quantitative evaluation of atherosclerosis, particularly in progression/regression studies, my reaction was that I didn't know enough about the area to do it justice. I still don't. (Of course, I knew about least squares regression but least squares progression was not in my statistical vocabulary.)

As investigators, all of you have been dealing with problems of experimental design in your own special areas in one context or another. The U.S. Multicenter Trial for Assessment of B-mode Ultrasound Imaging and the Coronary Artery Surgery Study (CASS) are good examples of what experimental design is all about; they contain the elements of planning, implementation, execution, data collection, management, and analysis that should be part of every research effort.

EXPERIMENTAL DESIGN VERSUS EXPERIMENTATION (STATISTICIAN VERSUS INVESTIGATOR?)

One context in which to discuss experimental design problems is the statistical one. In this context, experimental design refers to a conceptual framework leading to an appropriate statistical analysis upon which to base inferences about some research question; that is, to the problems of designing experiments for statistical analysis and interpretation. These problems are independent of subject matter and are the concern of professional statisticians engaged in education, statistical research, and statistical practice.

In another context, perhaps the one represented by most of the investigators at this workshop, experimental design problems are problems of experimentation; that is, the problems of measurement, technique, instrumentation, and so on. These problems deal with who, what, where, when, and how to measure. We have seen ample demonstration of the ability of investigators at this workshop to solve some of these problems. Obviously, these problems are primary; their solutions are fundamental to making progress in any context. Each of these problems have components that require statistical concepts of design, analysis, and interpretation. Any statistician hoping to contribute in the statistical context would have to be thoroughly familiar with these problems and solutions and how they have an impact on the practice of designing experiments leading to appropriate statistical analyses and inferences. I would like to suggest that a reciprocal effort needs to be made by investigators to improve their understanding and use of the large body of statistical methodology available to them.

All of you are experts in one or more areas related to the quantitative evaluation of atherosclerosis. All of you collect data with an acute awareness of the subject-matter problems of experimentation. I would like to provoke you into a greater appreciation for the statistical aspects of experimentation, particularly the statistical analysis and interpretation of data. After all, data are subjected to statistical analysis and interpretation whether collected within an experimental design framework or gathered under various investigative strategies imposed by pragmatic or other seemingly logical considerations.

All of you are also pressured in one way or another to accompany reports of your investigative efforts with some evidence of statistical arithmetic (if not statistical reasoning). Thus, it is impossible to look at a journal today without being bombarded with $\bar{X} \pm SE$, p-values of various and often mysterious origins, and other statistical manifestations. (We have seen and heard evidence of this pressure during this workshop. For example, in response to a question from the floor, one respondent said, "We hope to get a statistically significant answer to your question." Another respondent stated, "We could not find a significant correlation." Both of these statements represent misunderstandings [or misuse] of basic statistical reasoning.)

I would like, by example, to illustrate other chronic disorders created by this pressure to be statistical and to suggest that serious attention to problems of experimental design *and* analysis by investigators could improve both the efficiency and effectiveness of experimentation and add considerably to the value of research findings (or at least their communication). Recent issues of the journals *Circulation* (1) and *Archives of Internal Medicine* (2) have addressed some of these disorders. These issues point out that from one-half to two-thirds of articles in the medical literature contain examples of poor statistical practice. In the spirit of provocation, I have selected a few examples from articles and manuscripts I read in preparation for this conference. The examples have been partially disguised to protect the identity of individuals.

In my experience, the two most frequent questions asked of statisticians are

1. What size sample should I take?
2. Is this significant? ("This" refers to some feature of collected data that lends itself to statistical manipulation, i.e., means, proportions, contingency tables.)

Usually, the proper answer to both questions is "it depends."

SAMPLE SIZE (GAMES INVESTIGATORS PLAY)

The sample size issue is obviously a good beginning for a discussion. (Only one investigator has directly addressed this issue in this workshop.) However, this issue alone demands much more time than can be given. Let me state that in my experience it is not

uncommon for statisticians to be told that a certain maximum
sample size is all that can be obtained (based on time, patient
load, money, etc.). They are then expected to manipulate alpha
(the Type I error), beta (the Type II error), the size of the
"critical difference," and guesstimates of measurement variability
into a cogent argument for the sample size. In these circumstances, the size of the "critical difference" is often determined
by the levels of alpha and beta that are commonly used. That this
is an unsatisfactory state of affairs should not need further
amplification. Investigators must learn to use alpha and beta
errors as meaningful guides to study design and decision making.
They should not allow a statistical methodology to usurp what is
basically their responsibility as subject matter experts.
Unfortunately, many investigators seem to completely ignore the
sample size issue in their work. I think that this leads to a lot
of wasted effort on "too small" or low-power experiments.

P-VALUE ADDICTION (HOOKED ON SIGNIFICANCE)

A concept intimately related to sample size is that of statistical
significance. It may be the most misunderstood and abused statistical concept. I won't bore you with the standard lecture on
practical significance versus statistical significance (or importance versus statistical significance). Misuse of the concept
creeps into many presentations and publications. For example,
consider the following quote taken from a manuscript presented
in this workshop:

> Correlation between (variable A and variable B) was
> found, but at marginal significance level (.068).
> Another measure called (variable C) was more highly
> correlated (.036).

I would suggest that the p-values reported are meaningless (worth-
less), since neither the sample sizes nor the actual correlations
were presented. Furthermore, to state that C "was more highly
correlated" with A than with B because one p-value was smaller

than the other is a gross distortion of the concept of statistical significance. This misuse of statistical significance is of epidemic proportions in medical literature. If investigators would make an effort to understand the nature of this abuse, it would be laughed out of existence. This example of p-value addiction is followed by the statement: "The search for the best... measure of coronary atherosclerosis is still underway." I hope that when they find it, it is statistically significant (otherwise no one will ever know).

STANDARD ERRORS (SE), STANDARD DEVIATIONS (SD), AND THE TYRANNY OF THE MEAN ($\bar{X}$)

It has always puzzled me why investigators rely so heavily on $\bar{X} \pm$ SD or, more frequently, $\bar{X} \pm$ SE as descriptive and inferential statistics. In my experience, SEs are chosen primarily because they are smaller (by $1/\sqrt{n}$) than their corresponding SDs; the choice seldom appears to be made on the basis of imparting relevant information. To illustrate this statistical disorder, I have selected an example (disguised) from a published article in which two groups are compared with the following summary statistics:

	$\bar{X}$	SE
Group I	16.7	1.80
Group II	10.6	1.33
	p < .01	

The variable being compared is percent intimal surface with raised lesions.

Now, all of us are rational thinkers. The results seem obvious enough. But take another look! What are the sample sizes? What are the SDs? How was the p-value determined? Do the data really support the author's contention? For this particular example, no indication was given about the origin of the p-value. However, sample sizes were available in the article and, with a little arithmetic, SDs can be calculated. The summary statistics can then be augmented as follows:

	X̄	SE	n	SD
Group I	16.7	1.80	114	19.2
Group II	10.6	1.33	77	11.7
		p < .01		

Now, the measurement under investigation can only take on non-negative values. Thus, X̄ ± SD does not adequately describe the data. To the statistically sensitive reader, however, the information imparted here is useful. Obviously, the data are from a highly skewed distribution. So skewed, in fact, that an inference based on a comparison of the means using a t-test (or a z-test) might be suspect. Without further information, this is as far as we can go.

To say the least, my conclusions from reading this article and examining the evidence presented would be summarized with somewhat less conviction than the authors. They may be correct but they have been tyrannized by the mean and bludgeoned by the standard error. Examples of this kind are widespread in medical literature.

NON-SIGNIFICANCE, NO DIFFERENCE, AND MAKING INFERENCES ANYWAY

It is often of interest in an investigation to "prove" that two methods of measurement are not different. One such investigation reported the following (the measurements were percentage of intimal surface with raised lesions on 10 samples of coronary arteries each assessed by two methods). The appropriate summary statistics available in the article are:

	X̄
Method I	16.70
Method II	19.25
Difference (II-I)	2.55 NS
SE (difference)	1.82

NS = not significant

Now, I will not quibble about the non-significance of the difference. I will take issue, however, with the conclusion that "these results indicate that comparisons of the extent of coronary atherosclerosis (by Method I and Method II) are not likely to be confounded by a large (method) bias."

A statistically sensitive reader might be moved to do some arithmetic. For example, if the standard error of the difference between two means of paired data is SE $(\bar{d})$ = 1.82, the standard deviation of the differences is SD (d) = $\sqrt{n}$ SE($\bar{d}$) = $\sqrt{10}$(1.82) = 5.76. If this sensitive reader were also in a Gaussian frame of mind, often a dangerous frame of mind to be in, he or she might assume that the mean difference (2.55) and SD(d) = 5.76 provide estimates of the mean and standard deviation of a normal distribution. Based on area calculations for a normal distribution, this sensitive reader might then conclude, for example, that 44% of such differences exceed 5 percentage points of intimal surface area or similarly that about 12% of such differences exceed 10 percentage points of intimal surface area. Since the bulk of the measurements will be made on specimens that have less than 10 percent of the intimal surface involved, one might thus question the comparability of the two "methods" of measurement. It appears to me that the non-significant difference between the two methods is not so much a reflection of their comparability but of their dissimilarity. It would be useful to see a scattergram of the paired data (or at least know the correlation coefficient) but the sensitive reader is left hanging. In a sense, I agree with the author's conclusion "that comparisons of the extent of coronary atherosclerosis...are not likely to be confounded by a large (method) bias." Instead, they will be totally obscured by the large variability of the differences between the two methods.

SUMMARY AND CONCLUSIONS

From the above examples, I hope that investigators will become sensitized to the need to critically evaluate and present their own research data. None of the statistical disorders discussed involve sophisticated arithmetic, complex experimental designs,

involve sophisticated arithmetic, complex experimental designs, or advanced inferential techniques. They are chronic, epidemic disorders that deserve your serious attention. Subject matter investigators must bear the responsibility for improvement.

In conclusion:

If it's knowledge you seek
You shouldn't be meek
In choosing your sample size
With alpha and beta you can see what n buys
And finish your work in a week

The problems of experimental design are few
Only the area of application is new
Your designs are commendable
Your statistics amenable
To what you already know is true

Seekers of truth think they are done
When the p-value is .001
But if what they've computed
Is oft ill-reputed
The value is really next to none

If from your data you would glean
A statistic with significant lean
It's not the design
That should be on your mind
If the n doesn't justify the mean.

REFERENCES

1. Glantz SA (1980) Biostatistics: how to detect, correct, and prevent errors in the medical literature. Circulation 61:1-7
2. Sheehan TJ (1980) The medical literature: let the reader beware. Arch Intern Med 140:472-474

DISCUSSION: C. ALEX McMAHAN

I would like to mention two misuses of statistics that I encounter frequently in my role as a consultant. The first is related to the problem of sample size and occurs when there are multiple measurements on the same subject. Suppose we have 10 subjects per experimental group and three observations per subject. What is the effective sample size? By effective I mean the number of subjects we would need if we observed each subject only once. If I may quote Dr. Hall, the answer depends. It depends on the within-subject correlation structure. We can say that the effective sample size is somewhere between 10, the number of subjects, and 30, the total number of observations. In general, the effective sample size will be much closer to the number of subjects than to the total number of observations. The mistake occurs when an investigator uses the number of observations without examining the question of effective sample size. The choice of the number of subjects and the number of observations per subject depends on the chosen significance level, the desired power, the true difference, the variances and the within subject correlation. There is an optimal choice of the number of observations per subject. Generally, we don't have sufficient information actually to achieve the optimum value, but with the information we usually have we can approach the optimum. Particularly in these times, it is important to give careful thought to the allocation of limited resources.

The second misuse of statistics is the use of a correlation coefficient in situations where the investigator has manipulated or controlled one of the variables. There is a tendency to control a variable in validation studies or in method comparison studies because we often desire to make the comparison over a wide range. However, in order to obtain a valid estimate of the correlation coefficient, both variables must be uncontrolled. If one variable is controlled, we find ourselves in a situation where regression methods need to be applied rather than correlation methods. If an investigator computes the correlation coefficient in the situation where one of the variables is controlled, that correlation coefficient is very likely to be higher than it should be, that is, closer to +1 or to -1. The overestimation of the correlation coefficient occurs also when one examines the correlation coefficient between two variables across selected population groups (1).

Several speakers in this workshop have mentioned identifying bimodal distributions. This is a difficult statistical problem, but there are several methods that are much better than just graphical impressions. Associated with this problem of identifying bimodality is the problem of identifying subgroups that respond differently to experimental treatments. Suppose we are in the situation where only a subgroup responds. The classical statistical methods such as the t-test or analysis of variance are not powerful in this situation, as they assume the entire group responds. Some alternative to these classical methods should be used. There are limited statistical methods for analyzing such data and this area needs more investigation (2).

Many of the comments made by Dr. Hall and myself concern misuse of statistics and the articles that he quoted from Circulation and Archives of Medicine were concerned with this issue. There is another aspect that needs to be considered. This was expressed in a recent editorial in the American Journal of Physiology (3), which reported the results of an examination of articles in that journal by a committee concerned with the use of statistics. This committee concluded that there were few actual errors in the use of statistics, but there were many situations in which the most efficient statistical methods were not applied. That is, the method of analysis used by the investigator did not obtain all the information available in the data. As we anticipate spending large amounts of money and effort to gather data on atherosclerosis, we should make certain that we use the best and most efficient statistical methods that are available to analyze these data.

REFERENCES

1. McGill HC, McMahan CA, Wene JD (1981) Unresolved problems
    in the diet-heart issue. Arteriosclerosis 1:164-176
2. Good PI (1979) Detection of a treatment effect when not
    all experimental subjects will respond to treatment.
    Biometrics 35:484-489
3. Fishman AP, Berne RM, Morgan HE (1981) By the numbers...
    Am J Physiol 241:C91-C92

Part 4
Summary

25

Universal Reference Standards for Measuring Atherosclerotic Lesions
The Quest for the "Gold Standard"

WILLIAM INSULL, JR.

My purpose is to review the current state of reference standards for atherosclerotic lesions, reference standards that can be applied to the quantitative measurement of lesions and their changes by techniques currently available or under development. The aim of the measurements of lesions is to detect and characterize the lesions, and to measure the lesions once, for diagnosis, or serially, examining for changes that may occur with further natural progression, or for regression or stabilization induced by treatment. To achieve the highest quality measurements, each investigator must be assured that his measurements are being performed by valid techniques yielding reproducible results that are diagnostically accurate and that may be compared with serial observations over time or with observations in other laboratories or clinics. The conclusion of this review is that while criteria for the reference standards are available, the quest for the reference standard has not been systematically undertaken nor successfully completed. Hence, this review will describe the current state of the quest.

This review addresses the need for reference standards, the definition of a reference standard, the pertinent methods of pathology examination, the major pathology of the atherosclerotic lesion, the kinds of information about atherosclerotic lesions obtained from pathology studies and clinical methods, and criteria for the ideal reference standards. I have reviewed the proceedings of this workshop for pertinent information and am indebted to the workshop participants for their helpful reviews and comments.

NEED FOR REFERENCE STANDARDS

All investigators have reported the need for some form of reference standard. All investigators have used uniform procedures with the objective of obtaining measurements valid for comparisons and significant as measures of lesions. Glagov and Zarins in their definition of the problem of atherosclerosis measurement have emphasized the need for correlative studies between pathology and clinical methods (see Chap. 2). They emphasized the ideal goal that methods be capable of serial examination of lesions to assess prevention or therapy, and to determine how treatments affect the composition of lesions and the occurrence of complications. They stated that the goal of the pathologist is to describe and measure the lesions as they appear in vivo, an unusual requirement for pathology.

DEFINITION OF REFERENCE STANDARD

The definition of the term reference standard helps us focus on our goal. A standard is defined as "a means of determining what a thing should be" and "an acknowledged measure of comparison for quantitative or qualitative value" (1,2). From these a reasonable definition of the standard we seek is "a means of measuring and comparing atherosclerotic lesions which is acknowledged and used by those who evaluate and study atherosclerotic lesions." Such a reference standard would have two major parts: (1) accurately and precisely defined preparations of the various kinds of atherosclerotic lesions, and (2) a method, procedure, or instrument for the quantitative measurement of specific characteristics of these lesions. Such a standard is used by currently measuring and then comparing the standard lesion preparations, having known

characteristics, with study lesions having unknown dimensions and
characteristics. Similar values for the reference standard and
the unknown study lesions indicate a strong probability that the
study lesion has characteristics and dimensions similar to the
reference standard. These measurements also document whether the
methods are providing appropriate values for the reference preparations, i.e., provide calibration and quality control. Standards
may consist of phantoms constructed to mimic one or more selected
characteristics of lesions. Standard procedures may require the
selection of appropriate lesions in target arteries. The statistical precision of measurements of reference standards and study
lesions must be established and the requirements for precision in
routine use defined. The situation with reference standards for
atherosclerotic lesions is similar to the preparation and use of
national and international standards and reference preparations
of significant biological materials by a variety of laboratories
and clinics.

METHODOLOGY OF PATHOLOGY

Any measurements of atherosclerotic lesions must recognize and
accommodate four problems with pathology, methodology, and knowledge. Any pathology method proposed as a reference standard must
be evaluated with consideration for these problems.

First, significant tissue shrinkage and conformational change
during fixation and histological preparation for pathology examination results in measurements from these preparations being
significantly different from values in vivo (see Chap. 19).
Corrections for shrinkage due to removing the unfixed artery from
its adventitial attachment or due to tissue processing must be
made before comparing measurements from pathology preparations and
clinical techniques.

Second, specimens of arteries for pathology examination should
be fixed while distended by pressure or at greater than the normal
diastolic value. Arterial lesions in these distended preparations

show a flattened, concave configuration resembling their in vivo configuration, in contrast to lesions naturally bulging into the lumen frequently encountered in arteries fixed in the collapsed, undistended state.

Third, arterial dilatation at the site of stenotic lesions may obscure both the lesions' mass relative to other tissues of the artery, and the effects of the lesion mass on the artery lumen. Bond et al. have demonstrated this convincingly in several species of nonhuman primates exposed to a single risk factor for athero-sclerosis, i.e., hypercholesterolemia (see Chap. 19) and Zarins et al. have also shown this to occur in successive segments of a human carotid artery with narrowing of the lumen and simultaneous dilatation of the artery (see Chap. 13).

Fourth, a broad spectrum of changes occurs during regression of advanced atherosclerotic lesions, many of which could be potential indices of lesion regression. Wissler observed five major changes during regression of experimental advanced lesions in monkeys: decrease in lesion size, decrease in lipid content, decrease or disappearance of the necrotic center, an increase in the density of cells and of collagen in the fibrous cap, and a decrease in focal damage of the endothelium (3). Currently, most clinical methods measure the decrease in lesion size indirectly by a reduction of its invasion into the lumen.

PATHOLOGY DESCRIPTION OF LESIONS

The most extensive characterization of atherosclerotic lesions is currently obtained by pathology methods. Most of the qualitative characteristics can be described by quantitative measurements. The elements of the pathology characterization are: the lesions' locations; the lesions' extent in number of lesions, length, width, bulk and size; smoothness or roughness of the surface; severity by diameter and length of stenosis; composition of lesions and normal tissues using histological, cytological, and chemical features; and occurrence of complications such as lesion mineralization, necrosis, hemorrhage, ulceration, thrombosis and other changes in texture and organization (see Chap. 2). All these elements may undergo change during regression, but one is used almost exclusively, degree of stenosis. Many of the pathology methods are being developed further and promise to provide new characterizations that may be incorporated into reference standards. The elements of lesions described by pathology methods provide a list for evaluating clinical methods of lesions measurement.

Lesion characteristics based on local functional effects have not been developed for lesions with moderate or lesser grades of stenosis. However, as knowledge of these effects increases, it may become significant, and should be incorporated into criteria for reference standards.

CLINICAL IMAGING OF LESIONS

Clinically applicable methods for characterizing and measuring lesions have developed rapidly in recent years, and important problems unique to these methods have been identified. Many of these problems have been formulated in terms of requirements for optimal performance of serially imaging lesions, since almost all the clinical methods depend upon generating and examining images of lesions in lieu of direct examination of arterial tissue. Any imaging methods proposed as reference standards must be evaluated with consideration of these problems. The requirements for optimal performance of serial imaging noted by Selzer (see Chap. 3) and others include: multiple views, replicable exposure geometry for all views (since plaques are rarely axisymmetric), controllable vasospasm and vasodilatation, correction for arterial pulsation effects, use of discrete and symmetrical lesions, and measurement precision that satisfies needs for clinical diagnosis or evaluation of treatment in a clinical trial. These requirements apply to all clinical methods using images, contrast angiography, B-mode ultrasound, Doppler ultrasound, nuclear magnetic resonance, scintigraphy, and positron emission tomography.

COMPARISON OF PATHOLOGY AND CLINICAL METHODS

The search for the universal reference standard is aided by systematic comparison of the techniques currently available for their capability to qualitatively and quantitatively characterize lesions. Pathology methods, which provide the most comprehensive description and measurements, have been compared with contrast angiography and B-mode ultrasound, the two most highly developed methods applicable to lesions causing minor grades of stenosis (Table 1). Both angiography and B-mode ultrasound measure the severity of lumen stenosis at focal sites and in longitudinal display. Ultrasound has the capability of demonstrating the artery in cross-sectional views. Angiography may be able to do this with appropriate data analysis. The extent of lesions cannot be assayed by angiography; their evaluation by ultrasound is yet to be defined. The composition of lesions cannot be measured by angiography, while the capabilities of ultrasound are not yet established. Major complications of lesions can be detected in

Table 1. Comparison of pathology, angiography, and B-mode ultrasound for current evaluation of atherosclerotic lesions.

Lesion Characteristics	Method		
	Path.	Angio.	Ultras.
Severity of lumen stenosis			
Cross-sectional display	+	?	+
Longitudinal display	+	+	+
Display of focal differences	+	+	+
Extent of lesions			
Lesion area	+	0	?+
Arterial wall thickness	+	0	?+
Lesion bulk	+	0	?+
Composition of lesions	+	0	?
Complications of lesions			
Surface irregularities	+	+?	?
Thrombus detection	+	+?	?+
Mineralization	+	+?	+

many situations by angiography. B-mode ultrasound can detect mineralization, while its evaluation of surface irregularities and thrombi is not known.

Thus, while neither angiography nor B-mode ultrasound evaluations is as comprehensive as pathology examination, each provides information that is useful, and each has the promise of more information. Overall, their strongest characterization is of lumen stenosis and they provide less information than pathology methods. Analysis of other clinically applicable methods presents similar results of less information, but this is due to current incomplete development of methods and the inherent characteristics of the methods. Doppler ultrasound may become an indirect yet sensitive indicator of changes in blood flow that reflects morphology and size of stenosis when dealing with low-grade stenosis. Nuclear magnetic resonance, scintigraphy and positron emission have potential, unique power for identification and quantitation of specific constituents of lesions.

The current best reference standard is the pathology examination utilizing techniques that overcome the problems of tissue shrinkage during fixation, distortion due to incomplete distension, and localized dilatation frequently associated with lesions.

PROPOSED REQUIREMENTS FOR REFERENCE STANDARDS

The requirements for the ideal reference standard to be used to measure changes in atherosclerotic lesions by clinically applicable serial imaging techniques, while not described elsewhere, can be derived from the analysis presented above. A provisional set of reference standard requirements would be: provision of a comprehensive pathology characterization using adequate histological preparations of standard reference arteries, measurement of the bulk size of lesions, measurement of severity of lesions by either degree of stenosis or reduction of blood flow, definition of lesion composition by the nature and distribution of its components, and definition and measurement of any complications.

Serial imaging procedures applied to the reference standard need to have multiple views, replicable exposure geometry for all views, controlled vasospasm and vasodilitation, correction for arterial pulsation effects, use of discrete and symmetrical lesions, determination of lesion change along the artery, and measurements that satisfy the study design by their accuracy, precision, sensitivity, and specificity. To be able to assure quality control over time and among different observers and laboratories, the measurement sequence using concurrent measurements of reference standards and study lesions should be easily replicable with sufficient frequency to be practical.

The ultimate requirements for the reference standards are the standards' relevance for assuring accurate detection and measurement of lesion progression, regression, and stabilization. The current major criteria for lesion progression are accurate measurements of increases in lesion size, decreases in lumen caliber, and development of complications such as ulceration and thrombosis. The current major essential criteria for lesion regression are accurate measures of decrease in lesion size, increase in lumen size, and/or remodeling of other lesion characteristics. The criteria for stabilization have not been determined, but may focus on demonstration of stable major characteristics of lesions for a specified time.

The preparation of reference tissues, of instruments and procedures for measurements can be devised from these requirements.

CURRENT REFERENCE STANDARDS

Three kinds of standard preparations have been noted during the workshop. Investigators have used arteries in situ, in vivo for measurement by clinical methods, followed by sacrifice and examination with optimal pathology methods. Freshly obtained arteries have been studied in vitro. These arteries provide the complex material essential for comprehensive characterization of lesions.

Several investigators have used phantoms for limited reference standards with clinical methods. The potential for phantoms has not been systematically explored. The construction of phantoms mimicking selected complex characteristics of tissues may be difficult.

CONCLUSIONS

Reference standards for quantitative measurements of progression and regression of atherosclerotic lesions in the clinic and laboratory are needed. Pathology methods, including recently improved preparation of arterial tissues, provide the most comprehensive and accurate description of lesions. The requirements for quality measurements of lesions by serial imaging with clinically applicable techniques have been identified and should be applied to reference standard procedures. Promising clinically applicable methods are available: contrast angiography, B-mode ultrasound, and Doppler ultrasound, and others are under development. A standard reference method for measuring normal arterial tissues and atherosclerotic lesions has not been developed and generally acknowledged, but the requirements for reference standards have become apparent. A variety of reference standards are needed to match the variety of atherosclerotic lesions. The systematic development of reference standards for use in research and clinical measurements of atherosclerotic lesions should be undertaken. The most valid standards appear to be tissues defined by pathology methods. The use of lesion phantoms as one form of reference standards should be evaluated where clinical methods measure limited characteristics of lesions.

REFERENCES

1. Webster's Collegiate Thesarus. (1976) G and C Merriam Company, Springfield
2. Webster's New Universal Unabridged Dictionary, 2nd edn. (1979) Dorset and Barber, Simon and Schuster, New York
3. Wissler RW (1978) Progression and regression of atherosclerotic lesions. Adv Exp Med Biol 104:77-109

26

Recommendations

DAVID H. BLANKENHORN

Quantitative evaluation of lesions has an established and important role in atherosclerosis research. Atheroma measurement procedures were first used by European pathologists to study the relative distribution of lesions in various parts of the vascular system. These efforts led eventually to the extensive geographic surveys of atherosclerosis with standardized autopsy measurements, which have contributed much to the knowledge of atherogenesis. Quantitation of experimental atherosclerosis began shortly after it was shown that atherosclerosis could be induced in animal models, and has been extensively used to compare the potency of various atherogenic stimuli. Quantitation of lesions now plays a central role in studies of atheroma regression in experimental animals.

In parallel with these developments in lesion quantitation, there has been an extensive and successful effort to develop in vitro systems for the study of atherogenesis. Elegant procedures for culture of endothelial cells and arterial smooth muscle cells allow ultrastructure and intermediary metabolism to be studied in detail. Quantitative data from in vitro studies have furnished a wealth of information on how the process of atherogenesis may occur and how it might be ameliorated. This information awaits in vivo testing in experimental animals and in controlled clinical trials on human subjects.

In the last 10 years there has been a third development, the attempt to quantitate atherosclerosis in living subjects using angiographic and ultrasound techniques. The physicists, electronic engineers, bioengineers, computer scientists, and clinicians involved in this effort constitute a new group of research workers in atherosclerosis. This workshop has brought together pathologists, cell biologists, clinicians, and imaging specialists for a review of progress, to exchange new ideas, and to make recommendations for the future.

SIX RECOMMENDATIONS

1. An organized program to improve existing procedures and develop new ones is recommended.

Quantitative measurement is a necessary tool to transfer information derived from molecular biology and ultrastructural study to research in atherosclerotic animals and therapy for human beings. Credible concepts of atherogenesis suggesting ways in which the process might be modified for human benefit now exist. A wealth of information suggesting what might be done needs to be transferred from isolated cell systems to studies in animal models and tests of therapy in humans. New and improved quantitative procedures are required to accomplish this.

It is generally acknowledged that therapy is difficult at late stages when atherosclerotic lesions are large and complicated. On the other hand, there is a great deal of evidence which suggests that early lesions are susceptible to therapy leading to regression and, in fact, some early lesions, such as the fatty streak, may undergo spontaneous regression. The message for therapists is clear; treat the disease at an early stage, try to prevent formation of more serious lesions. Quantitative evaluation of lesion morphology in living subjects and serial lesion tracking can make this approach possible. There is no other way to evaluate agents or procedures that may modify or retard human atherosclerosis at an early stage.

It follows that atherosclerosis research would be greatly facilitated by an organized program to develop methods of quantitative lesion evaluation. Current efforts to develop new methods or improve existing ones are, for the most part, focused on short-term goals designed to meet the needs of individual research projects. This occurs because resources available to develop new methods are severely limited and funding for development of diagnostic instruments usually comes as part of some other effort. The cooperative trial currently funded by the National Heart, Lung, and Blood Institute to evaluate ultrasound devices described by Dr. Toole during this workshop may indicate an encouraging and favorable new trend.

2. It is recommended that the nature of atherosclerosis as a process with rate and direction be explicitly recognized.

This new way to think about atherosclerosis may represent a change equal to the switch from a concept of a single atherogenic agent to a polycausal hypothesis for atherogenesis. At one time, many atherosclerosis research projects were designed to find "the" cause of atherosclerosis, but now very few are. A change can be seen in titles from the annual meeting of the Council on Arteriosclerosis. In early days many titles suggest that "the" cause for atherosclerosis was under investigation, but in recent years such titles have become few in number as a majority of scientists have moved away from a single agent concept of atherogenesis. A change of opinion of equal importance may now be in progress with a conceptual change from a static to a dynamic model for atherosclerosis. For example, a static model of atherosclerosis is implied by population surveys in which a risk factor analysis is applied to patients classified as atherosclerotic or non-atherosclerotic at one time in their life. A single determination of atherosclerosis state at one age cannot adequately characterize the life history of any individual's atherosclerosis and this should be considered in the design of experiments.

In this workshop, Drs. Bond and Hollander discussed in detail dynamic changes that occur in blood vessel dimensions as atherosclerotic lesions form. Lesion development and aging both are associated with change in luminal diameter, which can ameliorate or exacerbate the effect of lesions on blood flow. It is recommended that atherosclerosis be considered a dynamic process with rate and direction. The rate and direction of lesion change can vary from one lesion to the next and can be influenced by lesion type and vessel size, as well as age, sex, and species. It is recommended that these details be specified when lesion change rates are reported.

3. It is recommended that the accuracy of existing atherosclerosis measurements be determined against set standards.

There is inherent merit in using accurate methods of measurement; this is self-evident for atherosclerosis research and all other science. There is additional need for accurate measurement of atherosclerosis because clinicians require accuracy when high stakes are involved in decisions based on these measurements. Carotid endarterectomy and coronary bypass surgery are planned on the basis of angiographic and ultrasound images, which must be accurate. This point was emphasized by Dr. Barnes.

4. It is recommended that the precision of existing atherosclerosis quantitation methods be increased. Precise new methods should be developed.

Precise measurements are recommended to reduce the number of study subjects required for hypothesis testing. All animals for research are expensive and some are in short supply, but there are many promising leads in atherosclerosis research. Therefore, the number of animals used in each experiment should be no more than is optimal, and fewer animals are required when precise lesion measurements can be made.

The development of more precise measurements is also recommended to facilitate tests of human treatment. Trials of therapy

for atherosclerosis in man, such as the Coronary Drug Project,
which involved more than 8000 subjects--each studied for five
years, have become ruinously expensive. One of the great potential advantages for studies in which atherosclerotic lesions are
measured and their progress tracked over time is a significant
reduction in the number of subjects and length of observation
for each. The saving of effort and time is greater if precise
measurements are used. Robert Selzer discussed this potential
bonus from image processing and from the mathematics of sample
size for trial design. His comments apply equally to human and
animal studies and to any measurement procedure.

Cross-sectional autopsy data on the extent of coronary lesions can be used to estimate the average rate at which atherosclerosis change may occur spontaneously in a control group of
human subjects. The precision of current angiographic measures
is sufficient that reasonably small and short-term trials can
be planned to detect an agent that will significantly reverse
atherosclerosis. An agent causing significant regression is one
sufficiently potent that a test group will have a rate of atherosclerosis change equal to the control group, but in the opposite
direction. For example, between ages 20 and 40, raised coronary
lesions can be estimated from autopsy data to spread at a rate
which covers 2 to 3% more of the intimal surface each year (1).
A therapeutic agent which reverses this trend to an extent causing
elimination of lesions from 2 to 3% of the coronary surface each
year could be detected with a high degree of probability if 100
subjects in a control group were compared with 100 subjects in a
test group and the interval between lesion measurement was two
years. Animal data suggest that agents this potent in treating
induced atherosclerosis exist. What remains to be seen is whether
effects on human lesions are as great.

Another argument for improved precision in measurement of
living subjects' atherosclerosis is to facilitate search for
agents retarding plaque growth. Many students of atherosclerosis

believe that it will be easier to retard growth of human lesions than to cause significant reversal. Agents which retard the growth of lesions could have great value because the early stages of atherosclerosis produce no symptoms and are not immediately harmful. Agents with this lesser degree of effect will be difficult to detect until more precise measures for living subjects are developed. Assuming that spontaneous average lesion growth rates in the coronary artery produce 2 to 3% coverage of new intima per year, an agent that cuts this rate in half would reduce the new area covered to 1 to 1.5% per year. When conventional sample size calculations are applied to estimate the size of trials capable of detecting a change of 1 to 1.5% per year it becomes clear that improvement in precision of lesion tracking will be very helpful in the search for agents with this effect. Another approach will be to develop noninvasive or less invasive procedures, as recommended next.

5.   It is recommended that noninvasive and less invasive atherosclerosis measurement procedures continue to be developed.

Promising new developments in ultrasound imaging and venous angiography have been presented at this conference, but currently selective angiography remains the mainstay of atherosclerosis evaluation when precision is desired in living subjects. In this workshop, Dr. Kennedy presented a review of data from 24,000 coronary angiograms registered in the Coronary Artery Surgery Study (CASS), a national cooperative effort to evaluate coronary artery bypass surgery.

One obvious and widely recognized advantage of noninvasive and less invasive atherosclerosis assessment is to reduce the risk and cost to the patient. Another bonus from these less invasive, but precise atherosclerosis measurement procedures, will be improved experimental design. Atherosclerosis measurement error and variation in atherosclerosis growth rate between subjects are two major determinants of the number of subjects in a study of lesion change. Less invasive measurement procedures could allow experiments in which subjects are prescreened to select less variable groups. Less invasive procedures could also allow cross-over designs with each subject serving as his own control.

The most immediately probable way to achieve precise, but significantly less invasive lesion measurement in living subjects, is to both validate and improve the precision of ultrasound imaging and venous angiography. There is also need to extend the tissue range of high-resolution ultrasound to a point where coronary arteries can be imaged in adults. Instrument development can be extremely expensive and so the potential cost of this recommendation must be considered in light of the cost of what is now spent in treating late stages of atherosclerosis. It is possible that agents now available have unrecognized potential for retarding lesion growth. These might significantly improve human health and longevity at a fraction of the cost we now expend in treating late stages of atherosclerosis.

6. It is recommended that a new class of images be developed that display some function of blood vessel walls or metabolism of lesions.

Current imaging procedures furnish information about the morphology of blood vessels, and the only evaluation of blood vessel function that is imaged is the velocity of blood flow. Existing procedures should be augmented with techniques for imaging vessel wall functions involved in the immediate steps of atherogenesis; for example, the images of LDL infiltration developed by Dr. Lees and mentioned by Dr. Budinger. A second promising procedure of this sort is imaging of platelet aggregation or adherence. The potential for images of this sort is to examine in detail steps in atherogenesis as they occur. With procedures of this sort, strategies to interpret the process at specific points can be projected.

These new measurement tools will not replace morphologic images and should not be considered competitive alternatives. An

optimal approach to atherosclerosis evaluation should furnish
three image types: (1) vessel wall morphology; (2) vessel wall
function images; and (3) blood flow images. The information
content of these three image types will be independent, but
complementary. Dr. Chris Wood presented an interesting example
of how blood flow imaging may provide morphologic information
about the presence of ulceration in carotid atherosclerosis.

When new images are developed and integrated with the images
we now use, it will be important to relate the information each
contains to the nature of the physical process used to obtain the
new image. This is a difficult intuitive process because optical
images are the natural medium for human thought. "Seeing is
believing," and since birth we have all been trained to perceive
reality in images generated by optical light. The images of
atherosclerosis we now obtain by roentgenography or ultrasound
are presented to us as optical images from film transparencies
or from a cathode ray tube and this tends to reinforce the per-
ception. Image information in an angiogram is formed by
absorption of roentgen rays by the target of interest, and the
image formed by ultrasound is a result of reflected sound waves.
The physics involved in both of these processes differ significantly from that of light and the information contained in
roentgen or ultrasound images is different from that in an optical
image. Many workers, particularly in clinical research, approve
most highly of new imaging devices that faithfully replicate the
image from some older procedure. A common argument advocating
a new image is that it is highly correlated with an existing accepted technique. However, if the two techniques are perfectly
correlated, the new images will faithfully reproduce all flaws of
the old procedure, as well as any advantages. When new techniques
are developed the potential for each should be examined and the
information it contains related to information we desire about
atherosclerosis. The most useful new images will be those which
provide new information.

SUMMARY

1. An organized program to improve existing procedures and
    develop new ones is recommended.
2. It is recommended that the nature of atherosclerosis as a
    process with rate and direction be explicitly recognized.
3. It is recommended that the accuracy of existing
    atherosclerosis measurement be determined against set
    standards.
4. It is recommended that the precision of existing
    atherosclerosis quantitation methods be increased.
    Precise new methods should be developed.
5. It is recommended that noninvasive and less invasive
    atherosclerosis measurement procedures continue to be
    developed.
6. It is recommended that a new class of images be developed
    that display some function of blood vessel walls or
    metabolism of lesions.

REFERENCES

1. Restrepo C, Eggen DA, Guzman MA, Tejada C (1973) Postmortem
   dimensions of the coronary arteries in different geographic
   locations. Lab Invest 28:244-251

Index

(numerals in italics indicate figure)